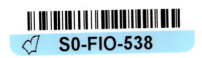

SOCIAL SUPPORT AND HEALTH

GARLAND LIBRARY OF SOCIOLOGY
General Editor: Dan A. Chekki
(Vol. 13)

GARLAND REFERENCE LIBRARY
OF SOCIAL SCIENCE
(Vol. 412)

GARLAND LIBRARY OF SOCIOLOGY
General Editor: Dan A. Chekki

1. *Conflict and Conflict Resolution: A Historical Bibliography*
   by Jack Nusan Porter

2. *Sociology of Sciences: An Annotated Bibliography of Invisible Colleges, 1972–1981*
   by Daryl E. Chubin

3. *Race and Ethnic Relations: An Annotated Bibliography*
   by Graham C. Kinloch

4. *Friendship: A Selected, Annotated Bibliography*
   by J. L. Barkas

5. *The Sociology of Aging: An Annotated Bibliography and Sourcebook*
   by Diana K. Harris

6. *Medical Sociology: An Annotated Bibliography, 1972–1982*
   by John G. Bruhn, Billy U. Philips, and Paula L. Levine

7. *The Clinical Sociology Handbook*
   by Jan M. Fritz

8. *Issues in the Sociology of Religion: A Bibliography*
   by Anthony J. Blasi and Michael W. Cuneo

9. *The Influence of the Family: A Review and Annotated Bibliography of Socialization, Ethnicity, and Delinquency, 1975–1986*
   by Alan C. Acock and Jeffrey M. Clair

10. *Jewish Family Issues: A Resource Guide*
    by Benjamin Schlesinger

11. *Social Stratification: An Annotated Bibliography*
    by Graham C. Kinloch

12. *Psychocultural Change and the American Indian: An Ethnohistorical Analysis*
    by Laurence French

13. *Social Support and Health: An Annotated Bibliography*
    by John G. Bruhn, Billy U. Philips, Paula L. Levine, and Carlos F. Mendes de Leon

SOCIAL SUPPORT AND HEALTH
An Annotated Bibliography

John G. Bruhn
Billy U. Philips
Paula L. Levine
Carlos F. Mendes de Leon

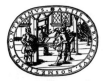

GARLAND PUBLISHING, INC. • NEW YORK & LONDON
1987

Library of Congress Cataloging-in-Publication Data

Social support and health.

(Garland library of sociology ; vol. 13) (Garland
reference library of social science ; vol. 412)
Includes indexes.
1. Social medicine. 2. Social interaction.
I. Bruhn, John G., 1934–   . II. Series.
III. Series: Garland reference library of social
science ; v. 412. [DNLM: 1. Health—abstracts.
2. Mental Health—abstracts. 3. Social Environment—
abstracts. ZWA 30 S678]
RA418.S6495 1987   016.3621   87-17796
ISBN 0-8240-8348-2 (alk. paper)

Printed on acid-free, 250-year-life paper
Manufactured in the United States of America

To Stewart Wolf, M.D.,

a leader in linking the behavioral sciences to clinical medicine, sensitive physician, imaginative researcher, challenging teacher, and friend.

CONTENTS

ACKNOWLEDGMENTS

We were extremely fortunate to have the superb resources of both works and people which made this project enjoyable. Mr. Emil F. Frey, Director of the Moody Medical Library, at The University of Texas Medical Branch at Galveston, and members of his library staff contributed to the success of this effort including: Mary Asbell, Deirdre Becker, Alex Bienkowski, Laura Cambiano, Pat Ciejka, Deborah Crawford, Cindy Hanak, Joseph Harzbecker, Patricia Lee, Carol Phillips, Robert Want, and Alice Wygant.

We also thank Marla Neely who assisted in locating and abstracting material in the early part of the project. Patsy Marullo supervised the production of the manuscript on the word processor. Debie Laycock is a highly skilled operator of the IBM 5520 and has patiently produced two annotated bibliographies in the last three years. We are grateful for her hard work and interest in the project.

The concept of social support has received much attention in the last decade. The loss or absence of familiar sources of social support has been linked to coronary disease, disorders of pregnancy, accidents, suicides, mental hospital commitments, school truancy, ulcers, cancer, scizophrenia, and longevity. Such findings suggest that the nurturing effects of social support may be good preventative medecine. The literature on the beneficial effects of social support also has its critics. The research base is weak and there are numerous studies in which the expected relationships do not hold, and some of the most positive findings are open to alternative interpretations. Some authors have questioned whether social support creates good health or whether good health makes a person more likely to receive social support.

It is difficult to measure and monitor social support since it has both qualitative and quantitative dimensions, has both positive and negative functions, and its mechanism or process varies throughout a person's life. In addition, studies of social support have been too limited in perspective, that is support and stress have usually been studied as they relate to a specific disease outcome. In order to make appropriate inferences about the impact of social support on health, however, we need to know how social support works when individuals are healthy as well as when they are ill.

The authors of this volume have spent the last two decades studying the phenomenon of social support among the sick and the well at the individual, family and community levels. A social epidemiological study of Roseto, Pennsylvania, an Italian-American community, found the community to have a remarkably low incidence of coronary heart disease. This study, carried out in the early 1960s, was one of the early efforts to revive interest in the relationship between health and social support. The authors of this volume are currently working with the principal investigator of the Roseto project, Stewart Wolf, M.D., in a 25-year follow-up of Rosetan residents, their relatives and off-spring.

In The Roseto Story: An Anatomy of Health, by John Bruhn and Stewart Wolf, (University of Oklahoma Press, 1979) the authors describe how Rosetans made choices about their lifestyle, and certain young Rosetans had heart attacks. They thought they were purposefully retaining the best of the Old World and gaining the benefits of the good life. By living in Roseto and attempting to live the good life, however, they deviated from Rosetan norms. They were not fully accepted either in Rosetan or in middle-class American society. Roseto is not a community one can return to as a former Rosetan, except to visit. The Rosetans who leave are changed persons. Those who remain in Roseto choose to do so. How we perceive and assess the life choices before us at any given time, and the choice we eventually make, will be easier or more difficult by the degree of social support we have. Our social ties can affect our resilience to change and both can profoundly influence our health.

Other researchers have also confirmed that supportive relationships from family, friends, and social organizations can act as buffers against stressful situations. Perhaps the most important lesson from Roseto for each of us personally is that close personal ties with others for whom we care and who care for us are important to our health and well-being. Social isolation can occur rather easily in our rapidly changing and mobile society. Change of any type has its costs and benefits. These choices must be weighed as decisions are made about the kind of lifestyle we want and the purpose and meaning of our lives.

Social support is an interdisciplinary topic. As such it is of interest to practitioners involved in programs designed to support or establish natural helping networks. It is also of interest to the large group of interdisciplinary research professionals concerned with the role of psychosocial factors in both physical and mental health. Social support is an integral part of the daily regimen of many intervention-ists and members of the helping professions and, therefore, is not a new or unique concpt to them. Nonetheless, there are always fresh ways to help create, enhance, or mobilize social support for individuals in need. This volume provides a wide range of information for a diverse audience. It is neither comprehensive nor current since information and data on social support are continually evolving. This volume is, however, a valuable compendium of what we have learned about support particularly during the 1970s and 1980s.

Professor John G. Bruhn, Dean, School of Allied Health Sciences, The University of Texas Medical Branch at Galveston, and his associates have provided a major reference work. I hope it will be very useful to all those involved in health and related professions.

Dan A. Chekki
University of Winnipeg

FOREWORD

It is a pleasure to prepare a Foreword for this timely and valuable book. There has been, in the last decade, an explosion in research dealing with the concept of social support. However, the results that have been generated by this outpouring have been difficult to interpret. There are many findings documenting the major importance of social support for health and well-being. There also are findings that show the opposite. On reflection, this is not surprising: a study of the natural history of new ideas reveals that this always happens. A new idea is proposed and the early research shows that it is indeed of potential importance. Following this demonstration, research is initiated to test the new hypothesis. If negative results emerge from these tests, it is important to recognize that they were generated only in response to the original positive finding. They would not have been of interest without the first research results. And this is exactly what is now happening in the field of social support.

Unfortunately, the literature on social support has grown at such a rate that it is difficult for even the most dedicated and informed scholar to keep up on the latest twists and turns. And it is for this reason that the present volume is so useful. Here, in one place, the results from over 1,000 recent studies on social support can be reviewed.

This book comes at just the right time. Enough research evidence has now accumulated dealing with the concept of social support that it is now possible to discern trends, reach generalizations, and come to conclusions. Enough data are now available that it can be sorted through to separate the important from the trivial. This is a crucial step in the history of science. It is only by confronting negative evidence and contradictory findings that clarification and progress can be achieved. The publication of such negative evidence is a welcome event and presents us with a special opportunity to think more carefully, selectively, and critically. Indeed, it is only from this process that true understanding can be achieved. In the field of social support, we now have enough positive, negative, and even neutral evidence to satisfy the most demanding historian of science.

To achieve a better understanding of the role of social support in our lives is important. That there has been such a proliferation of research and interest in the concept in recent years is no accident. It is almost as if we all had been waiting for an idea such as this and, when it was offered, we seized upon it immediately. There are, I think, several reasons for this. One is that the concept makes intuitive sense. Most of us know from personal experience that people need people. Indeed, it is, in some ways, a little embarrassing that we need to develop research projects to demonstrate what everyone already knows. While there probably is some truth to this, we all also know that "what everybody knows" often turns out not to be true. Nevertheless, an idea that makes intuitive sense certainly is appealing and it clearly needs to be taken very seriously. At a minimum, it would be good to know which elements of social support are important: is it the number of friends one has; how much one likes them; how often one sees them; what they do for one; or what one does for them?

A second reason for the great interest in the concept of social support is the evidence that it is related in some way to the likelihood of people getting sick or maintaining health. During the last 30 years, a massive research effort has been underway in this country to uncover the causes of such major diseases as coronary heart disease, cancer, stroke, arthritis, and diabetes. This research has resulted in the identification of many biomedical risk factors, but it has been disappointing that these risk factors have explained so little. For example, the three major identified risk factors for coronary heart disease (elevated serum cholesterol, hypertension, and cigarette smoking) account for less than half the disease that occurs. In the search for other risk factors to explain disease occurrence, the concept of social support was discovered (or re-discovered). Since earlier efforts to explain disease etiology were faltering, the identification of this new risk factor was of special and timely significance.

A third reason for interest in the concept of social support is that it may be of importance in treatment and rehabilitation programs. It has become increasingly clear over the years that the treatment of illness cannot simply be brought about by direct medical or surgical intervention. More and more, we ask people to change their behaviors and outlooks. We ask that people do more of some things and less of others. We ask that people change their priorities and perceptions. As we have come to realize this, we have come also to realize the power of self-help groups and of friends and family in helping to avoid disease and maintain health.

A fourth reason for the popularity of the concept of social support is that it may provide a parsimonious and convenient conceptual integration for a wide range of otherwise seemingly unrelated psychosocial risk factors. Researchers have, for 30 years, been looking for psychosocial risk factors to help us understand why some people get sick while others remain healthy. From this work, many possible psychosocial risk factors have been identified. The length of this list is both encouraging and distressing. It is encouraging because it supports the position that "something" about psychosocial functioning is important for health. It is distressing because the list seems to have no central theme or integrating concept. The concept of social support certainly could be considered that link. For example, when one examines the "stressful life events" that have been suggested as risk factors for disease, it turns out that the important events are those that involve disruption of social ties. Included here are divorce, job loss, death of a loved one, migration, and so on. Similarly, people with type A behavior pattern (and with higher rates of coronary heart disease) have difficulty in maintaining ties to other people. People who are married have better social ties (and lower mortality rates for almost all causes of death) than those who are single, widowed, or divorced. Members of such religious groups as Seventh Day Adventists and Mormons (with lower rates of coronary heart disease, cancer, and other diseases) have better social support networks than those who are not members. It is impressive and worthy of special attention that one concept can provide a parsimonious integration of a wide body of seemingly diverse findings.

It is impressive, when considering the body of research that has been developed around the concept of social support, to note that this has been achieved without a clear definition or understanding of the concept. The research that has been done on social support is remarkable because something important has been observed in so many studies in spite of this heterogeneity of definitions and in spite of the fact that different research methods have been used by different investigators in the study of different populations. This concept must be very rigorous, indeed, to withstand such crude treatment. To improve matters, some have suggested we move toward one definition of social support that all can use. Clearly, this would be of great value in comparing findings from so many different studies. While desirable, this proposal depends on picking the "right" definition and, on this issue, little agreement exists. Nevertheless, it clearly is time that we began to think about this issue. Enough research evidence has now accumulated to permit the observation of patterns, regularities, and consistencies.

For all these reasons, this book is of enormous value for all interested in health and well-being. It comes at a time when enough evidence is available for serious study, reflection, and review and it comes precisely at a time when we urgently need new approaches to the study of disease causation and treatment.

S. Leonard Syme, Ph.D.
Professor of Epidemiology
School of Public Health
University of California, Berkeley
Berkeley, California

PREFACE

The growing interest in social support in both the popular and scientific literature and the need for a reference source to assist researchers and scholars in screening the numerous works published in diverse sources provided the impetus for undertaking this project. Annotations provide a form of peer review and are, therefore, a resource for readers. Since social support is not a new concept and has existed under many labels, it is difficult to state that this work is comprehensive. We have attempted to include work which we felt was relevant to social support, even if the term social support was not explicitly used. The citations, we feel, provide an excellent coverage of social support literature through 1986.

Since social support is not a concept unique to any specific discipline, the book should be useful to teachers, researchers, clinicians, and students in numerous disciplines and subspecialties within the social and behavioral sciences, the health professions, humanities, religion, and education.

The bibliography includes mainly primary sources. It excludes reviews, reports, newsletters, and sources that are not indexed or available to most readers. The bibliography also includes works in languages other than English, in particular, those in French, German and Dutch. The work is organized into eight chapters representing major topic areas of the field, and each chapter is broken down into sub-topics. Books, journals, chapters in books, dissertations, and conference proceedings are kept separate, and sources are alphabetized within each sub-topic. This format, along with author and subject indices, facilitates the search for relevant material by the user. Sources are numbered and indexed using the source number.

We followed the thirteenth edition of the *Chicago Manual of Style* in compiling our references. Each reference contains a brief statement of purpose; a phrase noting what type of work it is (text, book of readings, editorial, theoretical, literature review and so forth); a few sentences describing the main theme(s) or finding(s); and a list of suggested audiences who may find the work useful. We edited the author's statement of purpose and findings to minimize jargon. Therefore, we are responsible for possible misinterpretations resulting from our editing.

In an undertaking of this magnitude, it is impossible not to offend someone who feels that their work has been overlooked, minimized by the number of citations, or the works selected not the ones they would choose as representative of their writing. Since social support is not a discipline with established boundaries, there may be work on social support available or published in sources unknown to the authors. We relied upon the expertise of reference librarians and the many computerized sources available to modern libraries to minimize important omissions.

A review of the references on social support has provided us with a perspective of ways to refine future work in this area. There is a need to sharpen and reach some consensus about the definition and meaning of the concept, scrutinize measurement techniques and how they might be enhanced, and there is a need for interdisciplinary studies of the concept. If social support research is to be meaningful, it needs to have practical applications and provide insight into how social support can be generated and changed when needed. There is also a need to learn more about the negative aspects of social support.

John G. Bruhn
Billy U. Philips
Paula L. Levine
Carlos F. Mendes de Leon
January 30, 1987

INTRODUCTION: Social Support:
A Rediscovered Concept

In the past decade, social support has become a popular concept in the research in both the health fields and the social and behavioral sciences. Social support is not a new idea. While a *Histline* search on social support was not productive, the earliest cumulative issue of *Social Science Citations* produced an abstract of a paper on social support and conformity presented at the 74th Annual Conference of the American Psychological Association in 1966. The *MESH* Vocabulary File yielded a long list of synonyms for the term social support. Examples include: social support network, social support systems, social network, social networking, community support, family networks, peer support, family support systems, group support, personal networks, mutual aid, psychosocial support systems, self-help groups, and social enforcement networks. The diversity of terms reflects the diversity in definitions of social support. The diversity in definitions, in turn, is reflected in numerous articles which debate the difficulties in measuring or assessing social support. No consensus about a definition of social support or how it should (or could) be measured exists. Nonetheless, social support has surfaced as a popular concept in research, especially as it relates to the risk of illness, the pace of clinical progress, and rehabilitation.

The impetus for the increasing current interest in social support is not entirely clear. Benjamin Gottlieb has traced some of the sources of contemporary interest in social networks and social support. John Cassel's proposal implicating the social environment in the origins and amelioration of stress, and Gerald Caplan's practical strategies for mobilizing social support systems are two sources which have stimulated a great deal of recent research. The study or development of natural support systems has offered a way of realizing the values placed on collaboration and cultural diversity. It offers insights into the way in which local sociocultural patterns, belief systems, and environmental forces set the conditions for deformities of social support. Research on the preferences people express for certain sources of social support in health protection have been favorably received because it has tied together recent formulations about the epidemiology of mental disorder and suggested a research agenda for understanding stress and coping.

The topic of social support has also provided a new focus for ecological methods of inquiry into life-span development and adaptation. A broad understanding of social support in coping and social adaptation requires the study of the interactions between sociocultural factors, the social and physical environment, and the personalities and competencies of people.

A third source of recent interest in social support is linked to current consumer criticisms of the way health sources are delivered and the gaps in service. Criticisms of a highly technological system of health care have highlighted the need to emphasize the patient's responsibility in maintaining and protecting his health and the role of family members and close friends in the course of treatment and rehabilitation. Additionally, social support has been shown to be important in the task of preventing or minimizing stress and facilitating adaptation to life change. Self-help groups have attracted a large number of people whose problems have not been completely addressed by the health care system. Finally, moral and ethical issues surrounding death and the quality of life have accentuated the need to examine the way we deal with death and dying in our culture and the resources available to dying persons and their loved ones.

SOCIAL SUPPORT AND HEALTH:

AN ANNOTATED BIBLIOGRAPHY

CHAPTER 1

SOCIAL SUPPORT

1. GENERAL, DEFINITIVE, AND THEORETICAL ASPECTS

a. Books

1. AIKEN, Linda H., and David Mechanic (Eds.). *Applications of Social Science to Clinical Medicine and Health Policy*. New Brunswick, NJ: Rutgers University Press, 1986.

This volume was initiated by the Medical Sociology Section of the American Sociological Association because it was believed that the contributions of the social sciences to clinical medicine and health policy are not well understood or appreciated by medical educators and practitioners, or by policymakers in various levels of government.

Book of Readings

The 25 chapters in this volume are grouped into five major sections: 1) social contexts of health care and health policy; 2) major medical problems and monitoring health outcome; 3) health and illness over the life cycle; 4) prevention and caring; 5) organization and delivery of health services.

Of special interest to medical sociologists and clinical sociologists, medical educators and administrators, and health care administrators.

2. ANDREWS, Frank M., and Stephen B. Withey. *Social Indicators of Well-Being: Americans' Perception of Life Quality*. New York: Plenum, 1976.

A study about perceptions of well-being specifically designed to investigate how these perceptions are organized in the minds of different groups of American adults, to find valid and efficient ways of measuring these perceptions, to suggest ways these measurement methods could be implemented to yield a series of social indicators, and to provide some initial readings on these indicators.

Book of Readings

The book is organized into three major parts. Part 1 describes the
methodological and conceptual explorations that provide the fundamental knowledge base on which one can begin to build a series of
perceptual indicators; Part 2 examines a large number of perceptual
indicators and what they tell about the well-being of the American
population; and Part 3 is concerned with the application of the
author's developmental efforts and is addressed to those who would use
the indicators explored to assess well-being in future studies.

Of interest to social and behavioral scientists, to health planners,
to demographers and geographers, and to statisticians.

3. BARKAS, Jan L.   *Friendship: A Selected, Annotated Bibliog-*
   raphy. New York: Garland, 1985.

An annotated collection of almost 700 citations of books, articles,
reports, audiovisual materials, and organizational resources that
focuses on friendship in its widest interpretation.

Annotated Bibliography

Most of the citations concentrate on the sociological literature.
There is no conceptual scheme for categorizing the material.
Summaries are provided. The breadth of materials cited is useful to
scholars and researchers interested in friendship.

Of interest particularly to social and behavioral scientists.

4. BUSCAGLIA, Leo.   *Loving Each Other*.   Thorofare, NJ: Slack,
   Inc., 1984.

A book about relationships and the complex nature of love.

Theoretical/Analytical

Contains the results of an extensive survey on relationships and
discusses the qualities of forgiveness, tenderness, communication,
honesty, and jealousy between husbands and wives and in the relationships between family, friends, and acquaintances.

Of interest to laymen and to social and behavioral scientists.

5. COHEN, Sheldon, and S. Leonard Syme (Eds.).   *Social Support*
   and Health. New York: Academic Press, 1985.

A guide for conducting research in social support and a source of
information on the implications of existing work for social policy.

Book of Readings

The 17 chapters comprise four parts. Section I provides a broad

definition of social support, discusses major theoretical, methodological, and practical issues, and shows the relationship of social
support to research and theory. Section II gives attention to the
meaning and functions of social support at different times in the life
cycle. Part III provides critical reviews and analyses of empirical
and theoretical work. The final chapters examine the effectiveness of
social support interventions and discuss the implications of existing
literature on social support for health policy.

Of use to social and behavioral scientists doing research in the area
of social support.

6. DERLEGA, Valerian J. (Ed.).   *Communication, Intimacy, and
      Close Relationships*. Orlando, FL: Academic Press, 1984.

A thorough exploration of intimate relationships, such as friendship
and love, which provide social support, a sense of belonging, and aid
in coping with life events.

Book--Readings--Theoretical

Addresses the development and maintenance of intimate relationships,
people's motives and goals in pursuing intimacy, the effects of
intimacy on self-concept, the nature of social exchange, and the
consequences of social isolation. Most chapters focus on the role of
communication, and all provide excellent reviews of theory and
research.

Important reading for anyone interested in social support, and could
serve as a text.

7. RUBIN, Zick (Ed.).   *Doing Unto Others*.   Englewood Cliffs,
      NJ: Prentice Hall, 1974.

An attempt to understand the ways in which people do unto others out
of curiosity and to come to terms with the problems and uncertainties
that pervade social life.

Book of Readings

The 14 papers in this book include a good deal of theorizing and
speculation about patterns of social behavior, but all of them remain
grounded in systematic empirical research. The five themes of
forming, molding, conforming, helping, and loving are explored as some
of the ways in which people relate to one another.

Of particular interest to social psychologists.

8. SARASON, Irwin G., and Barbara R. Sarason (Eds.).   *Social
      Support: Theory, Research, and Applications*.   Dordrecht,
      The Netherlands: Martinus Nijhoff, 1985.

Contains theoretical and research contributions, especially in regard

to the positive side of social interaction, those interpersonal ties
that are desired, rewarding, and protective.

Book of Readings

The book has five parts. Part One is concerned with several theoretical and methodological issues. The papers in Part Two look at
social support in a developmental context and consider some individual
variables, such as personality and sex. Part Three deals with what
happens when there are deficiencies in either the quality or quantity
of support. Part Four considers the interrelationship between stress
and social support in personal maladaptation. The chapters of Part
Five reflect the complexity of implementing interventions and putting
theory into practice.

Of importance to teachers and researchers of social support.

9. SARASON, Seymour B. *The Psychological Sense of Community:
    Prospects for a Community Psychology.* San Francisco:
    Jossey-Bass, 1974.

A book on the nature and significance of the psychological sense of
community.

Textbook

There is no formula for how to instill and maintain the psychological
sense of community. The thrust of this book has been that before we
indulge our tendency to develop formulas and techniques in our
endeavor to effect change, we need to understand better how the nature
of our culture produced the situation we wish to change. The one
thing of which we can be certain is, in our society, the absence or
dilution of the psychological sense of community is a destructive
force.

Of interest to social and behavioral scientists, especially community
psychologists, and psychiatrists.

10. WISPÉ, Lauren (Ed.). *Altruism, Sympathy, and Helping:
     Psychological and Sociological Principles.* New York: Aca-
     demic Press, 1978.

A variety of theoretical viewpoints on the general area of altruism,
sympathy, and helping.

Book of Readings

The authors attempt to explain and analyze helping behavior, presenting their individual research and theoretical assumptions
regarding man's impulse to concern himself with the welfare of his
fellows.

Should interest social and behavioral scientists.

b. Articles

11. BARRERA, Manuel, Jr. "Distinctions between social support concepts, measures, and models." *American Journal of Community Psychology* 14 (1986): 413-445.

The thesis of this review is that the global concept of social support should be abandoned in favor of more precise concepts that fit narrower models of stress-distress relationships.

Review and Analysis

Distinctions between measures of social embeddedness, perceived support, and enacted support are consistent with studies that find they are related only mildly. Six models are presented to illustrate important findings and to demonstrate how specific support concepts may fit unique models. The issues of confounds and future research directions are also discussed.

Of interest to teachers and researchers interested in social support.

12. ———, and Sheila L. Ainlay. "The structure of social support: A conceptual and empirical analysis." *Journal of Community Psychology* 11 (April 1983): 133-143.

Critically examines how social support has been presented in the literature.

Review and Theoretical

When social support is conceptualized as behavioral transactions provided by natural social support systems, these transactions can be classified into meaningful categories. The typology presented will lay the groundwork for investigating the buffering effects of specific types of support with respect to specific types of life stress.

Of interest to researchers of stress and social support.

13. BEISER, Morton, Jacob J. Feldman, Claudia J. Engelhoff. "Assets and affects." *Archives of General Psychiatry* 27 (1972): 545-549.

The relationship between positive and negative feeling states, selected personality assets, and certain sociodemographic characteristics in a group of rural adults is explored.

Research

Socially participant behavior and interpersonal reactivity are important for women, while the concomitants of contentment for men relate to the performance of instrumental activities associated with their roles as workers and providers. The data also suggest that, with increasing age, the cultivation of hobbies and formal social activities become more significant.

Of interest to social and behavioral scientists and mental health professionals.

14. BROADHEAD, W. Eugene, Berton H. Kaplan, Sherman A. James, Edward H. Wagner, Victor J. Schoenbach, Roger Grimson, Siegfried Heyden, Gosta Tibblin, Stephen M. Gehlbach. "The epidemiologic evidence for a relationship between social support and health." *American Journal of Epidemiology* 117 (May 1983): 521-537.

A review of published studies of social support and recommendations for future research.

Review

A discussion of the problems and research needs in studying social support as a modifier, a buffer, and a direct determinant of health or illness.

Of importance to researchers of stress and social support.

15. BROWNELL, Arlene, and Sally A. Shumaker (Eds.). "Social support: New perspectives in theory, research, and intervention. Part I. Theory and research." *Journal of Social Issues* 40, no. 4 (1984): Complete Issue.

Part I focuses on social support theory and research.

Theory and Research

The seven articles address several problems and gaps in the theory, research, and application of social support, and propose some solutions.

Of interest to social and behavioral scientists.

16. CLARK, Kenneth B. "Empathy: A neglected topic in psychological research." *American Psychologist* 35 (1980): 187-190.

An exploration of the topic, empathy.

Literature Review

This paper presents a definition of empathy, its determinants, form, limits, and scope. The author concludes that the blockage of functional empathy by power drives forms the basis of interpersonal, social, and other tensions and conflicts.

Psychologists and other social researchers will benefit from this thought provoking piece.

17. CUTRONA, Carolyn E. "Behavioral manifestations of social support: A microanalytic investigation." *Journal of Personality and Social Psychology* 51 (1986): 201-208.

This study was designed to examine the specific interpersonal behaviors that convey support from one person to another.

Research

Results showed that behaviors reflecting emotional support and informational support occurred as a specific response to stressful life events. Subjects who perceived themselves as having high levels of social support were more frequently the recipients of helping behaviors following stressful events than those who were low in perceived support.

Of interest to researchers of social support.

18. EISENBERG, Leon. "A friend, not an apple, a day will help keep the doctor away." *The American Journal of Medicine* 66 (April 1979): 551-553.

Assessing social connectedness is essential for accurate medical diagnosis and effective treatment.

Editorial

The point is made that social isolation is, in itself, a pathogenic factor in disease production. Mechanisms of social bonding, if disrupted, have a devastating impact. Good friends are an essential ingredient for good health.

Of interest to health professionals, social and behavioral scientists, and the general public.

19. ELL, Kathleen. "Social networks, social support, and health status: A review." *Social Service Review* 58 (1984): 133-149.

Reviews recent research suggesting that social ties increase immunity to physical illness.

Review

Study findings form a conceptual foundation for a social support system theory that includes social network structure, social support content, and behaviors and social conditions involved in mobilizing support, advancing knowledge about person-environment fit and health status. Social workers have a special opportunity to further refine social support system theory and intervention.

Of particular interest to social workers.

20.   FIORE, Joan, David B. Coppel, Joseph Becker, Gary B. Cox.
      "Social support as a multifaceted concept: Examination of
      important dimensions for adjustment." *American Journal of
      Community Psychology* 14 (1986): 93-111.

Four commonly used operations of the social support concept--
network contact frequency, satisfaction with support, perceived
availability of support, and use of support--were related to two
measures of psychological adjustment (Beck Depression Inventory) and
to one measure of physical adjustment (Cornell Medical Index).

Research

Satisfaction with support was the only significant prediction of
depression and general psychopathology. The set of four support
variables showed the strongest relationship to depression level, next
strongest to general psychopathology, and least to physical health.

Of interest to social and behavioral scientists.

21.   GOTTLIEB, Benjamin H. "The development and application of a
      classification scheme of informal helping behaviors." *Canadian
      Journal of Behavioral Science* 10 (1978): 105-115.

A study of the informal social supports provided to single mothers in
coping with child rearing, their need for emotional support, and their
financial stability.

Research

A set of 26 helping behaviors were classified into four areas of
informal social support based on the telephone interview responses of
40 single mothers. These four factors--emotionally sustaining
behaviors, problem solving behaviors, personal influences, and
environmental actions to effect social advising--are all suggested as
areas in which mental health services could be classified and
evaluated.

Researchers of social support may find this article helpful.

22.   _____. "Social support as a focus for integrative research in
      psychology." *American Psychologist* 38 (1983): 278-287.

The health protective effects of social support are examined in light
of the historical evolution of community psychology.

Literature Review

Proposes that social support systems are units of social structure in
much the same way as social networks and that they can be exploited to
provide primary prevention resources in community psychology.

Psychologists, social workers, and others working in communities or
with population groups may benefit from this paper.

23. _____, and Andrew Farquharson. "Blueprint for a curriculum
    on social support." *Social Policy* 15, no. 3 (1985): 31-34.

An outline of a generic curriculum on the topic of social support.

Theoretical

Outlines the components of a core curriculum on social support-
theory, intervention strategies, and general themes. The curriculum
directly addresses the tensions and prospects for a partnership
between professional and informal health and human services.

Of interest to educators, especially those in the health sciences.

24. HILBERT, Gail A., and Lois Ryan Allen. "The effect of social
    support on educational outcomes." *Journal of Nursing Educa-
    tion* 24, no. 2 (1985): 48-52.

A review of social support literature identified the theoretical
framework of this prospective correlational study.

Descriptive

The two hypotheses regarding social support in relation to outcomes
were not supported. The hypothesis regarding the relationship between
social support and self-concept was supported.

Of interest to social and behavioral scientists.

25. JACOBSON, David E. "Types and timing of social support."
    Journal of Health and Social Behavior 27 (1986): 250-204.

Describes several theories of stress and their related concepts of
support and illustrates the point that analyses of the temporal
dimension of support suggest that it be understood as an appraisal of
behavior.

Review and Analysis

Studies of social support timing contribute to an understanding of
support processes. By integrating different perspectives, it is
possible to answer questions about what support is and how it works,
and suggest new directions for research.

Of interest to social and behavioral scientists.

26. JUNG, John. "Bias in social support attributions." *Journal of
    Social Behavior and Personality* 1 (July 1986): 429-438.

Two studies investigate the hypothesis that a positive bias in favor
of social support may exist in lay explanations for successful coping.

Research

Social support may be receiving too much credit for positive outcomes and too little blame for negative events when observers attempt to make sense of outcomes. Findings of these studies challenge prevalent views about the extent to which social support produces beneficial effects. Overestimates of benefits may encourage positive social interaction, but could also promote false hope, undermine individual effort, and foster ineffective intervention programs. The ability to recognize situations where social support contributes to failure is important and could minimize the tendency to "blame the victim." Further research is needed to determine both the actual benefits and negative effects of social support.

An important article for social science researchers of social support.

27. _____. "Social support and its relation to health--a critical evaluation." *Basic and Applied Social Psychology* 5 (1984): 143-169.

Conceptual, methodological, and theoretical shortcomings of research on the relationship of social support to mental and physical health are presented.

Review and Analysis

Attention is directed toward the interactive process between provider and recipient of social support. Identification of factors involved in the receipt and offering of social support is essential for theory development. Recognition of individual differences in the giving, as well as taking, of social support is needed.

Of interest to researchers of social support.

28. KAPLAN, Berton H., John C. Cassel, Susan Gore. "Social support and health." *Medical Care* (Supplement) 15 (1977): 47-58.

Unravels some important dimensions of the social support concept and helps to clarify the place of the study of social support in biomedical research.

Theoretical

The areas included in this paper are: psychosocial factors in disease etiology, mechanisms of social support, social networks as support availability, and policy implications of medical care.

Useful to teachers and researchers concerned with the relationship between stress and social support.

29. LA ROCCA, James M. "Theoretical distinctions between causal and interaction effects of social support." *Journal of Health and Social Behavior* 24 (1983): 91-92.

A comment on Peggy A. Thoits' "Conceptual, methodological, and theoretical problems in the study of social support as a buffer against life stress," *Journal of Health and Social Behavior* 23, 1982 (Chapter 6).

Comment

Argues against Thoits' use of marital status as an indicator of social support, her theoretical discussion of the relationship between causal effects and main vs. interactive effects of social support, and her statement and discussion supporting the direct relationship of social support to psychological well-being. States that the fact that significant relationships exist between measures of social support and indicators of psychological well-being, even in the absence of stressors, and the fact that support can be a causal factor in the stress process are not relevant to the issue of buffering, and discusses the reasons for this argument.

Should be of interest to social science researchers who are interested in social support.

30. LIEBERMAN, Morton A. "Social supports--the consequences of psychologizing: A commentary." *Journal of Consulting and Clinical Psychology* 54 (1986): 461-465.

This commentary suggests that the term social support is too broad and provides some suggestions for conceptualizing it in its various component parts.

Theoretical

The author uses his own studies to describe areas of research need to better define and understand social support. The mechanism and transformation of the concept is tuned and critiqued.

Should interest social science researchers and others interested in social support.

31. LIU, William T. "Culture and social support." *Research on Aging* 8 (1986): 57-83.

Raises theoretical questions concerning the use of culture and support groups in mental health research on cultural minorities.

Theoretical

The concepts of culture and social support are treated by investigators as separate and independent phenomena, rather than as interactive and interdependent elements in the social environment of the individual patient. However, the attributes and structure of network support systems cannot be described apart from the cultural blueprint of a society. While the role of culture in mental illness is important, more rigorous research on social structure is needed before it can be understood.

Of interest to social and behavioral scientists, especially mental health researchers.

32. MacELVEEN-HOEHN, Patricia, and Sandra J. Eyres. "Social
    support and vulnerability: State-of-the-art in relation to
    families and children." *Birth Defects* 20 (1984): 11-43.

This paper reviews the concepts of social support and vulnerable
families and children, proposes a theoretical model on coping and
adaptation, and ascertains any significant implications for the
delivery of health care services and research.

Review and Analysis

The review of the literature indicates that major problems persist in
the classification, conceptualization, empirical investigation, and
clinical application of social support due to a lack of clarity
regarding the definition of social support and how it works. The
literature strongly suggests that the interactions of adults and
children with supportive members of their social networks are
important in the development of essential cognitive and social skills,
as well as for the promotion of security and comfort. Supports from
individuals, families, and groups are also associated with more
successful adaptation and favorable outcomes.

Of interest to social workers, developmental psychologists, nurses,
and family sociologists.

33. MINKLER, Meredith A., William A. Satariano, Carol Langhauser.
    "Supportive exchange: An exploration of the relationship
    between social contacts and perceived health status in the
    elderly." *Archives of Gerontology and Geriatrics* 2 (1983):
    211-220.

Six-hundred and seventy-eight elderly residents of Alameda County,
California, participated in this survey research study which examined
social ties, supportive exchange, and health status.

Research

A strong relationship was found between a key dimension of supportive
exchange--the giving and seeking of advice--and self-reported health
status.

Of interest to social and behavioral scientists.

34. MURAWSKI, Benjamin J., Doris Penman, Madeline Schmitt.
    "Social support in health and illness: The concept and its
    measurement." *Cancer Nursing* (October 1978): 365-371.

Documents past efforts to conceptualize social support, suggests some
conceptual refinements, and proposes some guidelines for developing
instruments for the measurement of social support in health and
illness.

Literature Review

The dynamics of social support during the illness experience and its potential role in facilitating coping with disease need exploration. The lack of an adequate instrument to measure social support remains a serious problem for research of this variable in disease etiology and coping with disease.

Useful to researchers in the area of stress and social support.

35. NORBECK, Jane S. "Social support: A model for clinical research and application." *Advances in Nursing Science* 3 (July 1981): 43-59.

A model is suggested for building a body of knowledge about the patient's social environment for clinical practice.

Review and Theoretical

Research that incorporates person and situation variables will lead to an accumulation of knowledge that will be helpful in determining what types of social networks are most useful for particular individuals in the light of specific issues and environmental conditions.

Of interest to nurses and health professionals in direct patient care.

36. ROSENTHAL, Karen R., Ellis L. Gesten, Saul Shiffman. "Gender and sex role differences in the perception of social support." *Sex Roles* 14 (1986): 481-500.

This study examined the relationships among support types, gender, sex role orientation, and stress level among 253 college undergraduates.

Research

Sex differences were found in emotional support, with men reporting less need, perceived availability, and satisfaction than women. Traditional sex-typed men reported less need for emotional support than traditional women, but there was no difference between androgynous men and women. Although gender differences do exist in need for emotional support, the effects of sex role orientation on perceptions of social support seem to be somewhat circumscribed.

Of interest to researchers of social support.

37. SARASON, Barbara R., Irwin G. Sarason, T. Anthony Hacker, Robert B. Basham. "Concomitants of social support: Social skills, physical attractiveness and gender." *Journal of Personality and Social Psychology* 49 (1985): 469-480.

Investigates the naturally occurring relationship between self-reported social support and social skills, on one hand, and behavioral measures and rated physical attractiveness on the other.

Research

Significant differences were found in the social skills of subjects who were high and low in social support. Women were found to be significantly more socially skilled, and were rated as being more physically attractive than men. The results help to delineate more clearly the dimensions of social support, demonstrating the relation between social support and social skills.

Of interest to social and behavioral scientists, especially social psychologists and sociologists.

38. SARASON, Irwin G., and Barbara R. Sarason. "Concomitants of social support: Attitudes, personality characteristics, and life experiences." *Journal of Personality* 50 (1982): 331-344.

Examines several personal characteristics of people who receive high or low levels of social support.

Research

Subjects low in social support expressed more negative attitudes toward mental illness and reported more anomy than subjects receiving high levels of support. Absence of social support seemed to be related to less tolerance of behavioral deviation by others, and to more negative views of friends and community.

Useful to all researchers interested in social support.

39. SHONKOFF, Jack P. "Social support and the development of vulnerable children." *American Journal of Public Health* 74 (1984): 310-312.

An important summary of the main body of knowledge regarding social support.

Editorial

Contributes 14 significant questions regarding a research agenda for social support.

Essential reading for anyone interested in contributing to a better understanding of social support and its relationship with stress and disease.

40. SHUMAKER, Sally A., and Arlene Brownell (Eds.). "Social support: New perspectives in theory, research, and intervention. Part II. Intervention and policy social support interventions." *Journal of Social Issues* 41, no. 1 (1985).

Provides a broad understanding of the concept of social support and its viability as a target for intervention.

Special Journal Issue

Seven articles by social psychologists and social workers address the design and implementation of interventions to improve the quality of people's lives.

Should interest social workers, psychologists, psychiatrists, and social scientists.

41. STARKER, Joan. "Methodological and conceptual issues in research on social support." *Hospital and Community Psychiatry* 37 (1986): 485-490.

A review and analysis of the literature on social support addressing the lack of clear definitions, lack of uniform and reliable assessment instruments, failure to consider negative and conflictual aspects of support relationships, and inattention to the confounding effects of life events, individual differences in needs, and environmental factors on social support.

Review and Analysis

A growing body of literature suggests that an individual experiencing stressful life events will be less susceptible to illness if social support is available. There is also some evidence that social support has a more pervasive function in its ability to regulate an individual's mental health. However, there is a need for greater consensus on the definition of social support and for the development of uniform assessment instruments. One must be cautious in the clinical applications of social support. A social support component to a clinical service or mobilization of community social support is not necessarily helpful.

Of interest to researchers of social support.

42. THOITS, Peggy A. "Main and interactive effects of social support: Response to La Rocca." *Journal of Health and Social Behavior* 24 (1983): 92-95.

Discusses La Rocca's comments in "Theoretical distinctions between causal and interaction effects of social support," a commentary on Thoits' earlier article, "Conceptual, methodological, and theoretical problems in the study of social support as a buffer of life stress" (Chapter 6), especially their disagreement over the importance of disentangling the main and interactive effects of social support.

Comment

Addresses points of disagreement with LaRocco concerning the measure and implications of social support. Closely addressed are the buffering effects of social support and the influence of social support on stress.

Of interest to social science researchers.

43. TILDEN, Virginia Peterson. "Issues in conceptualization and
     measurement of social support in the construction of nursing
     theory." *Research in Nursing and Health* 8 (1985): 199-206.

Reviews the present development of social support to assist nurses
toward an adequate understanding of the concept. Theoretical
frameworks underlying definitions are examined, and issues of
measurement and clinical assessment are discussed.

Theoretical

Clinical assessment instruments need to be developed, hypotheses on
the effect of social support on health status must continue to be
tested, and protocols for clinical intervention need to be developed
and tested.

Of particular interest to nurses.

44. TRIPATHI, Rama C., Robert D. Caplan, R.K. Naidu.
     "Accepting advice: A modifier of social support's effect
     on well-being." *Journal of Social and Personal Relationships*
     3 (1986): 213-228.

Tests hypotheses regarding conditions under which the beneficial
effects of social support will and will not occur.

Research

Evidence suggests that the freedom to reject advice is particularly
important in obligating relationships because the donor and recipient
of advice are likely to differ in their diagnoses of the cause of
problems. Attention is given to the costs and benefits which the
advice-giver may incur by encouraging the recipient to feel free to
reject advice.

Of interest to social psychologists and other social scientists.

45. VEIEL, H.O.F. "Dimensions of social support: A conceptual
     framework for research." *Social Psychology* 20 (1985):
     156-162.

Argues that the fallacious assumption of a single commodity, "social
support," lies at the root of present confusion about the nature and
consequences of social support, and that a multi-dimensional conceptual framework is necessary for developing assessment and intervention
strategies.

Theoretical

A differentiated framework is presented and shown to be consistent
with the present state of empirical and theoretical knowledge.

Of interest to social and behavioral scientists and mental health
professionals.

46. WINEFIELD, Helen R. "The nature and elicitation of social support--some implications for the helping professions." *Behavioral Psychotherapy* 12 (1984): 318-330.

Discusses the attributes of the individual who reports inadequate levels of social support.

Discussion and Analysis

A model of support elicitation skills has been proposed, which draws on the empirical literature concerning patterns of social interaction distinctive to depressed and lonely people. This analysis has several implications for clinical practice. Research needs are also pointed out.

Of interest to mental health professionals and practicing psychotherapists.

c. Chapters

47. ANTONUCCI, Toni C., and Charlene E. Depner. "Social support and informal helping relationships." *In* Thomas Ashby Wills (Ed.). *Basic Processes in Helping Relationships.* New York: Academic Press, 1982.

Supports the premise that social support has far-reaching implications for people's adaptation to the stresses they experience over their life course.

Theoretical

A discussion of the structural, functional, and reciprocal properties of social networks; the positive and negative effects of social networks; individual differences in the effect of support; and on-going methodological and conceptual issues in the study of social support.

Of interest to researchers of stress and social support.

48. CAPLAN, Robert D. "Social support, person-environment fit, and coping." *In* L.A. Ferman, and J.P. Gordus (Eds.). *Mental Health and the Economy.* Kalamazoo, MI: W.E. Upjohn Institute for Employment Research, 1979.

Presents a framework based on the premise that coping is probably a function of characteristics of both the person and the environment. Social support plays an important role in this framework because it is viewed as an aid (or hindrance) in helping people cope effectively.

Theoretical

The framework presents social support as a hypothesized determinant of people's perceptions of their environments and of their own abilities and needs, motivation to respond by coping and by defensive processes, mental and physical well-being, and available objective environmental resources. Although the framework is based on previous theory and research, it is largely untested. The model should suggest intermediate goals of social technologies that attempt to increase social support, coping, and environmental mastery.

Of interest to social and behavioral scientists.

49. COBB, Sidney. "Social support and health through the life course." *In* Matilda White Riley (Ed.). *Aging from Birth to Death*. Boulder, CO: Westview Press, 1979.

Defines social support and explains where it fits in the scheme of support systems, summarizes the literature relating this concept to various aspects of health, and discusses a possible theoretical explanation of the way in which social support acts to promote the health of individuals.

Review

Social support is defined as the sum of emotional, esteem, and network support, which has beneficial effects on a wide variety of health variables throughout the life course and on the bereaved after a death. Suggests that training in supportive behavior, at home and in school, and institutionalization of support workers' roles would be extremely desirable.

Of interest to mental health professionals and social scientists.

50. HAMBURG, Beatrix A., and Marie Killilea. "Relation of social support, stress, illness and use of health services." *In* Report to the Surgeon General on Health Promotion and Disease Prevention by the Institute of Medicine, National Academy of Sciences *Healthy People: The Surgeon General's Report on Health Promotion and Disease Prevention. Background Papers, 1979.* Washington, DC: U.S. Department of Health, Education, and Welfare, Public Health Service, Office of the Assistant Secretary for Health and Surgeon General. DHEW (PHS) Publication No. 79-55071A, 1979.

Examines the relationships between life stress, illness, patient behavior, and social support systems.

Review

Ample evidence shows an interdependent relationship between stress, illness, social support, and the utilization of medical services, but many research questions remain unanswered and need to be addressed. Social support and community support systems are clearly relevant to all levels of health care, and health professionals need to educate themselves about the value and complementarity of professional helping systems and natural social support systems and how they can be used differentially for maximum individual and social benefit. A variety of formal and informal preventive, supportive, and remedial services should be available to all people, provided in ways that assure availability and access and preserve the dignity and privacy of the individual.

Important to all health care providers, planners, and policymakers.

51. HELLER, Kenneth. "The Effects of Social Support: Prevention and Treatment Implications" *In* Arnold P. Goldstein, and Frederick H. Kanfer (Eds.). *Maximizing Treatment Gains: Transfer Enhancement in Psychotherapy.* New York: Academic Press, 1979.

An objective review of the evidence concerning social support, highlighting unanswered questions and the directions that research might take.

Review

Points out the need for understanding the ingredients of social support, the conditions under which its positive effects are facilitated, and the persons for whom it is beneficial or contraindicated.

Should be of particular interest to social scientists engaged in research regarding social networks and social support and to mental health professionals.

52. SINGER, Jerome E., and Diana Lord. "The role of social support in coping with chronic or life-threatening illness" *In* Andrew Baum, Shelley E. Taylor, Jerome E. Singer (Eds.). *Handbook of Psychology and Health, Volume 4.* Hillsdale, NJ: Erlbaum, 1984.

An overview of current research on social support with recommendations for future research.

Review of the Literature

Discusses hypotheses that have been examined in studies of the effects of social support, an explicit working definition of what is to be studied as social support, and how social support should be measured. Authors point out the need for more research on the extent to which social support does or does not aid recovery and coping with a long-term or life-threatening, and perhaps terminal, illness, and suggest the use of instruments that make explicit choices along the three dimensions of objectivity/subjectivity, formal/informal measurements, and disease specificity.

Should interest social scientists, especially those engaged in research on social support.

53. TURNER, R. Jay, B. Gail Frankel, Deborah M. Levin. "Social support: Conceptualization, measurement, and implications for mental health." *In* J.R. Greenley (Ed.). *Research in Community Mental Health: A Research Annual.* Greenwich, CT: JAI Press, 1983.

This paper has two purposes: it reports on efforts aimed toward achieving measures of social support, and examines the relationships between measures of social support and mental health.

Review and Analysis

The authors argue that while the measurement of social intimacy, social integration, or the nature of social networks is both important and indispensable, it is also insufficient. In the authors' view, social support can usefully be regarded as a personal experience rather than a set of objective circumstances or interactional processes. Accordingly, social support and social support resources should be viewed as related, but distinct concepts.

Of interest to social and behavioral scientists and researchers of social support.

c. Dissertation

54. BLAZER, Dan G. "Social support and mortality in an elderly community population." Ph.D. dissertation, University of North Carolina at Chapel Hill, 1980.

Development of a conceptual model of social support, which was used to test the social support-mortality relationship.

Research

Three parameters of social support were found and demonstrated to be independent but complementary. The three parameters significantly predicted 30 month mortality after controlling for potentially confounding variables.

Useful for social scientists, especially those interested in measurement of the concept of social support.

2. MEASUREMENT

a. Books

55. DONALD, Cathy A., and John E. Ware, Jr. *The Quantification of Social Contacts and Resources.* Santa Monica: Rand, 1982.

Prepared for the U.S. Department of Health and Human Services as part of the Rand Health Insurance Experiment (HIE), which was designed to investigate the effects of health care financing arrangements on the use of personal medical services, quality of care, health status, and satisfaction with care. Describes empirical studies designed to yield a set of scoring rules for HIE questionnaire items measuring social contacts and social resources.

Theoretical

The best conception of health may define individual health status in terms of the physiologic, physical, and mental status of the individual. The concept of social well-being extends measurement beyond the individual to focus on the quantity and quality of social contacts and social resources. The authors prefer a model of health status that defines these social factors as external to an individual's health.

Of interest to researchers of social support.

56. KANE, Rosalie A., Robert L. Kane, Sharon Arnold. *Measuring Social Functioning in Mental Health Studies: Concepts and Instruments*. U.S. Department of Health and Human Services, Public Health Service, Alcohol, Drug Abuse, and Mental Health Administration, National Institute of Mental Health Division of Biometry and Epidemiology. Rockville, MD: DHHS Publication No. (ADM) 85-1384, 1985.

Designed to provide a stimulus for the selection of items and scales to measure social functioning in mental health.

Government Report

A review of research design issues and concepts and research instruments to measure social functioning in mental health.

Of interest to mental health professionals and social and behavioral scientists, especially researchers in these areas.

b. Articles

57. BARRERA, Manuel, Jr., and Pamela Balls. "Assessing social support as a prevention resource: An illustrative study." *Prevention in Human Services* 2 (1983): 59-74.

Discusses approaches to measuring social support that might be adopted in needs assessment research. A prospective study of 74 young mothers is described, illustrating the use of multiple measures of support in investigating their relationship to birth outcome measures.

Research

Direct relationships were found between birth outcome indices and measures of both prenatal negative life events and psychological distress. Social support network size showed a stress moderating effect. Implications of findings for needs assessment designed for planning preventive interventions are discussed.

Of interest to health professionals interested in prevention and intervention.

58. BEELS, C. Christian. "Social support and schizophrenia." *Schizophrenia Bulletin* 7, no. 1 (1981): 58-72.

An introduction to a review of the literature on measurement of social support in schizophrenia.

Literature Review

Outlines the natural history of the career of the schizophrenic in his social networks and clearly identifies the dimensions of social support specific to schizophrenics.

Psychiatrists, social psychologists, and other mental health researchers would find this work useful.

59. BROWN, Marie Annette. "Social support during pregnancy: A unidimensional or multidimensional construct?" *Nursing Research* 35 (1986): 4-9.

The purpose of this study was to empirically test a conceptually derived multidimensional formulation of social support.

Research

Findings from this study raise questions about all currently used social support scales. Results suggest that research needs to systematically evaluate the multiple dimensions of social support.

Of interest to nurses and researchers of social support.

60. BRUHN, John G., and Billy U. Philips. "Measuring social support: A synthesis of current approaches." *Journal of Behavioral Medicine* 7 (1984): 151-169.

Definitions and concepts of social support are reviewed in an attempt to develop a theoretical structure for future research. Fourteen techniques for measuring social support are assessed to ascertain the degree to which they reflect common theoretical elements.

Review and Analysis

A paradigm is proposed to help focus research efforts on the construction of a systematic knowledge base about social support. A broad theoretical framework for studying social support is needed to understand how social support works when individuals are healthy as well as when they are ill.

Of interest to researchers of social support.

61. CARVETH, W. Bruce, and Benjamin H. Gottlieb. "The measurement of social support and its relation to stress." *Canadian Journal of Behavioral Science* 11 (1979): 179-188.

Focuses on the empirical relationship between three measures of social support and several stress indices among 99 mothers who completed questionnaires approximately eight weeks after their newborns were taken home from the hospital.

Research

Correlational analyses revealed a consistent pattern of weak to moderate associations between social support and stress. Discussion of the meaning of the pattern of correlations centers on the distinction between the role of social support in the coping process and its bearing on health outcomes.

Of interest to researchers of stress and social support.

62. PEARSON, Judith E. "The definition and measurement of social support." *Journal of Counseling and Development* 64 (February 1986): 390-395.

Examines definitions, constructs, and theories of social support and summarizes studies concerning recently devised scales for measuring social support and analyzing social network morphology.

Literature Review

Implications for counselors are discussed. One way to help clients improve their coping skills is to teach them to identify and use social supports and establish networks of helpful relationships that facilitate the coping process.

Of interest to social and behavioral scientists and counselors.

63. ROBERTS, Susan Jo. "Social support--meaning, measurement, and relevance to community health nursing practice." *Public Health Nursing* 21 (1984): 158-167.

Reviews recent advancements in the development and measurement of social support, the research that relates support to a variety of health outcomes and behaviors, and the relevance of the concept of social support to the practice of community health nursing.

Theoretical and Review

Suggestions are made for the use of new information in clinical practice and for the development of research within the practice area.

Of particular interest to nurses.

64. ROBSON, R.A.H.   "The effects of different group sex
     compositions on   support rates and coalition formation."
     Canadian   Review   of   Sociology   and   Anthropology   8 (1971):
     244-262.

An attempt to see whether differences between the behavior of men and
women occur in three person groups operating under the research
conditions of Mills, and to ascertain the effects of such differences
on the resulting group structure.

Research

From a comparison of the rates of support for three-male and three-
female groups, it was concluded that: 1) rates of support output are
almost three times as great for females as they are for males;
2) females distribute support more equally between the other two women
in the group than do males between the other two men; 3) females form
more coalitions than males; and 4) the least active member of the
group becomes an isolate in the three-male groups, but receives more
support than anyone else in the three-female group.

Of special interest to social psychologists and sociologists
interested in small groups.

65. TARDY, Charles H.   "Social support measurement." *American
     Journal of Community Psychology*   13, no. 2 (1985): 187-202.

Attempts to facilitate the study of social support through clarification of the decisions of researchers and increasing awareness of
the capabilities and limitations of available instruments.

Literature Review

The strengths and weaknesses of measures of social support are
addressed along with characteristics of the social support they
measure and priorities for the development of new measures. The most
pressing concern is the development of instruments that delineate
types of social support and assess the provision of support.

Of interest to social support researchers.

3. INDICES AND SCALES

a. Articles

66. ABBEY, Antonia, David J. Abramis, Robert D. Caplan. "Effects
     of different sources of social support and social conflict on
     emotional well-being." *Basic and Applied Social Psychology*
     6 (1985): 111-129.

Examines the effect of social support on emotional well-being during
social conflicts.

Research

Describes the development and testing of an instrument to measure sources of social support and social conflict. Social support and social conflict were not correlated, except when occurring between people closest to the respondents; then social support was correlated with measures of emotional well-being. The results are interpreted in light of the "buffer hypothesis."

Social science researchers may benefit from this article.

67. BARRERA, Manuel, Jr. "A method for the assessment of social support networks in community survey research." *Connections* 3, no. 3 (1980): 8-13.

A structured interview for identifying social support network membership was developed and its reliability evaluated.

Research

Results from several reliability indicators suggested that total network membership was reliably assessed. The interview method, therefore, appears feasible for use in survey research, and might be useful in studies of the relationship between social support variables and psychological adjustment. Future research in the development of this instrument is discussed.

Of interest to researchers of social support.

68. _____, Louise M Baca, Jon Christiansen, Melinda Stohl. "Informant corroboration of social support network data." *Connections* 8, no. 1 (1985): 9-13.

This study determines how well the self-reports of subjects examined by the Arizona Social Support Interview Schedule (ASSIS) can be corroborated by their network members.

Research

A sample of 36 community mental health outpatients and identified members of their networks (informants) were interviewed on items concerning the provision of support to the subjects by the informants and vice versa over the preceding month. With the exception of the category "Intimate Interaction," the self-reports of these subjects were corroborated by informants with a moderate to high degree of accuracy. It is important to recognize the limitations of the subject and informant samples, but the results of the study suggest that these network data reflect more than just the cognitive activity of subjects. The supportive exchange assessed by the ASSIS can largely be confirmed by the network members who provide support and receive it in return.

Of interest to researchers of social support.

69. _____, Irwin N. Sandler, Thomas B. Ramsay. "Preliminary
    development of a scale of social support: Studies on college
    students." *American Journal of Community Psychology*
    9 (1981): 435-447.

A 40 item scale, the Inventory of Socially Supportive Behaviors
(ISSB), in which respondents report the frequency with which they were
the recipients of supportive actions, was developed.

Research

Results suggest that the ISSB has adequate test-retest and internal
consistency reliability and is significantly correlated with network
size and perceived support of the family. The ISSB is seen as a
promising tool for understanding natural helping processes.

Of use to researchers of social support.

70. BEELS, C. Christian, Linda Gutwirth, Janet Berkeley, Elmer
    Struening. "Measurements of social support in schizophrenia."
    Schizophrenia Bulletin 10 (1984): 399-411.

Presents a selective review of methods and instruments that hold
promise for investigations of social support in the course and
treatment of schizophrenia.

Literature Review

Reviews social and psychological questionnaires, anthropological
network studies, ethnographies, and clinical epidemiological studies.
Concludes that social support measures designed for the general
population have limited usefulness in schizophrenia research.

Psychiatrists, psychologists, social workers, and others dealing with
schizophrenic patients may find this review useful.

71. BLAKE, Robert L., Jr., and David A. McKay. "A single-item
    measure of social supports as a predictor of morbidity."
    Journal of Family Practice 22 (1986): 82-84.

As part of a study of social risk for health impairment, a single-item
measure of social supports was evaluated as a predictor of six-month
self-reported morbidity.

Research

Women who had no one or only one person available for assistance in
times of difficulty had higher self-reported morbidity than women who
had such tangible assistance. For men there was a trend in the same
direction.

Of interest to social and behavioral scientists.

72. BLAZER, Dan G. "Social support and mortality in an elderly community population." *American Journal of Epidemiology* 115 (1982): 684-694.

A community sample of 331 persons, 65 years of age and older, was assessed for adequacy of social support along three parameters: roles and available attachments, perceived social support, and frequency of social interaction.

Research

The three parameters of social support significantly predicted 30-month mortality in both crude and controlled analyses in a community sample of older adults.

Of interest to researchers of social support.

73. BRANDT, Patricia A., and Clarann Weinert. "The PRQ--a social support measure." *Nursing Research* 30 (September/October 1981): 277-280.

A description of the development of the Personal Resource Questionnaire (PRQ)--a two-part measure of the multidimensional characteristics of social support.

Research

The PRQ was developed to measure social support in a study of the stress of long-term illness, social support of the "well" spouse, and the functioning of the family system. Evaluation of the PRQ supported its internal consistency, content validity, and predictive validity.

Of use to researchers of social support.

74. CAUCE, Ana M., Robert D. Felner, Judith Primavera. "Social support in high-risk adolescents: Structural components and adaptive impact." *American Journal of Community Psychology* 10 (1982): 417-428.

Examines the structure of social support and its relationship to adjustment for adolescents from high-stress, lower socioeconomic class, inner-city backgrounds.

Research

Factor analyses revealed three distinct support measures: family, formal, and informal support. Analyses of variance showed differences in the perceived helpfulness of the support dimensions as a function of the adolescent's age, sex, and ethnic background as well as in the relationship of each source of support to the adjustment indices.

Of interest to teachers, administrators, and mental health professionals.

75. DOHRENWEND, Barbara Snell, Bruce P. Dohrenwend, Margaret
     Dodson, Patrick E. Shrout. "Symptoms, hassles, social
     supports, and life events: Problem of confounded measures."
     Journal of Abnormal Psychology 93 (1984): 222-230.

Examines judgements by a sample of 371 clinical psychologists of the
extent to which items in leading stress instruments are likely to be
symptoms of psychological disorder.

Review and Analysis

Results indicate that each of the stress measures is confounded with
measures of psychological distress. This is more true of the Kanner,
Coyne, Schaefer and Lazarus Hassles Scale and the Lin, Dean, and Ensel
Social Support Scale than of the Holmes and Rahe Scale of Life Events.

Of particular interest to researchers of stress.

76. DUNCAN-JONES, Paul. "The structure of social relationships:
     Analysis of a survey instrument. Part 1." *Social Psychiatry*
     16 (1981): 55-61.

Discusses the development of the Interview Schedule for Social
Interaction (ISSI), an interview procedure for the assessment, for
research purposes, of the current state of a person's social
relationships.

Research

The interview schedule emphasizes a natural conversational style
rather than a more rigid list of questions. The instrument contains
items on six types of relationships: acquaintances, friends,
attachment, opportunity for nurturance, reassurance of worth, and
reliable alliance. Both availability and adequacy of sources of
support can be measured with this instrument.

Of particular interest to social scientists.

77. ————. "The structure of social relationships: Analysis of a
     survey instrument. Part 2." *Social Psychiatry* 16 (1981):
     143-149.

A test of the psychometric properties of the Interview Schedule for
Social Interaction (ISSI).

Research

Basically two underlying factors were found for the six original
dimensions of the ISSI (see Part 1): attachment and social integration. The availability and perceived adequacy of these two factors
could be measured with sufficient reliability, although the two
adequacy measures seem largely to be overlapping. The measures of
availability of attachment and availability of social integration were
more independent of each other.

Of particular interest to social scientists.

78. EVANS, Ron L., Sue Pomeroy, Margaret C. Hammond, Eugen M. Halar. "Family Resource Questionnaire: Reliability and validity of a social support measure for families of stroke patients." *Psychological Reports* 56 (1985): 411-414.

Describes the development of an interview instrument (Family Resource Questionniare) designed to measure dimensions of social support after stroke.

Research Report

This study of 48 stroke victims during rehabilitation identified 17 items associated with social support. Moderate validity and high reliability were found with adjustment to rehabilitation.

Physical and occupational therapists and other rehabilitation workers will benefit from this article, which describes a useful clinical tool.

79. FLAHERTY, Joseph A., F. Moises Gaviria, Dev S. Pathak. "The measurement of social support--the Social Support Network Inventory." *Comprehensive Psychiatry* 24 (1983): 521-529.

This report presents the rationale, design, and psychometric testing of one instrument in the Social Support Network Inventory (SSNI).

Research

The SSNI provides a reliable instrument to quantitatively measure social support in patients and the general population.

Of use to researchers of social support.

80. GARRISON, V., and Judith Podell. "Community support systems assessment for use in clinical interviews." *Schizophrenia Bulletin* 7, no 1 (1981): 101-108.

Presents a practical, economically efficient method for assessing a patient's social support system in a routine intake interview.

Clinical Review

Focuses on the Community Support System Assessment, an instrument sensitive to the subcultural and clinical variations that influence social supports.

Psychiatrists, social workers, community psychologists, and other mental health clinicians may find this a helpful clinical tool.

81. HENDERSON, Scott, P. Duncan-Jones, D.G. Byrne, Ruth Scott.
     "Measuring social relationships. The Interview Schedule for
     Social Interaction." *Psychological Medicine* 10 (1980): 723-
     734.

Describes the development and validation of a survey instrument to
measure social relationships.

Research Note

The Interview Schedule for Social Interaction (ISSI) assesses the
availability and perceived adequacy of social relationships and the
social support they provide. A general population test of the
instrument indicated good validity and reliability.

Researchers may find this a useful tool in clinical and epidemiological studies in psychiatry and general medicine.

82. HOLAHAN, Charles J., and Rudolf H. Moos. "Social support
     and adjustment: Predictive benefits of social climate indices."
     American Journal of Community Psychology 10 (1982): 403-
     415.

Estimates the relationship between social support and physical and
psychological adjustment, using measures that afford a qualitative
assessment of social support.

Research

Qualitative indices of social support in family and work environments
were derived from available social climate measures. Results from a
randomly selected community sample support hypotheses that qualitative
measures of support in family and work environments predict psychosomatic complaints and depression after variance due to negative life
change and quantitative measures of social support is accounted for.

Of interest to social and behavioral scientists, especially
researchers of stress and social support.

83. ———. "The quality of social support--measures of family
     and work relationships." *British Journal of Clinical Psy-
     chology* 22 (September 1983): 157-162.

Describes the development of indices of the quality of social support
in the family and work environments.

Research

The family and work scales were found to have a high reliability and
good concurrent and construct validity. The family scales and work
scales for males were negatively related to physical and psychological
symptoms, and both scales showed moderate positive relationships to a
traditional measure of social support.

Of interest to researchers of social support.

84. JENKINS, R., A. H. Mann, E. Belsey. "The background, design, and use of a short interview to assess social stress and support in research and clinical settings." *Social Science and Medicine* 15E (1981): 195-203.

A brief, standardized and semi-structured social screening interview, designed to identify and quantify social stresses and supports, is described.

Research

Validity and reliability are assessed and discussed. The use of the interview is described in a prospective study of 100 identified men and women with non-psychotic disorders where it proved to be a significant predictor and correlate of psychiatric outcome.

Of particular interest to mental health professionals and researchers of stress.

85. JENSEN, Peter S. "Risk protective factors, and supportive interventions in chronic airway obstruction." *Archives of General Psychiatry* 40 (1983): 1203-1207.

Fifty-nine patients with chronic airway obstruction completed the Schedule of Recent Experiences and Social Assets Scale to measure life stress and social supports.

Research

High risk control patients were hospitalized more often than low risk control patients and for more days than high risk patients in rehabilitation and self-help support groups. Measurements of stress and social supports can help identify high-risk patients. In turn, professionals might assist those patients by increasing their supports.

Of interest to mental health professionals.

86. LIN, Nan, Alfred Dean, Walter M. Ensel. "Social support scales: A methodological note." *Schizophrenia Bulletin* 7 (1981): 73-89.

Conceptualizes social support and assesses the reliability and validity of its various measures. Evaluates the ability of social support, along with stressors, to explain psychiatric symptoms.

Research

Representative data from a community survey of adults, ages 17-70, suggest that social support measures show strong relationships to depression and other psychiatric symptoms. Longitudinal studies are suggested to verify the causal relationship between social support and illness.

Of interest to researchers of stress and social support.

87. LINN, Margaret W. "Modifiers and Perceived Stress Scale."
     Journal of Consulting and Clinical Psychology 54 (1986):
     507-513.

The purpose of this study was to determine the interrelations between perceived stress and its modifiers and total or averaged scores, and obtain data on reliability and validity of the scale.

Research

The scale shows acceptable reliability as a measure of perceived stress related to recent events and to potential modifiers of stress perceptions. The perceived stress scores correlated significantly with clinical assessments of how much stress would be expected to be experienced in similar situations, and also with psychological and physical parameters generally thought to be associated with stress. Although the ratings were correlated with such measures as state anxiety and depression, they were not so highly correlated as to suggest that perceived stress ratings were simply reflections of mood.

Of interest to researchers of stress and social support.

88. LYON, Keith E., and Robert A. Zucker. "Environmental
     supports and post-hospital adjustment." *Journal of Clinical
     Psychology* 30 (1974): 460-465.

Investigates which specific environmental support variables produce successful community adjustment among former psychiatric patients.

Research

The Environmental Support Questionnaire was developed to assess informal sources of interpersonal support to ex-psychiatric patients. Two factors, derived by cluster analysis, appeared to have a positive effect on post-hospitalization symptomatology--a stable home environment and the presence of benign visitors.

Of interest to psychiatrists, psychotherapists, and social workers.

89. McFARLANE, Allan H., Kelly A. Neale, Geoffrey R. Norman,
     Ranjan G. Roy, David L. Streiner. "Methodological issues in
     developing a scale to measure social support." *Schizophrenia
     Bulletin* 7 (1981): 90-100.

Describes efforts to evaluate the properties of a Social Relationship Scale (SRS) that was developed as part of a prospective study of psychosocial influences on the health status of a population.

Research

Findings from the development, validation, and application of the SRS form a picture of a scale that is a reasonably reliable and valid instrument to use in assessing the extent and quality of social networks.

Of use to researchers of social support.

90. MILLER, Rickey S., and Herbert M. Lefcourt. "The assessment of social intimacy." *Journal of Personality Assessment* 46 (1982): 514-518.

The development of the Miller Social Intimacy Scale (MSIS), a 17-item measure of the maximum level of intimacy currently experienced, is presented.

Research

The MSIS is a reliable and valid measure of social intimacy. Evidence for internal consistency and test-retest reliability, as well as discriminant and construct validity is discussed.

Of special interest to researchers of the topic of social support.

91. NORBECK, Jane S. "The Norbeck Social Support Questionnaire." *Birth Defects* 20, no. 5 (1984): 45-57.

Summarizes the development and testing of the Norbeck Social Support Questionnaire (NSSQ).

Evaluative

Very high levels of internal consistency and test-retest reliability were found. At a seven-month retesting, medium levels of stability were found. The instrument has been found to be free from the response bias of social desirability. Medium levels of concurrent validity were shown with two other social support instruments. Construct validity has been demonstrated, and predictive validity was tested. Normative data are available as well as descriptive data about sources of support.

Of interest to social and behavioral scientists.

92. _____, Ada M. Lindsey, Virginia L. Carrieri. "The development of an instrument to measure social support." *Nursing Research* 30 (September/October 1981): 264-269.

Describes the development of the Norbeck Social Support Questionnaire, designed to measure multiple dimensions of social support.

Research

The instrument demonstrated high test-retest reliability, internal consistency, and apparent freedom from the social desirability response bias, suggesting that the NSSQ may be useful as a research and, perhaps, a clinical tool.

Of interest to researchers studying social support.

93. _____. "Further development of the Norbeck Social Support Questionnaire--normative data and validity testing." *Nursing Research* 32 (1983): 4-9.

Describes an instrument designed to measure multiple dimensions of social support.

Research

This second phase series of studies were conducted to provide a normative data base and to further test the validity of this proposed measure of social support. Test-retest and construct validity were found to be stable over a seven month period. Predictive validity of sub-scales was around 20%.

Nurses and others interested in a multidisciplinary social support measure will find this a useful instrument and method.

94. O'CONNOR, Pat, and George W. Brown. "Supportive relationships: Fact or fancy?" *Journal of Social and Personal Relationships* 1 (1984): 159-175.

The very close relationships of a sample of married women living in London are described, using a new instrument (SESS) measuring self-evaluation and social support.

Research

Only a third of the women had a "true" relationship with someone identified as very close, yet living outside the home. It is argued that recent research has failed to differentiate between those qualities of relationships which are actively supportive and those which simply reflect a search for attachment, and that this is the source of the failure to find an association between social support and psychiatric state. In the current survey, there is an association between the type of very close relationship and both the respondents' positive evaluations of themselves and their psychiatric states.

Of interest to mental health professionals.

95. ORITT, Eric J., Stephen C. Paul, Jay A. Behrman. "The Perceived Support Network Inventory." *American Journal of Community Psychology* 13 (1985): 565-582.

The development and psychosomatic investigation of the Perceived Support Network Inventory (PSNI), a measure of perceived social support, is described.

Research

A group of 146 introductory psychology students participated in a test-retest study design that collected reliability, internal consistency, and construct, convergent, and discriminant validity data on the scale. In addition, a contrast group of 28 counseling center clients was administered the PSNI. Test-retest reliability of the PSNI total score and subscale scores ranged from .72 to .88. Internal consistency for the PSNI was .77.

Of interest to researchers of social support.

96. POLLACK, Linda, and Rachel Harris. "Measurement of social support." *Psychological Reports* 53 (1983): 466.

Presents the preliminary development stage of a general social support measure.

Abstract

A 23 item, general social support instrument, which had a test-retest reliability of .90 in a sample of 12 is presented.

This instrument may be of use to researchers interested in social support.

97. PROCIDANO, Mary E., and Kenneth Heller. "Measures of perceived social support from friends and from family: Three validation studies." *American Journal of Community Psychology* 11 (1983): 1-24.

Three studies, in which measures of perceived social support from friends and from family were developed and validated, are described.

Research

The measures were internally consistent and appeared to measure valid constructs that were separate from each other and from network measures.

Of interest to researchers of social support.

98. ROCK, Daniel L., Kathy E. Green, Barbara K. Wise, Rachelle D. Rock. "Social support and social network scales: A psychometric review." *Research in Nursing and Health* 7 (1984): 325-332.

This review of 29 behavioral science studies published between 1967 and 1982 indicates many of these scales are developed by applying state-of-the-art psychometric approaches.

Review Article

Social support and social network scales were found to be deficient in
terms of their scaling techniques, reliability, and validity. The
dearth of psychometric data on these popular instruments has been
suggested as harmful to theory development and research efficiency.

Social support researchers should read this article.

99. SARASON, Irwin G., Henry M. Levine, Robert B. Basham,
     Barbara R. Sarason. "Assessing social support: The Social
     Support Questionnaire." *Journal of Personality and Social
     Psychology* 44 (1983): 127-139.

A measure of social support, the Social Support Questionnaire (SSQ),
is described, and four empirical studies employing it are presented.

Research

The research suggests that the SSQ is a reliable instrument. Social
support appears to be more strongly related to positive than to
negative life changes, negatively related to psychological discomfort
among women more than men, and an asset in enabling a person to
persist at a task under frustrating conditions.

Of interest to researchers of stress and social support.

100. SCHAFER, Lorraine C., Kevin D. McCaul, Russell E. Glasgow.
      "Supportive and nonsupportive family behaviors: Relationships
      to adhere and metabolic control in persons with Type I
      diabetes." *Diabetes Care* 9 (1986): 179-185.

The development and validation of the Diabetes Family Behavior
Checklist (DFBC), designed to assess both supportive and nonsupportive
family behaviors specific to diabetes self-care, is described.

Research

The DFBC is concluded to be a promising measure of family interaction
related specifically to the insulin-dependent diabetes mellitus
regimen. For adults, higher levels of nonsupportive family behaviors
may be related to reduced regimen adherence and poor control.

Of interest to family physicians, internists, and nurses.

101. SCHNEIDER, Lawrence J., and Nancy Polk. "Reliability note
      on the Social Support Scale." *Psychological Reports*
      59 (1986): 469-470.

Investigates the internal reliability of Pollack and Harris' Social
Support Scale and reports norms for 352 college males and 443 females.

Research

While the scale appears sufficiently reliable for research purposes, additional considerations of reliability and validity need to be addressed before clinical applications are appropriate.

Of interest to researchers of social support.

102. SOKOLOVE, Robert L., and David Trimble. "Assessing support and stress in the social networks of chronic patients." *Hospital and Community Psychiatry* 37 (1986): 370-372.

A discussion of show the social support network of deinstitutionalized chronic mentally ill patients can help moderate life stresses and reduce the need for rehospitalization.

Descriptive

The authors have developed a list of questions that can be used in assessing the various characteristics of a patient's social network, including the number of people in the network, the types of roles assumed in each relationship, and the nature of behavioral exchanges in each relationship. They believe that research on the social networks of chronic patients may provide information that will lead to more effective intervention.

Of particular interest to mental health professionals.

103. SPIEGEL, David, and Terry Wissler. "Family environment as a predictor of psychiatric rehospitalization." *American Journal of Psychiatry* 143 (January 1986): 56-60.

The Family Environment Scale scores and demographic characteristics of 108 discharged psychiatric patients were used to predict outcome at three months and one year.

Research

Higher ratings of family expressiveness predicted fewer days of rehospitalization. Higher family cohesion scores predicted better family-rated patient adjustment. Family environment was a better predictor of rehospitalization than baseline ratings of clinical status, indicating the importance of family support in the community adjustment of chronic psychiatric patients.

Of interest to mental health professionals.

104. STOKES, Joseph P., and Diane Grimard Wilson. "Inventory of Socially Supportive Behaviors: Personality, prediction, and gender differences." *American Journal of Community Psychology* 12 (1984): 53-69.

Describes the development of an inventory of socially supportive behaviors.

Research and Development

This instrument validates much of what has been found to be associated with social support in the literature, especially the number and quality of the interactions with others in the social network. Psychologists and other mental health professionals working in community mental health settings may find this helpful.

105. VAUX, Alan, Jeffrey Phillips, Lori Holly, Brian Thomson, Deirdre Williams, Doreen Stewart. "The Social Support Appraisals (SS-A) scale: Studies of reliability and validity." *American Journal of Community Psychology* 14 (1986): 195-219.

A scale of subjective appraisals of support (SS-A) was developed.

Research

Data from five student and five community samples indicated that the 23 item scale had good reliability, had adequate concurrent, convergent, and divergent validity with other perceived support measures, and showed predicted associations with measures of theoretically related antecedents (support network resources) and consequences (psychological well-being).

Of interest to social and behavioral scientists.

106. WEINERT, Clarann. "Evaluation of the Personal Resource Questionnaire: A social support measure." *Birth Defects* 20, no. 5 (1984): 59-97.

A study to further the psychometric evaluation of the Personal Resource Questionnaire (PRQ).

Evaluative

There is sound evidence to rule out the explanation that the respondents' answers on the PRQ reflect a reporting simply of socially desirable answers. There were no significant differences between the scores for women and the scores for men on either Part 1 or Part 2 of the PRQ. Evidence was provided to substantiate criterion-related validity. The validity and reliability of PRQ are sufficiently established to permit the continued use of the tool.

Of interest to social and behavioral scientists.

b. Dissertation

107. LIBERO, Peter. "The development of a social support measure and its relationship to physical illness, psychological symptoms, and medical care utilization." Ph.D. dissertation, California School of Professional Psychology, San Diego, 1983.

Construction of a new social support scale and the application in a study of the relationship between daily hassles and health outcomes.

Research

The new scale proved to have three dimensions: emotional support, instrumental support, and intimacy. Intimacy was positively but marginally associated with psychological problems, and there was a low, inverse relationship between emotional support and doctor's office visits. Self-reported somatic health and social support were not related to each other.

Of interest to social and behavioral scientists, and researchers of utilization of health care services.

4. EVALUATION

a. Articles

108. BAKER, Frank, and James Intagliata. "Quality of life in the evaluation of community support systems. *Evaluation and Program Planning* 5 (1982): 69-79.

Reviews the reasons for focusing on the quality of life as a desired outcome for this type of mental health program, some of the problems in quality of life evaluation research, the definition of methods for measurement of quality of life, a conceptual model, and the results of a pilot study of quality of life.

Research

As a result of their experience in conducting an evaluation of the community support system program in New York State, the authors have identified five reasons for focusing on the quality of life as a desired outcome of programs for the chronically ill.

Of interest to social and behavioral scientists.

109. GOTTLIEB, Benjamin H. "Assessing and strengthening the impact of social support on mental health." *Social Work* 30 (July/August 1985): 293-300.

Provides suggestions for preventive interventions that social work practitioners can initiate to enlarge the fund of support from the social network, to promote its utilization, and to supplement it with meaningful relationships.

Research

Offers a set of guidelines to assess the sources and types of social support that people use as first and direct lines of defense in coping with life events and chronic hardships. Highlights how these direct ties mediate people's access to other supportive peer relationships.

Of interest to social workers and health professionals providing direct patient care.

110. HENDERSON, Scott, and Donald Byrne. "Towards a method for assessing social support systems." *Mental Health and Society* 4 (1977): 165-170.

Evidence is presented documenting the stress-producing and protective qualities of the social environment, especially those of social bonds.

Review

An instrument is needed to assess the support available to an individual in order to further research on the affective component of the social network and its role in mental illness. Presents examples from the literature of the components of support as they are presented in an assessment package.

A useful article for social science researchers because of the transcultural nature of the instrumentation proposed.

111. MORGENSTERN, Hal, George A. Gellert, Stephen D. Walter, Adrian M. Ostfeld, Bernard S. Siegel. "The impact of a psychosocial support program on survival with breast cancer: The importance of selection bias in program evaluation." *Journal of Chronic Diseases* 37 (1984): 273-282.

A study of a psychosocial support program for breast cancer patients, with particular emphasis on selection bias in program evaluation.

Research

The psychosocial support program seemed to have a beneficial effect on survival with breast cancer. These results, however, were biased by the failure to match the group that was participating in the support program with one that was not participating in such a program for the duration of the lag period between diagnosis and entry.

Of special interest to cancer rehabilitation specialists and cancer epidemiologists.

112. WHITE, Michael J. "Determinants of community satisfaction in Middletown." *American Journal of Community Psychology* 13 (1985): 583-597.

Residents of Middletown were asked to evaluate characteristics of their community.

Research

Factor scores defined by aesthetic qualities of the community, "belongingness," social support, and personal control best predicted variance in community satisfaction.

Of interest to social and behavioral scientists.

CHAPTER 2

SOCIAL NETWORKS

a. Books

113. BIEGEL, David E., Ellen McCardle, Susan Mendelson. *Social Networks and Mental Health--An Annotated Bibliography.* Beverly Hills: Sage, 1985.

A compendium of information on the subject of social networks and mental health.

Bibliography

A listing and annotation of 1,340 references covering the period, 1962-1982. Divided into five major categories as follows: Overview and Theory, Research--Physical Health, Research--Mental Health, Intervention, and Professional Roles and Policy.

An essential resource for mental health professionals, social scientists, and others interested in social networks and social support.

114. BIEGEL, David E., and Arthur J. Naparstek (Eds.). *Community Support Systems and Mental Health: Practice, Policy and Research.* New York: Springer, 1982.

A book for caregiving professionals with little knowledge of the existence or identity of supportive networks in their community, to increase their understanding of support systems in the community and their use in the prevention of illness.

Book of Readings

It is important for health professionals to understand the supportive social matrix in which they and their clients live. Practitioners and program planners can prevent illness and promote health by building up mutually respectful partnerships with community supporters.

Useful to professionals and students in public administration, social work, the social and behavioral sciences, and community health.

115. GOTTLIEB, Benjamin H. (Ed.). *Social Networks and Social Support*. Beverly Hills: Sage, 1981.

The essays in this volume offer a variety of perspectives on the role of social support in the coping process and the contribution of laypersons to the provision of human services in our communities.

Book of Readings

Unified by its focus on the health consequences arising from the interplay between people and the social orbits in which they participate.

A volume for many audiences--researchers in search of sharper distinctions, new conceptions, and innovative applications; administrators and evaluators concerned with service design that is responsive to community needs; and clinicians and program developers interested in providing care that mobilizes the natural support systems of clients.

116. MITCHELL, J. Clyde (Ed.). *Social Networks in Urban Situations*. Manchester, England: Manchester University Press, 1969.

A collection of papers from a symposium examining the potentiality of social networks as a tool for studying the structure of social relationships in modern societies.

Book of Readings

Includes discussions on the concept and use of social networks; networks and political process; networks and urban social organization; gossip, norms, and social networks; voluntary associations and personal networks in the political process; norms and manipulation of relationships in a work context; personal crises and the mobilization of social networks; and "home-boy" ties and political organization.

Of interest to social and behavioral scientists.

117. PILISUK, Marc, and Susan Hillier Parks. *The Healing Web: Social Networks and Human Survival*. Hanover and London: University Press of New England, 1986.

A book about caring--about social support and health, loneliness, friendships, and families--bringing together a number of interdisciplinary approaches to the study of supportive connections.

Resource Book

An understanding of human interdependence is critical to the health, sense of belonging, and even the survival of the human community. The movement toward autonomy in modern society must be balanced with a conscious movement toward interdependence if we are to build a strong supportive social fabric while preserving the advantages of individual development.

Written for diverse audiences: scientists interested in the study of social support and health, professionals in health and human services, and any person concerned about society and the nature and development of the human bond.

118. SARASON, Seymour B., Charles F. Carroll, Kenneth Maton, Saul Cohen, Elizabeth Lorentz. *Human Services and Resource Networks*. San Francisco: Jossey Bass, 1977.

Deals with social networks and their importance in the provision of human services, a form of institutional support.

Text

The authors present a good foundation for detailing the rationale, work, functions, and characteristics of institutionalized social support networks.

Of interest to anyone concerned with human relationships.

b. Articles

119. ASHER, Cheryl Carleton. "The impact of social support networks on adult health." *Medical Care* 22 (1984): 349-359.

Knowledge of the determinants of adult health offers important implications for planning policy that may affect the overall level of health and, thus, the costs of health care. One potentially important factor is the amount of information individuals possess regarding health care or methods of preventive care.

Research

Social support networks were found to have virtually no impact on health outcomes of illnesses over which the individual has little control. However, when a broader range of illnesses was considered, social support networks played a role in producing better health.

Of interest to social and behavioral scientists and health administrators.

120. BERARDO, Felix M. "Social networks and life preservation." *Death Studies* 9 (1985): 37-50.

Examines the connections between social ties, health status, and death.

Review and Theoretical

Discusses the importance of social ties or social support to health
status, mortality, and survivorship. Several aspects of this
relationship are reviewed, including social isolation and mortality,
loss of a significant other, bereavement and mortality, and remarriage
after widowhood and survivorship. Some empirical evidence in each of
these areas is reviewed.

Useful for anyone interested in social factors' contributions to
change in health status and premature death.

121. BERKMAN, Lisa F. "Social networks, support, and health:
      Taking the next step forward." *American Journal of Epi-
      demiology* 123 (April 1986): 559-562.

A literature review and critique of research with respect to Type A
behavior pattern.

Review and Commentary

One of the common threads running through nearly all of the published
articles is the association of social support with a broad array of
diseases and causes of death. Building on this finding, studies
focusing on the relationships of social networks and support to risk
factors with multiple disease outcomes and to physiologic processes
that vary with age, seem particularly promising. We need much more
information on the relationship of these social factors to disease
incidence and case fatality.

Of interest to social and behavioral scientists and cardiologists.

122. ———, and S. Leonard Syme. "Social networks, host resis-
      tance, and mortality: A nine-year follow-up study of Alameda
      County residents." *American Journal of Epidemiology* 109,
      no. 2 (1979): 186-204.

A study of the relationship between social and community ties and
mortality in a random sample of 6,928 adults in Alameda County,
California and a subsequent nine-year mortality follow-up.

Research

Modest support for the notion that people lacking social and community
ties have higher mortality is provided. The relationship between
social isolation and mortality is found to be independent of a number
of factors, including socioeconomic status, health practices, and use
of preventive services.

Useful to epidemiologists interested in social isolation and
mortality, social researchers interested in social support and
illness, and community health surveyors.

123. BRIANCON, S., F. Blanchard, M. Cherrier-Baumann, C. Guenot-Gosse, E. Calés-Blanchard, J.P. Deschamps, R. Senault. "Isolement, support social, événements de vie et état de santé." (French) *Revue Epidémiologique et Santé Publique* 33 (1985): 48-65.

A general overview of the research relating social network and social support factors to health status.

Literature Review

Several aspects of the research on the social support/health status relationship are discussed, including the effects of isolation and loneliness on health, measurement issues of social support, effects of social networks and social support on health service utilization, and methodological problems in the study of the association of social support, life events, and health outcomes. Some questions for future research are formulated.

Of value to epidemiologists and social scientists.

124. BRUGHA, T., R. Conroy, N. Walsh, W. Delaney, J. O'Hanlon, E. Dondero, L. Daly, W. Hickey, G. Bourke. "Social networks, attachments and support in minor affective disorders: A replication." *British Journal of Psychiatry* 141 (1982): 249-255.

A replication of a study of the social networks and social support in nonpsychotic psychiatric out-patients and a group of controls.

Research

Patients reported spending less time in social interaction, but more time in unpleasant interaction during the previous week; they also had fewer attachment figures, close relatives, and good friends and fewer social contacts than controls.

Of interest to mental health professionals.

125. CROTTY, Patrick, and Regina Kulys. "Social support networks: The views of schizophrenic clients and their significant others." *Social Work* 30 (July/August 1985): 301-309.

This study compared the perceptions of schizophrenic clients concerning their social support networks with those of their significant others, regarding size, composition, and level of interaction.

Research

It was found that the schizophrenic clients reported having networks that were larger, more supportive, and more often composed of nonkin than were those reported by their significant others.

Of interest to mental health practitioners.

126. FIORE, Joan, Joseph Becker, David B. Coppel. "Social
     network interactions: A buffer or a stress?" *American
     Journal of Community Psychology* 11 (1983): 423-440.

Views and assesses the social network as a potential source of both
stress and support. In a population at high risk for depression, a
systematic attempt was made to assess the perceived supportiveness of
the network separate from the stress perceived when the network does
not provide wished-for support.

Research

The principal finding of this study was that the extent of upset with
the social network, either as a result of unmet expectations of
support or of negative input from important others, was the best
predictor of depression in a chronically stressed population. The
perceived supportiveness of the network did not relate to depression.

Of interest to social and behavioral scientists.

127. GOTTLIEB, Benjamin H. "Social networks and social support:
     An overview of research, practice, and policy implications."
     Health Education Quarterly 12 (1985): 5-22.

Highlights the role of social support as a resource for resisting
stress-induced illness and disability.

Theoretical and Analytical

Three different connotative meanings of the social support construct
are identified, and their empirical operationalization in several
recent studies is discussed. A review of possible mechanisms whereby
social support accomplishes its health-protective impact is also
offered, and two types of planned interventions involving the
mobilization of social support are detailed.

Of interest to social workers, social and behavioral scientists, and
community health workers.

128. HENDERSON, Scott. "The social network, support, and
     neurosis: The function of attachment in adult life." *British
     Journal of Psychiatry* 131 (1977): 185-191.

This essay, written from the point of view of attachment theory, deals
with the psychological function of the social network in the provision
of social support.

Literature Review

Illustrates the fact that humans require affectively positive
interactions with others to maintain health, but raises the question

whether depleted primary group interactions are causally linked to morbidity or merely an associated factor in disease etiology.

Research oriented psychiatrists, social psychologists, and medical sociologists will find this a thought-provoking article.

129. HIBBARD, Judith H. "Social ties and health status: An examination of moderating factors." *Health Education Quarterly* 12 (Spring 1985): 23-34.

Assesses the relationship between social ties and health status.

Research

The findings show that increased social ties, trust, and perceived control are related to better health. A large social network is important to those less able to utilize resources available to them, whereas size is less important to those who are able to mobilize support from their networks.

Of special interest to health professionals and social scientists.

130. HIRSCH, Barton J. "Adolescent coping and support across multiple social environments." *American Journal of Community Psychology* 13 (1985): 381-392.

Examines research on stress, social support, and coping mechanisms of adolescents and the importance of social ecological perspectives.

Research

Two case studies examining contrasting coping strategies of adolescents are presented. One strategy involves the use of a strong peer network, while the other focuses on school involvement. Preventive social-community interventions are suggested that may prevent potential trouble areas associated with these strategies.

Of particular interest to adolescent psychologists.

131. HUESSY, Hans R. "Social support networks--some added dimensions." *American Journal of Public Health* 74 (1984): 1169.

A response to an editorial on social support and the development of vulnerable children.

Editorial Response

Clarifies the ideas that social support can both create and abate stress, that natural mechanisms rather than institutional support have been studied, and that social support or the lack of same may be a response of others to temperamental and character traits.

A helpful reminder of three key factors often overlooked in social support research, and therefore valuable to most researchers interested in the subject.

132. KÄHLER, Harro D. "Das konzept des sozialen netzwerks: Eine einfuhrüng in die literatur." (German)   *Zeitschrift fur Soziologie* 4, no. 3 (1975): 283-290.

An introduction to the concept of the social network in German social anthropological literature.

Literature Review

The definition and origins of the concept of the social network are discussed, followed by a description of the most important dimensions of this concept. Some suggestions are made about the potential utility of the concept.

Of interest to social scientists.

133. KELNER, Merrijoy. "Community support networks: Current issues." *Canadian Journal of Public Health* 76, Supplement 1 (1985): 69-70.

Commentary on the Conference *Beyond Health Care*, sponsored by the City of Toronto, to develop strategies for creating a healthy society.

Commentary

Community support networks are seen to operate at two distinct levels. At the most general level, support networks can serve to counteract and buffer the noxious stresses in the social environment. They can also mediate between the individual and the social structure, thereby reducing the negative impacts of isolation and anomie.

Of general interest to researchers of social support.

134. KUO, Wen H., and Yung-Mei Tsai. "Social networking, hardiness and immigrants' mental health." *Journal of Health and Social Behavior* 27 (1986): 133-149.

An examination of factors that protect voluntary immigrants from psychological impairment.

Research

The immigrant can live separated from the larger society and not necessarily suffer from severe social isolation. Success of reestablishing a social network in the new society greatly reduces psychological distress and the detrimental effect of uprooting. The hardy personality can avert stresses associated with migration.

Of interest to social and behavioral scientists.

135. ROSEL, Natalie. "The hub of a wheel: A neighborhood support network." *International Journal of Aging and Human Development* 16 (1983): 193-200.

A neighborhood network and its functions are described in detail.

Descriptive

In a neighborhood where elderly residents have known each other for years, a closely-knit network of mutual assistance and support has developed among a few of the oldest residents. First, the "old-old" people help each other on a daily basis, and second, the routine nature of the assistance is taken for granted by all concerned. The implications are both theoretical and practical.

Of interest to gerontologists.

c. Chapters

136. HANSSON, Robert O., Warren H. Jones, Bruce N. Carpenter. "Relational competence and social support." *In* Phillip Shaver (Ed.). *Review of Personality and Social Psychology 5: Emotions, Relationships and Health*. Beverly Hills: Sage, 1984.

Explores the role that personality processes may play in allowing people to access and benefit from supportive social relationships.

Literature Review and Analysis

Reviews the assumptions that have guided the social support literature and the situations in which support appears to be important; presents examples from the literature of the nature of the primary and secondary relationships that constitute a person's social support network; introduces the construct of "rotational competence," and explores the manner in which personality may affect a person's ability to construe, construct, access, and maintain important supportive relationships.

Of interest to social and behavioral scientists.

137. HIRSCH, Barton J., and E. Ann Jolly. "Role transitions and social networks: Social support for multiple roles. *In* Vernon L. Allen, and Evert van de Vliert (Eds.). *Role Transitions*. New York: Plenum, 1983.

Considers the effect of the interplay of social role and social network factors on success in coping with role transitions, particularly focusing on the importance of obtaining social support for multiple roles and on how multiple role phenomena can affect the provision of social support.

Theoretical and Analytical

Highlights the importance of multiple role phenomena to understanding role transitions, the importance of social support to transition outcomes, and the potential importance of studying multiple role phenomena to the development of social support theory and research.

Should interest social scientists.

138. MITCHELL, J. Clyde. "The concept and use of social networks." *In* J. Clyde Mitchell (Ed.). *Social Networks in Urban Situations*. Manchester, England: Manchester University Press, 1969.

A discussion of the concept of the social network and its use in research.

Theoretical

Because social networks extend across and between institutions, they provide a means of examining interrelationships of people's behavior in different contexts. Networks and institutional analyses, by their different assumptions and procedures, complement one another.

Of interest to social and behavioral scientists.

139. MOOS, Rudolf H., and Roger E. Mitchell. "Social network resources and adaptation: A conceptual framework." *In* T.A. Wills (Ed.). *Basic Processes in Helping Relationships*. New York: Academic Press, 1982.

A discussion of social network resources and their determinants and effects.

Theoretical

Presents a conceptual framework to help guide planning for future research and intervention, which enables the researcher to explore the relative importance of social network resources on adaptation and to examine the way in which such resources are linked to and mediate the influences of environmental and personal variables.

Of interest to researchers of social support and stress.

140. REIS, Harry T. "Social interaction and well-being." *In* Steve Duck (Ed.). *Personal Relationships V: Repairing Personal Relationships*. London: Academic Press, 1984.

A discussion of the methodological and conceptual needs in research on those aspects of social relationships that are beneficial and of useful theoretical models.

Theoretical

The central thesis of this chapter has been that we have yet to discover what it is about social participation that is beneficial for

health and well-being. Two primary questions remain to be answered.
One concerns the gap between social interaction and social support:
How does the availability and existence of social contact lead to the
perception of support? The second pertains to the question of
underlying cause: By what mechanism do interaction and support
influence health?

Of interest to teachers and researchers interested in social support.

1. NETWORK ANALYSIS

a. Books

141. BOISSEVAIN, Jeremy, and J. Clyde Mitchell (Eds.). *Network
     Analysis Studies in Human Interaction*. The Hague: Mouton,
     1973.

A major work on the study of social relations and processes using
network analysis.

Book of Readings

Part I of this book consists of several chapters discussing theoretical and methodological issues relevant for this method of social
analysis. The other two parts are based on empirical material: Part
II focuses on social networks as a system of relations that influence
individuals and their behaviors, and Part III contains several
articles describing social networks as a series of relations which
persons use to achieve their ends.

Especially helpful for social and cultural anthropologists and
sociologists interested in network analysis.

142. FISCHER, Claude S., Robert Max Jackson, C. Anne Stueve,
     Kathleen Gerson, Lynne McCallister Jones with Mark
     Baldassare. *Networks and Places: Social Relations in the
     Urban Setting*. New York: Free Press, 1977.

Several empirical studies are addressed, largely to the question of
how people's structural situations affect their social relations and
the character of those relations. Concerned throughout with understanding how the structural circumstances that individuals face
influence the formation and maintenance of social ties.

Theoretical and Research

Provides a specific theoretical perspective on human behavior,
particularly on how people form personal networks; examines the
components of "community;" and attempts to provide a precise way of
analyzing social relations.

Of interest to sociologists and anthropologists.

143. PERRUCCI, Robert, and Dena B. Tarb. *Mental Patients and Social Networks.* Boston: Auburn House, 1982.

The social networks in which mental patients are involved were studied in an attempt to shed light on how people become mental patients and what happens to them once they are patients.

Research

Analysis of data were related to the following stages in the patient career: the identification and reaction to initial unusual behaviors; the decision to hospitalize; the hospital response to patients and their networks; the hospital experience; and release. Networks were found to influence the ways in which problem behaviors are defined and dealt with, and to provide a variety of social and emotional resources for supporting members in times of need.

Of interest to mental health professionals.

144. WELLMAN, Barry, Paul Craven, Marilyn Whitaker, Sheila DuToit, Harvey Stevens. *The Uses of Community: Community Ties and Support Systems. Research Paper No. 47.* Toronto, Ontario: Centre for Urban and Community Studies, University of Toronto, 1971.

This extensive study examines the integration of adult, urban Canadians into their community, spatial, and social support systems.

Research

This research uses network analysis to describe the informal inter-personal support systems of high density, high rise, urban environments. Support was found to be available primarily during times of emergency, even though it was suggested that the routine, daily stresses appeared to have the greatest effect on coping and well-being, especially when the frequency and quality of interaction was high.

A very well prepared, thorough report with an exceptional review of literature.

b. Articles

145. ANGERMEYER, Matthias C., and Beate Block. "Das soziale netzwerk alcoholkranker." (German) *Psychotherapie Psychosomatik Medizinische Psychologie* 34 (1984): 1-9.

A study of the social networks of a group of alcoholics.

Research

Data were analyzed with particular emphasis on gender differences and differences in marital status and family composition. Married persons generally reported attachment to another person, particularly a spouse, and better social integration. Married alcoholic men relied almost exclusively on their spouses for emotional support, whereas married alcoholic women were also able to rely on close friends and relatives. Single men generally relied on their mothers for emotional support, but single women did not rely on a particular person for fulfillment of similar needs.

Of interest to psychiatrists and social scientists, especially those working with alcoholics and their families.

146. BEELS, C. Christian. "Social networks and schizophrenia."
      Psychiatric Quarterly 51 (1979): 209-215.

A discussion of the relationships between social networks and the course of schizophrenia.

Descriptive

Taking the dimensions of natural network structure, types of ideology, patterns of initiative, and subtypes of diagnosis and history, typologies of specific intervention and networks can be constructed for different groups of patients.

Of interest to mental health professionals.

147. BELL, Wendell, and Marion D. Boat. "Urban neighborhoods
      and informal social relations." *American Journal of Sociology*
      62 (1957): 391-398.

The purpose of this paper is to contribute to the determination of particular urban conditions under which impersonal social relations arise most and those other conditions under which they arise least.

Research

Interviews with men in four neighborhoods of different social types in San Francisco reveal that informal relationships within the neighborhood are fairly frequent and likely to be personal, close, and intimate.   The frequency and nature of informal participation vary with the economic and family characteristics of the neighborhoods.

Of interest to social and behavioral scientists.

148. BELLE, Deborah E. "The impact of poverty on social networks
      and supports." *Marriage and Family Review* 5 (1982): 89-
      105.

A discussion of the ways in which poverty constrains, disrupts, and facilitates social support.

Review and Analysis

Future research should pay more attention to the costs as well as the benefits of social networks. Since the natural helping networks of the poor are often emotionally costly, they should not be viewed as a substitute for formal helping networks or for economic security. While social support is a powerful buffer against stress, many social networks are no buffer at all, and actually contribute to the stress their participants experience.

Of interest to social and behavioral scientists.

149. BERKMAN, Lisa F. "The assessment of social networks and social support in the elderly." *Journal of the American Geriatrics Society* 31 (1983): 743-749.

Provides some background on the epidemiologic work being done on social networks among the elderly, especially those with disabilities.

Review and Analysis

Little evidence supports the idea that the elderly are particularly fragile and vulnerable to the effects of social isolation. Social networks have been most often conceptualized and measured in static terms as if they were a stable property of an individual. It is likely that networks both influence, and are influenced by, physical and mental health. While social and community ties are probably important to the maintenance of health, we do not, as yet, have straightforward questions that clinicians can use to predict disease risks.

Of interest to social and behavioral researchers of social support.

150. BRANDT, Patricia A. "Clinical assessment of the social support of families with handicapped children." *Issues in Comprehensive Pediatric Nursing* 7 (1984): 187-201.

An analysis of the properties of social networks is conducted to enable a better understanding of the conditions under which support is provided, as well as the negative effects of network ties. Guidelines for obtaining a comprehensive assessment of family support are also provided.

Research

The assessment suggestions outlined offer the nurse a working guide. Interventions evolve from the assessment information and the nursing diagnosis. Knowledge of each family's competencies and personal and economic coping resources will usefully supplement the information obtained from the support assessment.

Of interest to nurses.

151. BRIM, John A. "Social network correlates of avowed happiness." *Journal of Nervous and Mental Diseases* 158 (1974): 432-439.

Describes a technique for gathering data pertaining to the correlations between social network characteristics and psychological avowed happiness, and discusses the data.

Research

Significant correlations were obtained between women's avowed happiness and the social network dimensions of assistance, value similarity, and concern. The patterns of correlation differed for married and unmarried women, possibly as a result of the presence of a stable relationship.

Of interest to social and behavioral scientists and social workers.

152. BRODY, Julia Green. "Informal social networks--possibilities and limitations for their usefulness in social-policy." *Journal of Community Psychology* 13, no. 4 (1985): 338-349.

Attempts to disentangle some elements of social networks that offer new approaches to persistent problems and some which simply disguise a repudiation of public responsibility for those in need.

Theoretical

The author argues that social networks are valuable in providing emotional resources, but that they are inherently limited in their ability to meet other needs and may impose severe social controls on their members.

Of interest to social and behavioral scientists.

153. COCHRAN, Moncrieff M., and Jane Anthony Brassard. "Child development and personal social networks." *Child Development* 50 (1979): 601-616.

The framework of network analysis is used to assess the social ecology of the parent and child in relation to its possible effects upon child development.

Theoretical

A model for understanding possible relationships between parents' personal social networks and the development of children. The model has 5 basic elements: 1) the network itself; 2) lines of influence transmission; 3) network-related developmental processes; 4) the child's stage of development; and 5) network-related developmental outcomes in the child. Directions for future research, using this model, are offered.

Of interest to child development specialists.

154. COE, Rodney M., Fredric D. Wolinsky, Douglas K. Miller, John M. Prendergast. "Complementary and compensatory functions in social network relationships among the elderly." *Gerontologist* 24 (1984): 396-400.

An analysis of the relationship between family and neighbor network systems for elderly persons with respect to complementary or compensatory functions.

Research and Analytical

The greatest health needs and highest rates of use of formal health services were found to be among those elderly persons who were dissatisfied with their network relationships. Both complementary (simultaneous participation in family and neighbor network) and compensatory (participation in either family or neighbor network only) network relationships provided support for the elderly.

Of interest to social scientists.

155. ———. "Social network relationships and use of physician services: A reexamination." *Research on Aging* 6 (1984): 243-256.

Reexamines the concept of social network relationships in both theoretical and empirical contexts.

Research

The four types of social network relationships originally proposed by Rundall and Evashwick (engaged, disengaged, trapped, and abandoned) were extended to include "discontented" and "alienated" relationships. Four hundred and one randomly chosen elderly residents in an urban area were interviewed to test hypotheses derived from the typology, using data on the use of physician services. The most common types found in the sample were the engaged, disengaged, and abandoned. The abandoned had the highest average number of physician visits. Possible avenues for further investigation are discussed.

Should interest social scientists.

156. COHEN, Carl I., and Jay Sokolovsky. "Health-seeking behavior and social networks of the aged living in single-room occupancy hotels." *Journal of the American Geriatrics Society* 27 (June 1979): 270-278.

Demonstrates how network techniques can be used to determine the extent to which sociability variables are correlated with the health states of single-room occupancy elderly and how network analysis can be profitably employed by gerontologists as a method for studying social variables.

Research

The assertion that elderly single-room occupancy residents lack a meaningful support system and that they rely on sheer will power to survive appears inaccurate. The data point to differences in network size, complexity, intensity, connectedness, and directionality based on varying degrees of physical and psychiatric health.

Of interest to gerontologists.

157. ———. "Social engagement versus isolation: The case of the aged in SRO hotels." *Gerontologist* 20 (1980): 36-44.

Utilizing network analysis techniques, the sociability levels of aged hotel residents were examined.

Research

Results indicated that older residents had viable personal networks which provided both material and nonmaterial support, although they were relatively isolated compared to other urban samples. Recognition of these networks has important ramifications for service providers and policymakers.

Of interest to gerontologists and community health workers.

158. COHEN, Carl I., Jeanne Teresi, Douglas Holmes. "Social networks, stress, and physical health: A longitudinal study of an inner-city elderly population." *Journal of Gerontology* 40 (1985): 478-486.

Using 19 network variables, the authors followed 133 elderly residents of mid-Manhattan hotels for one year.

Research

Findings indicate that social networks exert a direct effect on reducing subsequent physical symptoms. Social networks also reduce symptoms by buffering the effect of increased levels of stress.

Of interest to researchers of stress and social support.

159. ———. "Social networks, stress, adaptation, and health: A longitudinal study of an inner-city elderly population." *Research on Aging* 7 (1985): 409-431.

Describes a one year follow-up study of the role of social support in the lives of the elderly.

Research

This study of 133 elderly residents of mid-Manhattan hotels followed for one year, used 19 social network variables to predict the three outcome measures of need fulfillment, psychological symptoms, and physical symptoms. The findings indicate that social support networks exert a direct effect on symptom reduction and enhance an individual's ability to meet his/her personal needs. Social networks were found to buffer the stress of high risk subjects.

Sociologists and other community mental health researchers will find this a useful paper.

160. CRAWFORD, Gretchen. "A theoretical model of support network
      conflict experienced by new mothers. *Nursing Research* 34
      (1985): 100-102.

Describes sources of conflict which arise in the social support
network of new mothers, and presents a theoretical model describing
the interactions.

Theoretical-Research

Evidence is presented linking parenthood and social support networks.
Network conflicts are examined to identify variables appropriate for
nursing interventions.

Nurses and others working with new mothers will find this an
interesting study.

161. CRONENWETT, Linda R. "Network structure, social support,
      and psychological outcomes of pregnancy." *Nursing Research*
      34 (1985): 93-99.

Describes an investigation to determine whether perceived social
support, alone or in conjunction with specific network characteristics, was associated with self-evaluations of primagravida parents
on dimensions of postpartum adaptation to the parental role.

Research

An investigator-developed tool was used to measure social network
characteristics and perceived social support in 50 primagravida
fathers and mothers during the third trimester of pregnancy. At six
weeks postpartum, these same parents completed the Postpartum
Self-evaluation Questionnaire (PSQ). Relationships among network
factors, perceived support, and postpartum outcomes were documented
for four of the seven PSQ scales. A larger percentage of relatives in
the network and more overlap with the spouse's network were important
factors associated with positive postpartum outcomes for men, but not
for women. Emotional and instrumental support were important
variables in six-week postpartum outcomes, but information and
appraisal support were not significant. Men scored lower than women
on the PSQ scale measuring confidence in ability to cope with the
tasks of parenting.

Should interest pediatric researchers and social scientists.

162. ————. "Parental network structure and perceived support
      after birth of first child." *Nursing Research* 34 (1985):
      347-352.

Changes in the content and structure of social relationships following
the birth of the first child were studied in a sample of primiparous
couples.

Research

More women than men perceived an increased need for support post-partum, but no differences in satisfaction with available support existed. For men, network size decreased, but the percentage of network members with preschool children, the percentage of members offering emotional support, and the boundary density with wives' networks all increased. Women reported decreased frequency of contact with coworkers, but increased frequency with friends, and, as did fathers, named more members with preschool children.

Of interest to obstetricians, obstetrical nurses, and social workers.

163. ———. "Social networks and social support of primagravida mothers and fathers." *Birth Defects* 20 (1984): 167-203.

The objectives of this study were to describe the social networks of primigravida women and their husbands; to determine if there are any differences in social networks based on gender, education, or income; and to examine the relationships among network characteristics, demographic characteristics, and perceived availability of support from network makers.

Research

Findings indicate that men perceive as much access to support in their intimate social networks as women do. The individual variables of education and age were associated with men's emotional support and women's instrumental support. Age was also associated with women's information support. These findings support the notion that properties of the individual are related to perceived social support.

Of interest to obstetricians, pediatricians, family physicians, and nurses.

164. CUTRONA, Carolyn E. "Objective determinants of perceived social support." *Journal of Personality and Social Psychiatry* 50 (1986): 349-355.

The objective characteristics of the social networks of 50 elderly adults and 71 mothers of one-year olds were examined as determinants of the perceived availability of social support. Number of network members and frequency of contact with network members, computed separately for kin and nonkin, were examined as predictors of loneliness, overall social support, and the six components of social support proposed by Weiss.

Research

Kin were found to be more effective providers of some aspects of social support than nonkin. Network characteristics were better predictors of perceived social support for the elderly than for the mothers, but a maximum of 30% of the variance in perceived social support was attributable to the objective network characteristics in either sample. It is recommended that future research on the determinants of perceived social support consider actual interpersonal behaviors, their contexts, and personality characteristics that affect the facilitation and interpretation of supportive behavior.

Should interest social science researchers concerned with social support.

165. DEGENNE, Alain. "Sur les réseaux de sociabilité." (French) *Revue Francaise de Sociologie* 14 (1983): 109-117.

Deals with methods of network sampling.

Theoretical

Several methods of network analysis are discussed. The author argues that social relations between individuals could be conceptualized as individual cases within larger social circles or networks. Social relations research should employ methods that enable the description and analysis of these larger social structures.

Useful for sociologists, particularly those interested in network analysis.

166. ERICKSON, Bonnie H., T.A. Nosanchuk, Edward Lee. "Network sampling in practice: Some second steps." *Social Networks* 3 (1981): 127-136.

Report on a method for obtaining reliable estimates of the density of large networks.

Research

Describes two pre-tests of a network sampling instrument used in favorable settings. The results were positive, and suggestions for future applications were made.

Useful to researchers of social networks.

167. FELD, Scott L. "The focused organization of social ties." *American Journal of Sociology* 86 (1981): 1015-1035.

Essay based on Homan's concept of activities, interactions, and sentiments in friendship and other intimate interactional groups.

Essay--Theoretical

Presents a theory in contrast to Heider's balance theory, suggesting that social networks and personal interaction are transitory and are both flexible and responsive to extraordinary influences.

Sociologists and other social theorists will find this intriguing, especially as a basis for understanding the adaptive aspects of social support.

168. FROLAND, Charles, Gerry Brodsky, Madeline Olson, Linda
     Stewart. "Social support and social adjustment: Implications
     for mental health professionals." *Community Mental Health
     Journal* 15 (Summer 1979): 82-93.

Network analysis was used to examine differences in the social
networks of mental health clients in order to identify factors
associated with positive social adjustment.

Research

Subjects were selected from three different types of mental health
programs and from the general population of Marion County, Oregon.
Results revealed that subjects from the community sample more often
sought support from immediate family members. Better functioning
chronic clients emphasized professional contacts, whereas more poorly
adjusted chronic clients looked to friends for support. Implications
are drawn from the results regarding both understanding the nature of
support available to clients and mobilizing support resources of
existing networks to aid in adjustment to community living.

Of interest to social workers, mental health professionals, and
researchers of social support.

169. GALLO, Frank. "The effects of social support networks on the
     health of the elderly." *Social Work in Health Care* 8, no. 2
     (1982): 65-74.

A study of the relationship between social support networks and health
of the elderly. Specific dimensions of a social support network were
identified and measured to determine which had the greatest effect on
health status. The collective effect of all measurable dimensions of
the network on health status was examined.

Research

A high statistical correlation was found between the social support
network and health, providing evidence that knowledge about the social
support network is important in assessing health.

Should interest social workers, health care professionals, and
researchers in the social sciences.

170. GREENBLATT, Milton, Rosina M. Becerra, E.A. Serafetinides.
     "Social networks and mental health: An overview." *American
     Journal of Psychiatry* 139 (August 1982): 977-984.

Reviews selective research on the supportive and protective functions
of social networks, facilitative programs exploiting them, and network
interventions.

Review

Illuminates patterns and characteristics of social networks that
maintain health and help prevent illness, explores the relationship
between social networks and the course and outcome of treatment for
mental illness, describes clinical network interventions used to
facilitate inpatient care and maximize performance of expatients in
the community, and discusses the implications of research findings for
mental health practice.

Of interest to mental health professionals.

171. GREIDER, Thomas, and Richard S. Krannich. "Neighboring
      patterns; social support and rapid growth--a comparison
      analysis from 3 western communities." *Sociological Per-
      spectives* 28 (1985): 51-70.

Examines the data on neighboring phenomena in three small towns that
have recently experienced different rates of population growth.

Research

Results suggest that a rapid growth in population is accompanied by a
decline in neighbors as a source of social support. The data refutes
the notion that primary neighboring interaction declines with the
onset of rapid population growth. The decline in the amount of social
support from neighbors may therefore be indicative of an overall
decline in the mechanisms of social bonding.

Of interest to sociologists and social psychologists.

172. HAMMER, Muriel. "'Core' and 'extended' social networks in
      relation to health and illness." *Social Science and Medicine*
      17 (1983): 405-411.

Considers several models of the nature of the association between
characteristics of social networks and health.

Theoretical

The proposition is tentatively warranted that the social network is
directly and causally involved in health outcomes--perhaps through the
impact of social feedback, as mediated by the network. It is argued
that the social processes that affect the association between networks
and health involve a larger social unit than the small core networks
that have generally been the focus of study.

Of interest to social and behavioral scientists.

173. ——. "Social supports, social networks and schizophrenia."
      Schizophrenia Bulletin 7 (1981): 45-57.

Considers the meaning of "social support" and its relationship to
social networks, and discusses a structural approach to analysis of
social connections in the study of schizophrenia.

Theoretical

The concept of social support is seen as methodologically more problematic and less strategic than the more connotatively neutral and more structurally oriented concepts of social networks and social connections. It is argued that, in terms of a research strategy, if social connections are studied structurally as they change and develop over time, the impact of specific social processes can be better separated from that of personal characteristics.

Of interest to researchers of social support.

174. ———, Susan Makiesky-Barrow, Linda Gutwirth. "Social networks and schizophrenia." *Schizophrenia Bulletin* 4 (1978): 522-545.

An overview of the psychosocial factors associated with schizophrenia from the perspective of social network theory.

Theoretical

Three types of social networks are described—personal (first order) networks, family and friends (second order) networks, and extended social contacts (third order) networks. Evidence of the role of these social networks is presented from epidemiological, clinical, and sociological studies. Communications, stress, social isolation, social networks, and cultural supports are linked in their association to both the etiology of and recovery from schizophrenia.

Researchers, mental health professionals, and others interested in psychotic disorders and the social factors associated with them will find this article useful.

175. HAYS, Robert B., and Diana Oxley. "Social network development and functioning during a life transition." *Journal of Personality and Social Psychology* 50 (1986): 305-313.

Presents a 12-week longitudinal study of the development of social support networks among college freshmen.

Research

Eighty-nine male and female students, living either in university residence halls or at home with their parents, completed a series of questionnaires in which they described their social networks while attending college and their adaptation to university life. It was found that, in accordance with an ecological view of social support, the functional characteristics of the freshmen's networks varied with the individual's gender and living situation and the temporal stage of the network. Network characteristics were significantly associated with the freshmen's successful adaptation to college, though the relative adaptiveness of particular network characteristics varied over time.

Of interest to social scientists interested in social networks.

176. HENDERSON, Scott. "A development in social psychiatry. The
      systematic study of social bonds." *Journal of Nervous and
      Mental Diseases* 168 (1980): 63-69.

Discusses the effect of the social environment on the development of
neurosis.

Review and Theoretical

Social psychiatry is beginning to demonstrate that deficiencies in
social relationships may be associated with the development of
neurosis. The distinction of cause and effect in such relationships
remains a methodological problem. Particular study design and
statistical models are proposed to overcome this problem.

Of primary interest to social psychiatrists and epidemiologists.

177. ———, Paul Duncan-Jones, Helen McAuley, Karen Ritchie.
      "The patient's primary group." *British Journal of Psychiatry*
      132 (1978): 74-86.

The size and utilization of the primary group was examined in 50
patients with nonpsychotic psychiatric disorders and 50 matched
controls.

Research

Patients were found to spend the same amount of time as normals with
their primary group, but proportionately more of that time was
affectively unpleasant. They had fewer good friends and fewer
contacts with persons outside the household. They had fewer
attachment figures. The majority of patients considered that their
principal attachment figures gave them insufficient support.

Of interest to mental health professionals.

178. HENDRIX, Lewellyn. "Kinship, social networks, and integration
      among Ozark residents and out-migrants." *Journal of
      Marriage and the Family* 38 (1976): 97-104.

Research findings are reported which relate to how migration affects
primary ties and how these factors affect integration.

Research

The findings indicate a clear need to distinguish among types of
primary ties and to distinguish the characteristics of the individual's social ties from the characteristics of the networks that
are made up from those ties. The classical theoretical position seems
to be essentially correct in regard to kinship involvement. Kin ties
are weakened by migration and by urbanism, and do not contribute to
the integration of urban migrants.

Of interest to social and behavioral scientists.

179. HIRSCH, Barton J. "Coping and adaptation in high-risk populations: A social network approach." *Schizophrenia Bulletin* 7 (1981a): 164-172.

Clarifies the role of the social network in the coping process of groups at high risk of developing psychopathologies.

Research

Low density, multidimensional social supports were found, in two studies, to be associated with more satisfying emotional support and better mood, fewer symptoms of illness, and high self-esteem.

Researchers interested in mental health, social support and physical illness will find this useful.

180. ———. "Natural support systems and coping with major life changes." *American Journal of Community Psychology* 8 (1980): 159-172.

This study sought to identify natural support systems that enhance coping with major life changes.

Research

Less integrated and multidimensional friendships were significantly associated with better support and mental health. Discussion centers on delineating two prototypical support systems and developing a model for conceptualizing their differential impact on coping and adaptation.

Of interest to social and behavioral scientists, especially researchers of stress and social support.

181. ———. "Psychological dimensions of social networks: A multimethod analysis." *American Journal of Community Psychology* 7 (1979): 263-277.

Two exploratory studies, which sought to identify important psychological dimensions of social networks, are discussed.

Research

Results suggest that multidimensional relationships are an important source of social network satisfaction. Social networks also can provide considerable quantities of support to individuals under stress. Denser or more integrated social networks furnish substantially greater quantities of support, though less satisfying emotional support.

Of interest to social and behavioral scientists.

182. ———, and T. David. "Social networks and work/nonwork
      life: Action research with nurse managers." *American Journal
      of Community Psychology* 11 (1983): 493-508.

Explores the possibility of using social network analysis as a basis
for understanding and increasing the quality of work life.

Research

Presents a rationale for developing support groups in the workplace to
provide emotional support and facilitate group problem-solving and
participatory decision-making in order to enhance the quality of work.
Implications for developing support programs are discussed.

Of interest to mental health professionals and psychologists.

183. ———, and Bruce D. Rapkin. "Social networks and adult
      social identities: Profiles and correlates of support and
      rejection." *American Journal of Community Psychology* 14
      (1986): 395-412.

Concerned with the differentiation of social network dimensions linked
to important adult social identities.

Research

Network variables related to important adult social identities were
differentiated. Factor analyses revealed four network interaction
factors: work support, work rejection, general support, and general
rejection. Cluster analysis of these factor scores identified five
network profiles, which differed in the importance of the woman's work
to her nonwork ties, as well as the frequency and pattern of different
positive and negative interactions.

Of interest to psychologists.

184. ISRAEL, Barbara A., Carol C. Hogue, Ann Gorton. "Social
      networks among elderly women: Implications for health
      education practice." *Health Education Quarterly* 10 (1983):
      173-203.

The results of a study of the properties and distinctions between
social networks and social support and their relationship to health
status as these relate to health education practice are presented.

Research

This secondary analysis of data from 130 women, 60 to 68 years of age,
examined the relationship of psychological well-being and social
network characteristics. The study suggests that the quality of
social interactions were related to psychological well-being, while
quantitative characteristics were not related.

Health educators and other social researchers interested in social support will find this interesting.

185. KAZAK, Anne E., and Brian L. Wilcox. "The structure and function of social support networks in families with handicapped children." *American Journal of Community Psychology* 12 (1984): 645-661.

A sample of 56 families having a child with spina bifida were matched with 53 comparison families to assess the structural and relationship characteristics of their respective social support networks.

Research

The networks of families with handicapped children appeared to be smaller, particularly in regard to the mothers' total and friendship networks, and were also denser than those of comparison families, with greater boundary density in spousal networks. Families of handicapped children tended to rely more heavily on multidimensional network contacts for support than did comparison families. The results are discussed in light of the authors' understanding of stress, social support, and the social ecological context of families.

Of interest to social scientists.

186. KLOVDAHL, Alden S. "Social networks and the spread of infectious diseases: The AIDS example." *Social Science and Medicine* 11 (1985): 1203-1216.

Data related to AIDS are used to illustrate the potential usefulness of a network approach in evaluating the infectious agent hypothesis when studying a disease or disease outbreak of unknown etiology, and in developing strategies to limit the spread of an infectious agent transmitted through personal relationships.

Research

Illustrates the use of network data and network analysis in epidemiology. Suggests how a network perspective can help stimulate insights regarding some infectious diseases and assist in designing rational control strategies.

Of interest to social and behavioral scientists, public health professionals, and health professionals specializing in infectious diseases.

187. LANGLIE, Jean K. "Social networks, health beliefs, and preventive health behavior." *Journal of Health and Social Behavior* 18 (1977): 244-260.

Study investigating whether an individual's social/psychological attributes continue to have an impact on preventive health behavior when social group characteristics are held constant, and, if so, which specific attributes, independently or jointly with social network variables, account for observed differences in preventive health behavior.

Research

Indirect risk preventive health behavior was related, 1) to the perception that one has some control over one's health status, and that the benefits of preventive action are high and the costs, low, and 2) to belonging to a social network characterized by high socioeconomic status and frequent interaction between nonkin. In contrast, direct risk preventive health behavior was mainly associated with older age and female gender.

Of interest to social and behavioral scientists.

188. LEFFLER, Ann, Richard S. Krannich, Dair L. Gillespie. "Contact, support, and friction: Three faces of networks in community life." *Sociological Perspectives* 29 (1986): 337-355.

Discusses a method for distinguishing conflict, support, and simple contact network linkages.

Review and Analysis

The analysis offered here suggests that the under-emphasis on conflict in network analysis requires remediation. An effort was made to examine the structure of friction in communities mainly characterized as supportive. It was concluded that friction, as well as accord, is a regular aspect of community life, and that these relations overlap not only with each other, but also with general relations of routine contact. At the same time, friction, support, and regular contact are often separate. Thus, the three kinds of relationships must be investigated simultaneously, not separately.

Of interest to social and behavioral scientists.

189. LONGINO, Charles F., Jr., and Aaron Lipman. "The married, the formerly married, and the never married: Support system differentials of older women in planned retirement communities." *International Journal of Aging and Human Development* 15 (1982): 285-297.

Explores the nature of informal support given to older women, depending upon their marital status and presence of living children.

Research

Women who were presently, or who had been married, received more emotional, social, and instrumental support from their family members. The presence of a husband only assured the married woman of significantly more instrumental (task-oriented) support. It was the existence of living children that generated greater emotional, social, and instrumental support from her family. The greatest informal support deficits are among the never married, but are the result of the lack of children rather than the absence of a husband.

Of interest to mental health professionals.

190. McALLISTER, Lynne, and Claude S. Fischer. "A procedure for surveying social networks." *Sociological Methods and Research* 7 (1978): 131-148.

Describes and illustrates the methodology the authors have developed for studying personal networks by mass survey.

Theoretical and Review

The conceptual problem in network definition and measurement and the description and illustration for surveying personal networks is discussed.

Of interest to social and behavioral scientists.

191. McFARLANE, Allen H., Geoffrey R. Norman, David L. Streiner, Ranjan G. Roy. "Characteristics and correlates of effective and ineffective social supports." *Journal of Psychosomatic Research* 28 (1984): 501-510.

Investigates specific features of social relationships leading to help and support.

Research

Subjects with helpful social supports reported smaller social networks. Support was primarily received from the spouse and other family members. Subjects with the least helpful social supports reported a significantly larger number of life events, both in the past five years and in their childhood.

Of interest to all researchers of social support.

192. McPHERSON, J. Miller. "Hypernetwork sampling: Duality and differentiation among voluntary organizations." *Social Networks* 3 (1982): 225-249.

Describes a method to study organizations using survey data obtained from individuals.

Research

A mathematical model is offered to derive macro-level characteristics of affiliation to voluntary organizations. These characteristics include the number and size of organizations, links among organizations, links among individuals, and density of these links. An illustration of the method is provided.

Of interest for researchers of social networks, particularly within voluntary organizations.

193. MIRANDE, Alfred M. "Extended kinship ties, friendship relations, and community size: An exploratory inquiry." *Rural Sociology* 35 (June 1970): 261-266.

Deals with urban-rural differences in social relations.

Research

Examines the relative importance of kinship in rural settings as a principal source of social support, as opposed to more attenuated relationships in urban settings. Variables which have been found to affect these relations include community size, population density, and more complex divisions of labor.

Sociologists and others interested in family studies will find this an interesting study.

194. MITCHELL, Roger E. "Social networks and psychiatric clients: The personal and environmental context." *American Journal of Community Psychology* 10 (1982): 387-401.

Examines the extent to which characteristics of psychiatric clients and their families are associated with dimensions of clients' social networks.

Research

Individual and environmental variables were revealed to be significant correlates of social network dimensions. Results highlighted the need to examine individual and environmental processes that shape and are shaped by social network patterns.

Of interest to mental health professionals, especially social workers, community psychologists, and psychiatrists.

195. ———, and Edison J. Trickett. "Task force report: Social networks as mediators of social support. An analysis of the effects and determinants of social networks." *Community Mental Health Journal* 16 (1980): 27-44.

Presents a representative overview of the current literature on social networks, with an emphasis on research linking social networks to psychological adaptation.

Literature Review

Includes a review of social network concepts, an analysis of the multiple determinants and varied effects of social networks, and implications for policies and practices of community mental health centers. The authors adopt the view that the concept of social networks is a useful tool in examining the functional and dysfunctional influences of one's primary group on individual adaptation.

Of interest to students of social support.

196. MORGAN, Myfanwy, Donald L. Patrick, John R. Charlton. "Social networks and psychosocial support among disabled people." *Social Science and Medicine* 19 (1984): 489-497.

Analyzes the characteristics of social ties among physically disabled people living in a London borough.

Research

Social network size, rather than type, was found to be related to the availability of psychosocial support. Since large numbers of married people were found to lack emotional support, the authors suggest measures to promote the broadening of psychosocial networks and caution against the use of marital status as a proxy measure of support.

Of interest to social scientists and mental health professionals.

197. MOUSER, Nancy F., Edward A. Powers, Willis J. Goudy, Patricia M. Keith. "Widowhood for older men: A study of social network ties and support in bereavement." *Gerontologist* 24, Supplement 1 (1984): 299.

A study of 1,287 small-town and rural men over age 60, comparing the social network ties of men having three different marital statuses.

Research Abstract

There were no significant differences found in the subjects' levels of involvement with grandchildren, siblings, friends, confidants, or voluntary associations. Widowers were more involved with children than remarried men, and the difference existed at time of spouse's death. Widowers, more frequently than remarried men, reported never recovering from grief. Results support the "Functional Specificity of Relationships" idea and suggest that child and friend relationships do not fully compensate for loss.

Should interest social workers and social and behavioral scientists.

198. MUELLER, Daniel P. "Social networks: A promising direction for research of the relationship of the social environment to psychiatric disorder." *Social Science and Medicine* 14 (1980): 147-161.

Considers the role of personal social networks in the etiology and course of psychiatric disorders.

Literature Review

Evidence is presented linking network structure, the degree of supportiveness of networks, and recent disruption in social networks to the development of several specific psychiatric disorders, in particular, depression.

Psychiatrists, psychologists, and other counselors will benefit from this article.

199. NAKAO, Keiko, Laura J. Milazzo-Sayre, Marilyn J. Rosenstein, Ronald W. Manderscheid. "Referral patterns to and from inpatient psychiatric services: A social network approach." *American Journal of Public Health* 76 (July 1986): 755-760.

Examines interorganizational linkages in mental health service systems, with network of patient referral patterns as the basic unit.

Research

The results emphasize the issues of conceptual framework and methodology in assessing mental health service delivery systems. The applicability of network perspectives have been documented in the area of mental health source system assessment. The structure of interorganizational relations, measured by the number of referrals, is clearly patterned. The analysis distinguishes two structural characteristics of inpatient psychiatric services, i.e. public and private, and change over time in referral patterns. As a methodological issue, the present analysis documents the utility of multidimensional scaling techniques in distilling key features from large data sets and presenting the results in an easily interpreted visual representation.

Of particular interest to mental health professionals and researchers interested in health care delivery and utilization issues.

200. O'BRYANT, S.L. "Neighbors' support of older widows who live alone in their own homes." *Gerontologist* 24, Supplement 1 (1984): 300.

A comparison of neighbor support to 226 widows in three cate-gories--those with one or more children in the same city, those with children in other cities, and those with no children.

Research Abstract

Support received by childless widows was not significantly greater than that received by those who had children in the same city. Widows with children in other cities received the most support. Results are discussed in terms of hierarchical-compensatory and task-specific models, which have been proposed as predictors of primary support groups. Explanations are offered for the present results in terms of social activity patterns, work histories, family relationships, and neighbor attitudes.

Should interest social and behavioral scientists.

201. PATTISON, E. Mansell, and Myrna Loy Pattison. "Analysis of a schizophrenic psychosocial network." *Schizophrenia Bulletin* 7, no. 1 (1981): 135-143.

A social network paradigm is presented, focusing on intimate psychosocial networks as measured by the Pattison Psychosocial Kinship Inventory.

Research

Characteristics of normal networks are shown to differ from those of schizophrenic networks, which exhibit dynamics that generate and perpetrate psychotic behavior.

Psychiatrists, social workers, psychologists, and other mental health clinicians may find this paradigm useful.

202. PETROWSKY, Marc. "Marital status, sex, and the social networks of the elderly." *Journal of Marriage and the Family* 38 (1976): 749-756.

A study of the impact of sex and marital status on the social relationships of the elderly.

Research

No sex differences were found in terms of frequency of social interaction with kin and friends. Older males, particularly widowers, were somewhat less likely to participate in religious organizations. The widowed did not seem more isolated from their social environment than the married elderly.

Of interest to gerontologists and sociologists.

203. PHILLIPS, Susan L. "Network characteristics related to the well-being of normals: A comparative base." *Schizophrenia Bulletin* 7, no. 1 (1981): 117-124.

An efficient method of mapping social participation and social networks of the general population is described.

Research

Several characteristics of social network participation are related to reported well-being. The best predictor for men is the size of the social network, while the best predictor for women is the range of socializing across groups.

This is a must read article for researchers interested in social support measurement and health outcomes.

204. PILISUK, Marc, and Meredith Minkler.   "Supportive networks:
      Life ties for the elderly."   *Journal of Social Issues*   36
      (1980): 95-116.

Data showing detrimental effects to the health of the elderly
associated with the diminution of supportive interpersonal ties are
summarized, and findings from a study of six programs for elderly
persons that illustrate the range and diversity of tasks involved in
the provision of supportive associations are presented.

Research

The six programs that address the supportive needs of the elderly
underscore the great variety of ways in which social support among
older persons can be enhanced. They highlight, as well, the diversity
of needs of the elderly and the importance of an equally diverse set
of responses to meet support needs.

Of interest to social and behavioral scientists.

205. PILISUK, Marc, and Susan Hillier Parks.   "The place of
      network analysis in the study of supportive social associa-
      tions."   *Basic and Applied Social Psychology*   2, no. 2
      (1981): 121-132.

Discusses network analysis as a method for documenting transactions
within social units and among individuals.

Literature Review

Four studies are examined to illustrate the use of network analysis in
the study of social support and health.

Researchers using social support constructs should read this article.

206. RIGER, Stephanie, and Paul J. Lavrakas.   "Community ties:
      Patterns of attachment and social interaction in urban
      neighborhoods."   *American Journal of Community Psychology*
      9 (1981): 55-66.

Factors affecting residents' attachments to their communities are
investigated, using data collected from telephone interviews with
1,620 adults in three U.S. cities.

Research

Attachment to local community settings consists of two empirically
distinct, although related dimensions--social bonding and behavioral
rootedness. People's life circumstances, particularly their stage in
the life cycle, may play a critical role in determining their degree
of attachment to local community settings.

Of interest to health professionals working in community programs and
projects.

207. RILEY, Dave, and Moncrieff M. Cochran. "Naturally occurring childrearing advice for fathers: Utilization of the personal social network." *Journal of Marriage and the Family* 47 (1985): 275-286.

Ninety-six fathers were interviewed to map their personal networks and probe their reliance on network members for childrearing advice.

Research

Utilizers of childrearing advice had large networks, but a large network did not always lead to more childrearing advice. Twenty-seven percent of the fathers reported no one with whom they discussed childrearing, yet those fathers were embedded in supportive networks dominated by kinfolk and had wives who had significantly fewer sources of childrearing advice than other mothers. The men who had the greatest number of interpersonal sources of childrearing advice had large social networks, used a relatively high percentage of their network members for advice, were relatively inexperienced parents, were high in salience of the parental role, and tended to have more education, white-collar occupations, and relatively low work hours. The most common interpersonal source of childrearing advice was kinfolk; advice from kinfolk had fewer correlates and varied less than advice from non-kin, and was greater for men who had firstborns and who worked fewer hours. Non-kin advice was significantly related to aspects of social structural position, social network, work, and the father's attitudes.

Should interest social scientists.

208. SALZINGER, Suzanne, Sandra Kaplan, Connie Artemyeff. "Mothers' personal social networks and child maltreatment." *Journal of Abnormal Psychology* 92 (1983): 68-76.

The social networks of a group of mothers whose children had been severely maltreated were compared to the social networks of mothers in families where there was no known maltreatment occurring.

Research

Clinic mothers were found to be more isolated and more insulated from other people in their networks. Mothers' isolation reflected a deficiency, primarily in their peer connections, and their insularity served to separate their immediate families from their peer connections and from the rest of their families.

Of interest to mental health professionals and child protective workers.

209. SCHOENBACH, Victor J., Berton H. Kaplan, Lisa Fredman, D.G. Kleinbaum. "Social ties and mortality in Evans County, Georgia." *American Journal of Epidemiology* 123 (April 1986): 577-591.

In an attempt to replicate Berkman and Syme's study of social networks and mortality in Alameda County, California, the authors investigated the relation between a social network index and survivorship from 1967 to 1980 in the Evans County cohort.

Research

The social network effect among white females, black males, and black females was weak and clearly insignificant. Exploratory analyses suggested that marital status, church activities, and an alternate social network index predicted survivorship, but not in a close–response fashion. Reduced survivorship among older subjects with few social ties was the most significant feature of the data.

Of interest to social and behavioral scientists and cardiologists.

210. SEEMAN, Melvin, Teresa Seeman, Marnie Sayles. "Social networks and health status--a longitudinal analysis." *Social Psychology Quarterly* 48 (1985): 237-248.

Tests the proposition that network engagement, particularly in connection with a high sense of control, is associated with favorable health behavior.

Research

Favorable health behavior was found to be associated with a high sense of self control and high social network engagement. The poorest health practices were found in subjects with both low support and low sense of control. Other combinations of these factors were variable in their association with positive health practices.

Social psychologists, medical sociologists, and other health behavior researchers will find this a thorough study.

211. SELTZER, Marsha M. "Informal supports for aging mentally retarded persons." *American Journal of Mental Deficiencies* 90 (1985): 259-265.

Available data on the informal support networks of aging, mentally retarded persons was reviewed.

Review and Analysis

The number of retarded persons surviving to old age has grown substantially in recent years. There is an increasing need for the younger generation to assume responsibility for the elderly. A number of factors that might pose obstacles to the involvement of families and friends with aging retarded persons are discussed.

Of interest to gerontologists and to health care workers caring for the mentally retarded.

212. SILBERFELD, Michel. "Psychological symptoms and social sup-ports." *Social Psychiatry* 13 (1978): 11-17.

Explores the hypothesis that psychological symptom levels are moderated by the presence of social support.

Research

Psychiatric patients were found to be lacking in social networks, and particularly lacking in the total time spent in relationships, regardless of type. There is a general association between the presence of psychological symptoms and a tendency to have less extensive social networks for support.

Of interest to mental health professionals.

213. SINGER, Merrill. "Family comes first--an examination of the social networks of Skid Row men." *Human Organization* 44 (1985): 137-142.

This study assesses the character of the social networks of Skid Row men.

Research

Disjointed networks illustrate the disjointed character of Skid Row life. While the men in this study have comparatively few individuals in their social networks, most of them are not real social isolates. Because Skid Row alcoholics have been defined as social isolates, interactional patterns they maintain with family members that may contribute to their drinking habits have been ignored. While the links Skid Row men maintain with family members may play a role in the perpetuation of their drinking behavior, these links may also provide a pathway for their return to society.

Of interest to social and behavioral scientists.

214. STEPHENS, M.A.P., J.M. Kinney, V.K. Norris, S.W. Ritchie, T. Sbroceo, F. Moncher. "Informal networks of geriatric rehabilitation patients--social support or social stress." *Gerontologist* 25, Supplement 1 (1985): 97-98.

Examines negative and positive interactions between social networks and 48 elderly stroke patients to determine factors influencing patient outcomes following discharge from the hospital.

Research Abstract

Positive interactions were shown to be associated with less mental confusion, while negative interactions were associated with poorer morale and higher incidence of psychiatric symptomotology. Social networks may, therefore, impede or facilitate progress in the rehabilitation process.

Of interest to social researchers and theorists.

215. STEPHENS, Mary Ann Parris, and Murray D. Bernstein. "Social support and well-being among residents of planned housing." *Gerontologist* 24 (1984): 144-148.

Examines the extent and sources of social, psychological, and material support of the residents of two apartment complexes designed for self-reliant and healthy older people; the nature of these informal helping networks; and the relationships between the characteristics of these networks and the residents' well-being.

Research

Social support networks were documented for 44 residents of the planned housing facilities. Although other residents were often regarded as sources of support, it was with persons outside the housing facilities that the locus of these networks lay. Except in times of medical crisis, the less healthy residents of the facilities were socially more isolated. Individuals expressing lower levels of life satisfaction, as well as those who had experienced serious illness requiring hospitalization during the past year, had more relationships with other residents than did their more satisfied neighbors. Implications of the findings are discussed.

Of interest to social scientists.

216. STEPHENS, Mary Ann Paris, and Carolyn Norris-Baker. "Social support in college life for disabled students." *Rehabilitation Psychology* 29 (1984): 107-111.

This study examined the social support networks of 30 disabled students using wheelchairs on two university campuses.

Research

Results indicated that while friends outnumbered family members in disabled students' networks, family members were more highly valued. Disabled students' networks were more extensive, including more relationships with friends, than those of nondisabled students.

Of interest to social and behavioral scientists, student counselors, and rehabilitation therapists.

217. STOKES, Joseph P. "Predicting satisfaction with social support from social network structure." *American Journal of Community Psychology* 11 (1983): 141-152.

This predictive study attempted to clarify the relationship of social networks to satisfaction with social support.

Research

Satisfaction was related to number of confidants and network size, but network density was not predictive of satisfaction with social

support. This study fails to support the common notion that low
density and more intimate networks foster greater satisfaction.

Researchers interested in population studies of social support and
network analysis will benefit from this study.

218. STOLLER, Eleanor Palo.   "Exchange patterns in the informal
     support networks of the elderlv: The impact of reciprocity on
     morale." *Journal of Marriage and the Family* 47 (1985): 335-
     342.

Examines patterns of exchange of assistance within the informal
helping networks of the elderly through the analysis of interviews
with a sample of 753 noninstitutionalized older persons.

Research

It was found that most elders are involved in some type of exchange.
Those who receive help usually reciprocate in some way, with the
prevalence of unreciprocated assistance higher among family members
than among friends or neighbors.   Analyses of exchange patterns
suggested that the inability to reciprocate had a greater negative
effect on morale than the need for assistance. The data also showed a
negative relationship between the scope of formal service use and
reliance on the informal network.

Of interest to social and behavioral scientists.

219. STRUG, David L., and Merton M. Hyman.   "Social networks of
     alcoholics." *Journal of Studies on Alcohol* 42 (1981): 855-
     884.

Examines the social networks of a group of alcoholics treated on an
inpatient basis and a group of untreated alcoholics at a detoxication
center.

Research

The data seem to suggest that alcoholics who seek treatment at a
rehabilitation center generally have larger networks than those who
don't seek formal treatment, and that members of the larger networks,
particularly confidants, are effective in urging the alcoholic to seek
treatment.   However, there is also a subgroup of alcoholics who enter
rehabilitation in order to survive physically.

Of particular interest to professionals working with alcoholics and
public health officials.

220. THOMAS, Paula D., Philip J. Garry, Jean M. Goodwin, James
     S. Goodwin.   "Social bonds in a healthy elderly sample:
     Characteristics and associated variables." *Social Science and
     Medicine* 20 (1985): 365-369.

This study examined factors associated with social bonding in a sample of 256 healthy elderly people.

Research

Using state of the art measures, this study revealed that subjects involved in satisfying, supportive, interpersonal relationships, also tended to have higher incomes, were married, worked, and were in relatively good health. Emotional status, cognitive functioning, and memory were found to be independent of social bonds.

This paper is well done and suggests several areas for additional research by researchers interested in the well elderly.

221. TIETJEN, Anne Marie. "The social networks and social support of married and single mothers in Sweden." *Journal of Marriage and the Family* 47 (1985): 489-496.

The networks of 37 single and 43 married women were compared in an attempt to identify structural characteristics of social networks and contextual factors associated with high levels of social support for married and single mothers in Sweden.

Research

Single mothers received more instrumental and personal support than married mothers, although their networks did not differ substantially in structure. Those receiving the highest levels of support were employed full time, had few children, had networks composed mainly of friends, saw their network members frequently, and kept a balance of giving and taking in their relationships. Although results were similar for married mothers, reciprocity was less important for maintaining relationships and neighbors were more important as a source of support.

Of interest to social scientists.

222. TOLSDORF, Christopher C. "Social networks, support and coping: An exploratory study." *Family Process* 15 (1976): 407-417.

An investigation of the areas of stress, support, and coping, using the structural model of the social network.

Research

Compares the networks of samples of normal and schizophrenic males to identify differences in their relationships to social networks, the composition of the networks, and the coping styles and recent histories of the subjects. Suggests that greater attention should be paid to an individual's perception of his network, which affects his ability to function.

Of interest to mental health professionals.

223. TORO, Paul A. "A comparison of natural and professional help." *American Journal of Community Psychology* 14 (1986): 147-159.

This study investigated the process and effectiveness of three natural and professional groups who commonly provide help to persons experiencing the important critical life event of marital disruption.

Research

Lawyers did more overall talking, showed greater proportions of information giving and closed questions, and were more effective in the legal/financial domain. Additional analyses indicated that all helpers showed fewer information-gathering behaviors and more information-and-advice-giving behaviors as the helping interaction progressed.

Of interest to mental health professionals, social and behavioral scientists, nurses, lawyers, and other helpers.

224. TOWNSEND, Aloen L., and S. Walter Poulshock. "Intergenerational perspectives on impaired elders' support networks." *Journal of Gerontology* 41 (1986): 101-109.

Compares the reports of impaired elders and those of their adult children regarding the elders' care-giving and decision-making support networks.

Research

The two generations generally agreed on the primary person in each network and on the overall hierarchy of sources of support, but they differed on the network's size, specific composition, and the member's relative centrality. Decision-making networks were consistently smaller, more highly centralized, and more restricted to immediate family, suggesting the need to distinguish this network from the general caregiving network.

Of interest to gerontologists and to social and behavioral scientists.

225. VAUX, Alan, and Deborah Harrison. "Support network characteristics associated with support satisfaction and perceived support." *American Journal of Community Psychology* 13, no. 3 (1985): 245-268.

Investigates which support network characteristics are associated with perceptions of and satisfaction with support.

Research

Ninety-eight women students are studied for characteristics of five modes of support, satisfaction with each mode, and perceptions of support from family, friends, and others. Findings indicate that support perceptions and satisfaction are related to size of support

networks, closeness of support relationships, and composition of
networks, particularly the presence of a spouse and proportion of
close friends, social acquaintances, and immediate family.

Of interest to social psychologists.

226. WALKER, K.N., A. MacBride, M.L.S. Vachan. "Social support
     networks and the crisis of bereavement. *Social Science and
     Medicine* 11 (1977): 35-41.

Various models of support structure are assessed in terms of their
adequacy in meeting the needs of individuals under stress.

Literature Review

Suggests that there is often a discrepancy between an individual's
social and psychological needs during crisis and the normal stress
with which his social support network is adequate in helping him to
cope. Careful assessment of needs, resources, and skill is necessary
to bring about an effective adjustment between social needs and social
supports during times of crisis.

Of interest to mental health professionals.

227. WAN, Thomas T.H., and William G. Weissert. "Social support
     networks, patient status, and institutionalization." *Research
     on Aging* 3, no. 2 (1981): 240-256.

Research to identify the relationship of social support to the
patient's functional status and to whether he/she is institutionalized.

Research

This study demonstrates that social support plays an important role in
mitigating the effects of deteriorating health status associated with
aging. Subjects who had strong social support networks were less
likely to be institutionalized and more likely to improve in physical
and mental functioning.

Social scientists interested in aging research and social support will
find this a useful paper.

228. WEEKS, John R., and Jose B. Cuellar. "The role of family
     members in the helping networks of older adults." *Ger-
     ontologist* 21 (1981): 388-394.

Helping networks of older people in 10 different ethnic groups were
examined for the extent to which they included family members.

Research

Immigrants were more likely than native-born older people to have family members to turn to in times of need. Although older people are not generally abandoned, policymakers and senior providers need to be aware that major group differences exist in the helping networks of older people.

Of interest to gerontologists.

229. WELLMAN, Barry, and Barry Leighton. "Networks, neighborhoods and communities." *Urban Affairs Quarterly* 15 (1979): 363-390.

An attempt to sort out the merger of the concepts of "neighborhood" and "community."

Theoretical and Analytical

We must be concerned with neighborhood and community rather than neighborhood or community. The two concepts may or may not be closely associated.

Of interest to social and behavioral scientists.

230. YOUNG, Shiaomay. "Aspects of social support networks among institutionalized adolescents." *Adolescence* 16 (Spring 1981): 123-137.

Describes the social support networks within the adolescent units in two mental health centers and explores the possible existence and functions of informal peer support groups.

Research

Results indicate that some form of peer support network exists on the wards, as well as outside the institutions.

Of interest to mental health practitioners and administrators.

c. Chapters

231. GOTTLIEB, Benjamin H., and David M. Todd. "Characterizing and promoting social support in natural settings." *In* R.F. Munoz, L.R. Snowden, J.G. Kelley (Eds.). *Social and Psychological Research in Community Settings.* San Francisco: Jossey-Bass, 1979.

An account of the kinds of resources that are exchanged in primary group helping relationships, and a discussion of the structural features of social networks and their interaction with individual characteristics as they affect social support.

Research

Suggests a major shift from the more dominant view that coping with
stress is an individual and largely psychological process and that
help, when needed, is best provided by a trained professional.
Of interest to social and behavioral scientists.

232. GRANOVETTER, Mark. "The strength of weak ties--a network
theory revisited." *In* Peter V. Marsden, and Nan Lin
(Eds.). *Social Structure and Network Analysis.* Beverly
Hills: Sage, 1982.

Focuses on the impact of weak ties on individuals and the role of weak
ties in affecting cohesion in complex social systems.

Literature Review and Analysis

The importance of weak ties is asserted to be that they are likely to
be bridges between network segments as compared to strong ties. This
does not preclude the possibility that weak ties have no bridging
function. Systematic investigation of those ties that bridge, as
compared to those that do not, is needed.

Of interest to social and behavioral scientists.

233. HAMMER, Muriel. "The role of social networks in schizo-
phrenia." *In* Graham D. Burrows, Trevor R. Torman,
Gertrude Rubinstein (Eds.). *Handbook of Studies on
Schizophrenia. Part 2: Management and Research.*
Amsterdam: Elsevier, 1986.

Discusses the possible relationship between people's social support
systems and psychiatric and physical morbidity, and the potential
contribution of social network analysis to a resolution of the
methodological difficulties in determining the role of various social
variables in the etiology, course, and outcome of schizophrenia.

Review and Analysis

Discusses some key concepts of social network analysis. Summarizes
findings from studies of the networks of schizophrenic patients, and
considers how they should be interpreted. Discusses inferences that
can be drawn from a general knowledge of network processes and
possible implications of the findings on the relationship of social
networks to mental and physical health. Indicates research strategies
that may help to answer critical unresolved issues.

Of interest to researchers of social networks and social support and
of schizophrenia.

234. KEUPP, Heiner. "Soziale netzwerke." (German) *In* Heiner
Keupp, and Dodo Rerrich (Eds.). *Psychosoziale Praxis-
gemeinde-psychologische Perspectiven.* Munchen: Urban &
Schwarzenberg, 1982.

A critical analysis of the emergence of the concept of "social networks" in social psychiatry, community psychology, and medical sociology.

Review

A sociological analysis of the use of the concept, social networks, in research on health problems, particularly in psychiatry. Discusses how this research has influenced treatment, emphasizing less dependency upon medical professionals and more reliance on one's self or on close family and/or friends. Some recommendations for future (sociological) research on social support and health/mental health, treatment and prevention are offered.

Of particular interest to sociologists in general, medical sociologists, and social psychiatrists.

235. LA GAIPA, John J. "A systems approach to personal relationships." *In* Steve Duck, and Robin Gilmour (Eds.). *Personal Relationships 1: Studying Personal Relationships.* London: Academic Press, 1981.

A systems-based approach to personal relationships, characterized both by looking at a three-dimensional model for understanding relationships and by examining them in reference to the various real life contexts and systems in which they take place.

Theoretical

An underlying theme of this chapter has been the dialectics between the cultural-normative and behavior levels. Another theme has been the pervasive quality of tension and conflict. From a systems point of view, tension is a normal, ever-present dynamic agent which must be kept at an optimal level if the system is to remain viable. Structural analysis was used for locating and examining personal relationships within a three dimensional conceptual framework: level of analysis, support systems, and psychosocial satisfactions.

Of interest to teachers and researchers interested in social support.

236. ORTH-GOMER, Kristina, Britt-Marie Wallin, Anna-Lena Undén. "Social support and coronary risk factors. *In* Ulrich Laaser, Raoul Senault, Herbert Viefhues (Eds.). *Primary Health Care in the Making.* Berlin: Springer-Verlag, 1985.

An examination of the psychological aspects of the social support network system in 83 Swedish men, some of whom were healthy, some of whom had symptoms of heart disease, and some of whom had other types of chronic conditions.

Research

Two dimensions of social support--attachment and social integration--were examined. The instruments measuring these two dimensions did not yield data that distinguished the groups studied.

Of interest to researchers of coronary heart disease and social support.

237. WELLMAN, Barry. "Studying personal communities." *In* Peter V. Marsden, and Nan Lin (Eds.). *Social Structure and Network Analysis.* Beverly Hills: Sage, 1982.

Community network studies are related to fundamental concerns of both social network analysis and urban sociology. The current limitations of community network studies are discussed.

Research and Analysis

Data show that about one-quarter of East Yorkers' ties are with persons whom they do not like and with whom they would not voluntarily form a twosome. Such "structurally embedded" ties become involuntary parts of network membership packages. Most are ties to persons with whom the participants have to deal seriously in their neighborhoods, in a kinship group, or at work. Communities are not necessarily nice things.

Of interest to social and behavioral scientists.

238. ———, P. Craven, M. Whitaker, H. Stevens, A. Shorter, S. Du Toit, H. Bakker. "Community ties and support systems: From intimacy to support" *In* L.S. Bourne, R.D. McKinnon, J.W. Summons (Eds.). *The Form of Cities in Central Canada: Selected Papers.* Toronto: University of Toronto Press, 1973.

An examination of the conditions under which social support is provided by intimates outside the bounds of the household.

Research

This survey of 845 adults demonstrates several correlates of social support, including the composition of social networks, socioeconomic homogeneity, and a variety of contextual or environmental factors such as neighborhood characteristics.

Urban researchers and others interested in the human ecology of social support will find this a useful study.

d. Dissertations

239. BERKMAN, Lisa F. "Social networks, host resistance, and mortality: A follow-up study of Alameda County residents." Ph.D. dissertation, University of California, Berkeley, 1977.

The sample for this study was drawn from the population of adults living in Alameda County, California in 1965. From 1967 until 1974, when a follow-up survey was conducted, information was collected on those who died in the nine-year period following the survey. The survey and mortality follow-up provide prospective information on the impact of various social and environmental factors on mortality.

Research

The extent of a person's social and community ties was found to be associated with risk of mortality from all causes. Four sources of social relationships—marriage, contacts with close friends and relatives, church membership, and formal and informal group associations—were each predictive of mortality rates.

Of interest to social and behavioral scientists and mental health professionals.

240. BURGHER, Peter L. "Social network characteristics, social support and compliance to a chronic hemodialysis regimen." Ph.D. dissertation, University of Windsor, Canada, 1982.

A study of the relationship between support network characteristics and dialysis compliance.

Research

The main hypotheses were generally confirmed: compliant patients had larger, denser, and more family oriented networks than noncompliant patients. Based on the results, it was suggested that emotional support, empathy, and stable sense of self identity are important factors in compliance to a hemodialysis regimen.

Particulary useful to nephrologists and other professionals working with hemodialysis patients.

241. CRONENWETT, Linda R.H. "Relationships among social network structure, perceived social support, and psychological outcomes of pregnancy." Ph.D. dissertation, University of Michigan, 1983.

Examined social networks and perceived social support, their associations with gender and educational level, and their effects on adaptation to the parental role.

Research

Women were found to obtain most support from friends, whereas men received more from relatives. Satisfaction and coping with the parental role were related to network and social support variables for both men and women.

Should interest practitioners in neonatal care and young parents.

242. CROTTY, Patrick. "How schizophrenics and their significant others perceive their social support networks." Ph.D. dissertation, University of Illinois at Chicago, 1983.

Examines the differences between the way schizophrenics perceive their social support networks and the way their significant others perceive them, and which factors may account for these differences.

Research

In general it was found that schizophrenics reported a much more positive view of their support networks than did their significant others. The burden schizophrenics posed on their families was inversely related to a number of support variables.

Of special interest to mental health workers, social workers, and community health researchers.

243. FANDETTI, Donald Vincent. "Sources of assistance in a white, working class, ethnic neighborhood." D.S.W. dissertation, Columbia University, 1974.

Examines attitudes towards sources of assistance among residents in a working class, ethnic neighborhood.

Research

Interviews of 100 randomly selected neighborhood residents in east Baltimore disclosed that working class, ethnic Catholics prefer traditional structures such as the family, the church, and, to some extent, the ethnic voluntary organization for meeting needs in relation to child care, care of the aged, financial aid, and personal problems. Members of the extended family and traditional professionals such as the clergy and general physicians are the preferred sources of assistance. A substantial number of the respondents failed to identify mental health specialists as potential sources of assistance. Implications for policy and program development and delivery of health care services are drawn from the findings and discussed.

Of interest to social scientists and health and welfare planners, providers, and policymakers.

244. FROLAND, Charles G. "Improving the social adjustment of mental health clients: The case for social support networks. Ph.D. dissertation, University of California, Berkeley, 1978.

Examines how social networks of mental health clients contributed to their social adjustment through network analysis in a sample of 77 adult subjects.

Research

Results indicated that clients who could rely on primary kin for support and assistance in times of need reported the best psychological adjustment. The data suggested social support has three central characteristics: support has to be perceived as given voluntarily, supportive exchanges have to be reciprocal, and support should confirm the individual's competence in performing socially expected roles.

Of interest to social scientists, mental health professionals, and social workers.

245. GALLO, Frank T. "Social support networks and elderly health." Ph.D. dissertation, Boston University Graduate School, 1982.

Explores the impact of social support networks on health status and health care utilization among the elderly.

Research

Both network variables and demographics were moderately associated with health status and health care utilization in general, and combined, showed an incremental predictive effect over the effect of demographic variables. Social support network variables were most significantly associated with health outcomes.

Of interest to gerontologists and researchers of health care utilization by the elderly.

246. HEALY, James E. "The relation of social network structure variables to mental health and the breadth and quality of church support of single young adult members." Ph.D. dissertation, University of Illinois at Urbana-Champaign, 1985.

A study of the social support networks of young adult church members and their effects on mental health.

Research

An overall measure of availability of social support was significantly associated with a number of mental health outcomes. Social network structure variables were significantly related to "enhancement" mental health variables, but not to "deficiency" mental health variables.

Should interest social and behavioral scientists, in particular those who are interested in the quality and dimensions of social support.

247. MAXWELL, Mary B. "The impact of social networks on mortality, disease incidence, and disease progression." Ph.D. dissertation, Portland State University, 1985.

Attempts to determine the relationship between social network indicators and mortality in an urban sample, to investigate the relationship between networks and disease incidence and progression, and to investigate which specific networks were the best predictors of health related outcomes.

Research

The four social indices of network (scope, size, frequency of contact, and interaction) were predictive of future mortality. Marital, family, and kin relationships were not predictive, but ties of close friends, work associates, and social leisure activities were significantly predictive of death. No relationships were found for disease incidence or progression.

Of interest to social and behavioral scientists and public health officials.

248. MONTGOMERY, Mary B.H.   "Structure and attributes of social
       support networks that affect health of the aged."   D.S.W.
       dissertation, University of California, Berkeley, 1983.

An analysis of the relationship between social support and health conditions and health perceptions among noninstitutionalized elderly.

Research

A number of social network variables were found to have an impact on health, but the relative importance of the several indicators of network ties differed across socioeconomic and other relevant variables.

Useful for social scientists, in particular gerontologists.

249. ROOK, Karen S.   "Social networks and well-being of elderly
       widowed women."   Ph.D.   dissertation,   University   of
       California, Los Angeles, 1980.

A study of the contribution of social support to psychological health in a sample of 115 elderly widowed women.

Research

It was found that life satisfaction was better predicted by the number of negative exchanges, whereas loneliness was better predicted by the number of positive exchanges. Frequency of interaction was associated with both outcomes. Results were explained within the framework of social exchange theory.

Of interest to social scientists, gerontologists, and social policymakers.

250. STONE, Jeffrey D. "The influence of social networks and perceived social support on depressive symptomatology." Ph.D. dissertation, University of California, Los Angeles, 1981.

Investigates the buffering effects of objective social network characteristics and perceived supports on chronic strains.

Research

Perceived support was associated with larger social networks and more frequent self-initiated discussion of problems. Evidence was found only for an independent, protective effect, regardless of amount of stress, of social support on depressive symptomatology. No buffering effects could be demonstrated.

Useful for social and behavioral scientists, in particular stress researchers.

251. SWEARINGEN-ARCHER, Dolores J. "Social network support among veteran psychiatric patients." Ph.D. dissertation, University of Arizona, 1981.

An exploratory study of perceived support from social networks for psychosocial problems among 244 male veteran psychiatric patients.

Research

Only a small number of the available informal social networks were found to be used for support during periods of psychosocial problems--in particular, nuclear family, kin, or friends. Formal sources of support were also considered to be important in times of need. Factor analyses revealed five social network patterns, and a regression analysis yielded a number of important predictor variables for choice of support pattern, e.g. marital status and living situation.

Of interest to social scientists and mental health professionals, in particular, those working in VA hospitals.

2. NETWORK RESOURCES

a. Books

252. SAUER, William J., and Raymond T. Coward (Eds.). *Social Support Networks and the Care of the Elderly*. New York: Springer, 1985.

A collection of articles devoted to issues surrounding the development and use of social support systems that help the elderly person maintain independence and meet personal needs in time of crisis.

Book of Readings

The 13 chapters are divided into five major parts: the state of the
art, family relations, community relations, social networks under
special circumstances, and the applications of theory and research.

Of particular interest to students of gerontology and to health
professionals and service providers working with the elderly and their
families.

253. WHITTAKER, James K., James Garbarino, and Associates.
      *Social Support Networks. Informal Helping in the Human
      Services.* New York: Aldine, 1983.

Suggests ways in which formal and informal caregivers can create new
alliances to offer more effective responses to people in need of help.

Book of Readings

A conceptual framework for identifying and using a variety of social
support networks with different age groups in different practice
settings. Provides practical information on the best current uses of
social support in such areas as child and youth services, day care,
family services, mental health and mental retardation, schools, aging,
and health care delivery.

Of interest to social workers, community psychologists, mental health
professionals, and other human service providers.

b. Articles

254. ANTONUCCI, Toni C., and Barbara A. Israel. "Verdicality of
      social support: A comparison of principal and network
      members' responses." *Journal of Consulting and Clinical
      Psychology* 54 (1986): 432-437.

Examines the agreement and effect of social support on principals in
networks.

Research

Perceptions of support and closeness were highest among spouses,
somewhat high among family members and lowest among friends,
establishing a concept of verdicality. Verdicality was not
significantly related to life satisfaction, happiness, or negative
effect.

Useful to researchers.

255. BAKER, Frank. "The interface between professional and
      natural support systems. *Clinical Social Work* 5 (Summer
      1977): 139-148.

Examines the types and functions of natural support systems and discusses the nature of their relationships with professional support systems.

Literature Review/Theoretical

Natural support systems exist separately from a community's professional care-giving system. The two systems may compete with one another or one may attempt to engulf the other. However, under ideal conditions, the two systems may communicate, collaborate, and complement each other in meeting the needs of community residents. A hypothesis regarding the sequence of interdependent development of natural and professional helping systems is presented, and examination of the natural histories of support systems in a community is suggested to test this hypothesis.

Of interest to social scientists.

256. BRANCH, Laurence G., and Alan M. Jette. "Elders' use of informal long-term care assistance." *Gerontologist* 23 (1983): 51-56.

Investigates the nature and composition of the informal support network that provides long-term care assistance to elders in the community, the extent to which elders are influenced by network members to make use of such assistance, and the extent to which they actually do so.

Research

Over 80% of a sample of community-living elderly in Massachusetts, aged 71 and older, were found to be self-sufficient in performing the basic activities of daily living, but only 18% were self-sufficient in performing instrumental activities of daily living. Most elders who used long-term care assistance relied solely on their informal support networks in both instrumental (86%) and basic (50%) activities of daily living. The key predictor of the amount of informal assistance used was increasing physical disability. The only network characteristic consistently related to the use of informal services was the elder's living situation.

Of interest to social scientists and health planners and policymakers.

257. BURDA, Philip C., Alan Vaux, Thomas Schill. "Social support resources--variation across sex and sex-role." *Personality and Social Psychology Bulletin* 10 (1984): 119-126.

Assesses the influence of sex and the sex-role on college students' social support resources on three levels: network characteristics, availability of several modes of support, and perceived supportiveness of family and friends.

Research

On a composite measure of overall support resources, females were superior to males, and feminine and androgynous individuals were superior to masculine and undifferentiated individuals. Only some specific social support variables differed across these groups-- network size and homogeneity, emotional support, and perceived supportiveness of the family for the sex role.

Of interest to social and behavioral scientists.

258. CANTOR, Marjorie H. "Life space and the social support system of the inner city elderly of New York." *The Gerontologist* 15 (1975): 23-26.

Selected data from a cross-cultural survey of 1,552 elderly people living in New York City's 26 poorest neighborhoods was examined to determine the life space of the inner city elderly, the extent of their functioning social support system, and their perception of the strengths and weaknesses of city life.

Analytical

A majority of the respondents have relatively easy access to desired facilities and essential services, although medical services are frequently outside the immediate neighborhood and, thereby, less accessible. Two-thirds of the elderly have at least one living child and receive substantial assistance from their children. In addition, the presence of numerous persons living in the immediate vicinity provides a large reservoir to draw upon for intimate and supportive relationships. The majority of respondents considered New York City a viable place to live, despite its problems, because of availability of facilities and services, relationships with neighbors, and opportunities for work and a sense of privacy.

Of interest to social scientists.

259. ------. "Neighbors and friends: An overlooked resource in the informal support system." *Research on Aging* 1 (1979): 434-463.

Presents empirical findings concerning the extent to which older people in the inner city neighborhoods of New York City have an informal network of friends and neighbors and the nature of the interactions which occur.

Descriptive

Several theoretical models concerning the operation of the informal support system are considered, and the author presents a new model--the hierarchical-compensatory model--as best fitting the data at hand. The findings are from the largest cross-cultural study of the elderly in urban poverty.

Of interest to social and behavioral scientists.

260. CLARK, Alfred W. "Personal and social resources as correlates of coping behavior among the aged." *Psychological Reports* 51 (1982): 577-578.

Reports the results of a study of available resources to assist the elderly in coping with the problems of aging.

Research

A survey of 1,841 residents of Great Britain over the age of 60 indicated a strong correlation of coping effectiveness and the management of daily affairs with social resources. Those elderly who reported strong support from family, friends, and neighbors reported better adjustment.

An interesting article, which will be useful to gerontologists interested in social support.

261. COOKE, Kenneth, and Dorothy Lawton. "Informal support for the carers of disabled children." *Child Care and Health Development* 10, no. 2 (1984): 67-79.

This article draws on data from a nationally representative sample of disabled children to investigate the support which carers receive from spouses, relatives, friends, neighbors, and voluntary organizations.

Research

The results confirm the findings of previous studies that, within families, mothers bear the major burden of both child care and housework. However, the results indicate that families with disabled children generally do not receive as much support from relatives, friends, and neighbors as some previous studies of children with particular disorders have suggested, and that membership in voluntary organizations is very low.

Of interest to pediatricians, child care workers, and rehabilitation specialists.

262. CROOG, Sydney H., Alberta Lipson, Sol Levine. "Help patterns in severe illness: The roles of kin network, non-family resources, and institutions." *Journal of Marriage and the Family* 34 (February 1972): 32-41.

Examines patterns of support or assistance reported by men in an urban setting who had experienced a situation of severe crisis in the form of a first heart attack.

Research

Studies concerned with aid patterns and with response to crisis have paid inadequate attention to the total range of resources for support that are employed by persons in time of need. The role of friends and neighbors has not been given the scrutiny that it may deserve. There

is a paucity of cross-cultural comparisons of types of family systems
and their aid and resources in times of crisis.

Useful to researchers in the area of coronary heart disease as well as
rehabilitation specialists.

263. FINLAYSON, A. "Social networks as coping resources: Lay
help and consultation patterns used by women in husband's
post-infarction career." *Social Science and Medicine* 10
(1976): 97-103.

Examines how differences in families relate to differences in outcome
twelve months after the husband's myocardial infarction.

Research

Women whose husbands had favorable outcomes tended to acknowledge
support from a wide range of sources including non-kin and adult
children. Women whose husbands had less favorable outcomes showed
less support, which was often restricted to family members.

Of interest to physicians, social workers, and mental health
professionals.

264. GOODMAN, Catherine Chase. "Natural helping among older
adults." *Gerontologist* 24 (1984): 138-143.

A survey of neighbors in retirement housing was conducted to identify
the distinguishing characteristics and natural helping styles of the
members of a dynamic informal support system.

Research

Three distinct neighborhood exchange types were identified: those who
exhibit a quasi-professional style of helping without reciprocation;
those who share an interdependent style of give and take; and those
whose social ties and sources of help are primarily outside the
neighborhood. Natural helping styles suggest such service models as
volunteer programs and self-help group interventions.

Should interest social and behavioral scientists.

265. GRIFFITH, James. "Social support providers: Who are they?
Where are they met? and the relationship of network
characteristics to psychological distress." *Basic and Applied
Social Psychology* 6 (1985): 41-60.

Randomly selected adults living in one of three suburban communities
in southern California provided responses to a standardized measure of
psychological distress and named those persons on whom they depended
when personal problems arose.

Research

Friends and spouses accounted for the largest proportions of social support providers. Nonrelative support providers were generally same-sex friends whom respondents had known six years or more and were of similar age and ethnic/racial origin as respondents. Results reinforce the notion that qualitative aspects of support are better measures of the construct, social support. Quantitative measures of social support were unrelated to perceived well-being.

Of interest to social and behavioral scientists.

266. HORWITZ, Allen. "Family, kin, and friend networks in psychiatric help-seeking." *Social Science and Medicine* 12 (1978): 297-304.

Data regarding the help-seeking efforts in the community of 120 patients at a community mental health center are used to examine the different types of assistance provided to individuals with psychiatric problems by different sectors of the social network.

Research

Major findings are: 1) the type of husband-wife relationship is significantly related to help-seeking efforts; 2) friends and close kin are the most common sources of assistance; and 3) kin and friends provide certain specialized forms of assistance to help-seekers.

Of interest to mental health professionals, social workers, and social and behavioral scientists.

267. KOHEN, Janet A. "Old but not alone: Informal social supports among the elderly by marital status and sex." *Gerontologist* 23 (1983): 57-63.

An investigation of the frequency of social contacts and of confiding behaviors within informal relationships among the elderly respondents (55 and older) included in a national survey that focuses on differences in marital status and sex in these two dimensions of their social lives.

Research

The widowed elderly of both sexes generally had a significantly higher frequency of social contacts than did the married. Married men were less likely to report many/several close friends than women, but all respondents, regardless of marital status or sex, were more likely to report few or no friends or relatives as confidants. Women, however, were more likely to use family or friends as a resource when worried. Married people turned to their families more often, but widowed more often turned to friends. Women were more likely than men to talk to their families, but both sexes were equally likely to talk to friends. When serious problems arose, the widowed were more likely to turn both to children and friends than were the married, and women appeared to have closer relationships with their children than did men. Married men were least likely to turn to their families, whereas widowed men were most likely to do so. There was no reported difference between married and widowed women. Men and women were equally likely to assess their children as helpful in times of crisis.

Of interest to social and behavioral scientists, gerontologists, and geriatricians.

268. LEE, Gary R. "Kinship and social support: The case of the United States." *Aging and Society* 5 (March 1985): 19-38.

Deals with two related issues: the extent to which older persons requiring assistance in the tasks of or resources needed for daily living receive such assistance from informal networks; and the consequences of the receipt of this assistance for the older person.

Review and Analysis

Evidence is insufficient to prove that the provision of services by formal agencies is more beneficial than reliance on informal support networks; however, the author raises serious doubts about the reverse assumption.

Of interest to social and behavioral scientists, gerontologists, and public policymakers.

269. LEVITT, Mary J., Ruth A. Weber, M. Cherie Clark. "Social network relationships as sources of maternal support and well-being." *Developmental Psychology* 22 (1986): 310-316.

Describes the social networks available to mothers of infants, focusing on the contribution of specific relationships to maternal well-being.

Research

Mothers reported an average of 13 persons in their networks, but support was provided primarily by the husband, followed by the infant's maternal grandmother, and one or two other family members or friends. Maternal affect and life satisfaction were related to infant difficulty and to support from, and satisfaction with, the spouse. Negative maternal affect was related to anxious/resistant attachment.

Of interest to child development specialists and social and behavioral scientists.

270. LIPMAN, A., and C. Longino, Jr. "Support systems of women by marital status." *Gerontologist* 24, Supplement 1 (1984): 291.

Summarizes support system findings from the Midwestern Retirement Community Study.

Research Abstract

Family members were found to be the most prominent resources for instrumental social and emotional support. The type and amount of support received by women varied with their position in the family. Those with husbands and children tended to consider husbands their primary source of support, followed by children, siblings, other relatives, and friends. Widows tended to list siblings as their most important support resource. Voluntary social behavior was motivated by expectations of the returns it would bring.

Should interest social and behavioral scientists.

271. LIPMAN, Aaron, and Charles F. Longino, Jr. "I remember mama: Support network differentials of older married and nonmarried men and women." *Gerontologist* 19, Supplement (1979): 111.

Explores the nature of informal support by source (family, friend, other) and type (emotional, social, instrumental service) and how these measures differ by gender and marital status of the recipient.

Research Abstract

Four hundred and forty-eight noninstitutionalized residents of two life care retirement communities were interviewed. After adjusting for the effects of age, education, income, and self-assessed health, it was found that the greatest family support goes to the married, followed by the nonmarried (never married less than widows). In all marital status categories, women receive greater support than men. The greatest informal resource deficits are among nonmarried men.

Should interest gerontologists, geriatricians, and social scientists.

272. LITWAK, Eugene, and Ivan Szelenyi. "Primary group structures and their functions: Kin, neighbors, and friends." *American Sociological Review* 34 (1969): 465-481.

A theoretical discussion of the variety of primary group structures and their differential functions in an industrial society.

Theoretical

The processes of technological development have forced an increasing differentiation of primary group structures. At the same time, the level of technology permits the survival of forms of primary group structures that could not remain stable in some earlier stages. Thus, the neighborhood as a primary group must frequently exist with high membership turnover, and kinship structures must frequently exist without face-to-face contact.

Of interest primarily to sociologists and anthropologists.

273. LONGINO, C., and R. Garland. "Health, crime, and loneliness: Are people in retirement communities really better off?" *Gerontologist* 17, Supplement (1977): 93.

Distributions on background variables and assessment of problems of residents in probability samples of two retirement communities were compared with those of older people in the Harris survey to determine whether people in retirement communities have fewer serious problems with health, fear of crime, and loneliness than do older people in the general population.

Research Abstract

After controlling for variables of age, sex, number of living family members, and socioeconomic status, it was found that retirement community residents tend to see health, crime, and loneliness as being less seriously problematic than do older people in general. These findings imply that retirement communities may provide supportive environments, especially for those older people who are more vulnerable to problems of health, crime, and loneliness.

Of interest to gerontologists and social scientists.

274. LOPATA, Helena Znaniecki. "Support systems of elderly urbanites: Chicago of the 1970's." *Gerontologist* 15 (1975): 35-41.

A theoretical framework was developed for examining variations in the support systems of the Chicago area urban elderly and factors contributing to those variations, using data from two studies of metropolitan widows and the Chicago Needs Assessment Survey.

Analytical, Research

A lag was found between the city's social system and the personal abilities and resources of elderly urbanites. Many were from minority backgrounds, were born outside the city, and did not possess the personal resources, such as health, money, self-confidence, competence, knowledge, and ability to work out problems in the abstract and then carry on plans of action, which are necessary to the voluntaristic social engagement required for developing secondary support networks in the city. Social scientists and urban planners need to develop ways of helping elderly people who do not have initiating behavior habits to lead a more urban life when life circumstances bring about the dissolution of their primary support systems.

Of interest to social scientists, social workers, and urban planners.

275. ————. "Contributions of extended families to the social support systems of metropolitan area widows: Limitations of the modified kin network." *Journal of Marriage and the Family* 40 (1979): 355-364.

An examination of the economic, service, social, and emotional support systems of Chicago area widows.

Research

Children and, in the case of younger widows, parents are frequent contributors to the support systems. Siblings, cousins, nieces and nephews, and grandchildren contribute very infrequently and selectively, and most widows do not list such relatives at all.

Of interest to social and behavioral scientists, social workers, and marriage and family counselors.

276. LYNAM, M. Judith. "Support networks developed by immigrant women." *Social Science and Medicine* 21 (1985): 327-333.

Women with young children, who were immigrants to Canada, were interviewed to determine how they defined their needs and what resources they perceived to be available to meet their needs.

Research

All of the women described a need to feel as if they belonged in Canada and had people to turn to for personal support. The women identified general groups of people who they perceived to be capable of providing them with different forms of support. The three groups were labeled kin, insider, and outsider. The women also described how they used their sources of support and the feelings which resulted from their interactions with members of the support groups.

Of interest to social and behavioral scientists.

277. MORRIS, John N., and Sylvia Sherwood. "Informal support resources for vulnerable elderly persons: Can they be counted on, why do they work?" *Internaitonal Journal of Aging and Human Development* 18 (1983-1984): 81-98.

A study of the informal support systems of the vulnerable elderly and their operation and effectiveness.

Research

The majority of the elderly proved to have a responsive informal support system. There was a general acceptance of responsibility for the needs of the lonely elderly person among the informal network members. The required care was generally provided. It is suggested that this informal support system not be disturbed by a formal care system.

Of particular interest to gerontologists, policymakers, and planners of the health care and other needs of the vulnerable elderly.

278. PILISUK, Marc, and Charles Froland. "Kinship, social networks, social support and health." *Social Science and Medicine* 12B (1978): 273-280.

Discusses family and kinship ties and an individual's broader social

network.   Changes in society have placed different burdens on these
social forms, with resulting implications for the kind of support
available to individuals in times of need.

Review and Theoretical

Points out the general immunological value that may be obtained from
the nurturance of social support networks. Recommends examination of
the tools and concepts of network analysis, which could help in
understanding what is meant by reliable social support and how it is
related to health maintenance and the delivery of health services.

Of interest to researchers and teachers interested in social support.

279. SALLOWAY, Jeffrey Colman, and Patrick B. Dillon.   "A
      comparison of family networks and friend networks in health
      care utilization."   *Journal of Comparative Family Studies*
      4 (Spring 1973): 131-142.

Reports the results of a study that examined the relationship between
health care utilization and some selected aspects of family and friend
networks.

Research

The findings suggest that the larger the networks of friends that
people have, the less likely they are to delay in using health care
services. The larger their family networks, however, the more likely
they are to delay utilization of health care services.

Of interest to health administrators and social and behavioral
scientists.

280. STOLLER, Eleanor Palo, and Lorna L. Earl.   "Help with
      activities of everyday life: Sources of support for the
      noninstitutionalized elderly." *Gerontologist* 23 (1983): 64-70.

Explores the patterns and sources of assistance provided to
noninstitutionalized older persons with varying degrees of functional
capacity.

Research

A probability sample of 753 noninstitutionalized elderly living in
northeastern New York were interviewed. Analysis of the data suggests
that the primary source of help for married elders with impaired
capacity is the spouse. When a spouse is not present or provides
insufficient help, adult daughters are the major helpers.   As
functional capacity declines, older persons' helping networks increase
in both size and scope.

Of interest to sociologists, gerontologists, and geriatricians.

281. SULLIVAN, Deborah A. "Informal support systems in a planned retirement community: Availability, proximity and willingness to utilize." *Research on Aging* 8 (1986): 249-267.

Compares the informal support systems of residents in a planned retirement community with those of their national peers, focusing on the availability of friends and family to provide personal assistance in the event of a health problem, their proximity, and the extent to which respondents express willingness to utilize these support systems on a short- and long-term basis.

Research

Data indicate that residents form mutual assistance networks for short-term help in lieu of or in addition to distant or nonexistent kin. Only a minority expect long-term help from friends, and few rely on any primary group for long-term care. As the community ages, the residual population is made up of individuals with attenuated kin networks or strong reservations about informal support for long-term care. There is a need to develop formal support systems in retirement communities.

Of interest to community planners, gerontologists, and social scientists.

282. SWANN, William B., Jr., and Steven C. Predmore. "Intimates as agents of social support: Sources of consolation or despair?" *Journal of Personality and Social Psychology* 49 (1985): 1609-1617.

Concerned with the processes whereby members of people's intimate circles offer them support for their self-conceptions when these conceptions are under attack.

Research

Findings suggest that self-concept stability emanates from forces outside the person, from continuity in the manner in which people's social relationships are organized. Pivotal in such organizational schemes are people's friends and intimates.

Of interest to social and behavioral scientists.

283. TAYLOR, Robert Joseph, and Linda M. Chatters. "Church-based informal support among elderly blacks." *Gerontologist* 26 (1986): 637-642.

Examines sociodemographic and religiosity factors as predictors of the receipt of church-based support among a national sample of 581 elderly black Americans.

Research

Frequency of attendance was the most important predictor of both frequency and amount of support. The relationship between age and support was modified by the presence of children and church membership. The most prevalent form of reported aid was socioemotional support during illness.

Should interest social and behavioral scientists.

284. TIETJEN, Anne Marie, and Christine F. Bradley. "Social support and maternal psychosocial adjustment during the transition to parenthood." *Canadian Journal of Behavioral Science* 17 (1985): 109-121.

Questions whether support from social networks and/or support from husbands is associated with women's adjustment during pregnancy and/or postpartum. Levels of perceived stress, anxiety, depression, marital adjustment, attitude toward baby, and social support are assessed for 23 well-educated, middle to upper middle class women.

Research

Findings suggest that women who are experiencing a difficult adjustment turn to their networks for support. Network support is not effective in promoting better postpartum adjustment. Prebirth social support does not predict postpartum adjustment.

Of interest to obstetricians, nurses, and other health professionals providing care to pregnant women.

285. UNGER, Donald G., and Abraham Wandersman. "The importance of neighbors: The social, cognitive, and affective components of neighboring." *American Journal of Community Psychology* 13, no. 2 (1985): 139-169.

Broadens the concept of neighboring to include social interaction, symbolic interaction, and the attachments of individuals to the people around them and the place in which they dwell.

Literature Review

Examines three components of neighboring: the social component (emotional, informational, support, and social network); the cognitive component (the physical environment and symbolic communication); and the affective component (the sense of community and attachment to place). Neighboring, it is concluded, affects perceptions of neighbors, social interaction or social isolation, problem solving, and neighborhood viability.

Of interest to social scientists.

286. VAN FOSSEN, Beth E. "Sex differences in the mental health effects of spouse support and equity." *Journal of Health and Social Behavior* 22 (1981): 130-143.

Examines the relationship of sex differences in spouse expressiveness of emotional support on the morale, well-being, and mental health of employed husbands, unemployed wives, and employed wives.

Research

Findings suggest that depression emerges from the unsupportive relationships that people have with intimate others, and from everyday social roles that foster low self-esteem and role strain.

Sociologists, social psychologists, and other social researchers interested in role strain, social support, and mental health will benefit from this article.

287. WARD, Russell A., Mark LaGory, Susan R. Sherman. "Social ties and morale of the elderly." *Sociology and Social Research* 70 (October 1985): 102-105.

Presents detailed data on a sample of 1,185 persons, 60 years of age and over, in New York State, providing evidence that different social relationships are used in different ways for social support.

Research

Sub-group variations were found in the contributions of social networks to morale. The importance of neighborhood-based social ties and support for the more vulnerable elderly suggests that the accessibility of social support is important.

Of interest to social and behavioral scientists.

288. WOOD, Vivian, and Joan F. Robertson. "Friendship and kinship interaction: Differential effect on the morale of the elderly." *Journal of Marriage and the Family* 40 (1978): 367-375.

Examines the differential effects of kinship and friendship relationships on life satisfaction among older people.

Research

Involvement with friends contributed more to the morale of older people than involvement with grandchildren. Findings are discussed in terms of differences in the qualitative dimensions of friendship and kinship relationships.

Primarily of interest to gerontologists and family sociologists.

289. ZAUTRA, Alex J. "Social resources and the quality of life." *American Journal of Community Psychology* 11 (1983): 275-290.

Four social resource measures were distinguished based on their cognitive and affective properties and were tested in a survey of the quality of life of community residents.

Research

Positive measures of resources were associated with boosts in positive effect, but not reductions in negative affective states. A measure of negative aspects of social resources was associated with distress and negative effect, but not with a reduction in positive effect. Buffer effects did occur, but only when the resident was experiencing high levels of stressful life events. There were life cycle differences in the availability of social resources to residents of the community and evidence suggested that the value of some resources changed as a function of the resident's stage in life.

Of interest to social and behavioral scientists.

c. Chapter

290. RUBIN, Nissan. "Social networks and mourning patterns: Toward a sociological theory of mourning." *In* Andre deVries, and Amnon Cormi (Eds.). *The Dying Human.* Ramat Gan, Israel: Turtledove, 1979.

A sociological theory explains the connections between mourning practices and social networks.

Theoretical

Discusses how the type of social network to which people belong affects the type of social support that is readily available to them and the particular needs they have for support, thereby supporting the development of different mourning practices by various societies.

Should interest social scientists.

A. FAMILY SUPPORT

a. Books

291. BOTT, Elizabeth. *Families and Social Networks* Second Edition. New York: Free Press, 1971.

Describes the social and psychological organization of some urban families.

Research

A discussion of the variation in conjugal roles, in network-connectedness, in behavior towards kin, and in concepts of class and norms of conjugal roles. Based on intensive interviews with 20 families.

Of interest to anthropologists, sociologists, and social workers.

292. KINGSON, Eric R., Barbara A. Hirshorn, John M. Cornman.
Ties That Bind: The Interdependence of Generations. Cabin
John, MD: Seven Locks Press, 1986.

Identifies some of the more important demographic trends related to
the aging of America, and some key indicators of the economic and
health status of the elderly.

Monograph

Discusses the intergenerational inequity thesis and the role of
intergenerational transfers. Promotes the premise that, in an
interdependent aging society, all generations have a common stake in
family efforts and public policies, or intergenerational transfers,
that respond to the needs of people of all ages.

Of interest to gerontologists, demographers, and social and behavioral
scientists.

293. LEWIS, Robert A., and Robert E. Salt (Eds.). *Men in Families*
Beverly Hills: Sage, 1986.

Places the critical assessment and investigation of men within the
context of families, investigates, in depth, the major positions and
roles that men play in contemporary families, and attempts to
stimulate curiosity and encourage future research on the ways in which
contemporary men relate to other persons in their marital and familial
relationships.

Book of Readings

Focuses on the changes in values, expectations, and roles of men in
families in response to contemporary social conditions. The 16
chapters are divided into three sections dealing with men as husbands;
men as fathers; and men in family, kin, and friendship networks.

Of interest to social scientists, especially researchers of sex roles
and families.

294. MELBIN, Nona Glazer (Ed.). *Old Family/New Family.* New
York: D. Van Nostram, 1975.

This book of original articles focuses on interpersonal relationships
in the numerous lifestyles associated with love and sexual roles.

Book of Readings

Organized in four parts ranging from a broad overview of interpersonal
relationships within the institutional and compassionate forms of
family through discussions of pair relations, couple relations, and,
finally, communal and other group bondings and networks. While this
book tends to focus more on the psychosexual aspects of family, it
provides some useful insights into mechanisms basic to supportive
interactions in the myriad of lifestyles available in contemporary
society.

Sociologists and others who teach about or study the family will find this text helpful.

295. PRATT, Lois. *Family Structure and Effective Health Behavior: The Energized Family*. Boston: Houghton Mifflin, 1976.

An exploration of the type of structure the family needs in order to function effectively in contemporary society. Assesses the effect of alternative forms of family structure in the family's performance of personal health care.

Research

Evidence from the author's field research indicates that those families whose structure is based on a high degree of autonomy in relationships among members, encouragement of individual development, aggressive coping effort, dynamic relationships among members, flexible and nontraditional role patterns, egalitarian power, and energetic participation in external social systems, carry out their health activities quite effectively. These families are more likely than other types of families to sustain the level of health of their members, to achieve a high level of personal health practices in their members, and to use medical services appropriately.

A useful supplement for courses in sociology, health education, health administration, maternal and child health, and public health.

296. TOWNSEND, Peter. *The Family Life of Old People*. Glencoe: Free Press, 1957.

Provides extensive coverage of the family life of old people.

Research

Deals with relatives, family care giving, economics, children, social networks, social support, and state supported care. Based on intensive interviews with 200 elders in a suburban English town.

This book provides a classic study of family social support among the aged.

b. Articles

297. BANKOFF, Elizabeth A. "Aged parents and their widowed daughters: A support relationship." *Journal of Gerontology* 38 (1983): 226-230.

Examines the relationship between social support and psychological well-being among recent widows.

Research

Social support provided by aged parents was by far the most effective in helping their daughters adjust to widowhood. Support from other members in the informal social network was virtually ineffective, even in the absence of parental support. It was concluded that middle-aged and older children still depend in important ways on their elderly parents.

Of interest to gerontologists and other researchers of social supports in old age.

298. BARBER, Brian K., and Darwin L. Thomas. "Dimensions of fathers' and mothers' supportive behavior: The case for physical affection." *Journal of Marriage and the Family* 48 (1986): 783-794.

Focuses on physical affection as a separate and distinct dimension of parental supportive behavior.

Research

Factor analysis of 527 college students reveals four separate dimensions of parental support: general support, physical affection, companionship, and sustained contact. Fathers are shown to differentiate their expression of physical affection and sustained contact on the basis of the child's sex, giving more to daughters than sons. Both parents express more companionship to the same-sex child. Regression analysis reveals that daughters' self-esteem is best predicted by mothers' general support and fathers' sustained contact.

Of interest to researchers of social support.

299. BARKER, Chris, and Russell Lemle. "The helping process in couples." *American Journal of Community Psychology* 12 (1984): 321-336.

This study examined couples' informal helping interactions, how partners helped each other with their psychological problems.

Research

The important characteristic of the helper's communication was not the type of response used, but the evaluative quality of the response. Helpers who were more satisfied with their relationships tended to be more understanding and supportive. Interactions that were rated as more understanding and supportive tended to be experienced as more helpful by the disclosers.

Of interest to social workers, family therapists, and mental health professionals.

300. BEELS, C. Christian. "Social networks, the family and the schizophrenia patient." *Schizophrenia Bulletin* 4 (1978): 512-640.

Deals with the social supports and networks of the schizophrenic.

Special Journal Issue

Presents several papers describing studies of the family, kinship, ethnic differences in social networks, and community interventions, all dealing with schizophrenia.

Social and behavioral science researchers and mental health professionals will find this an excellent review of the literature on schizophrenia and social support.

301.   BELSKY, Jay, and Michael Rovine.   "Social network contact, family support, and the transition to parenthood." *Journal of Marriage and the Family* 46 (1984): 455-462.

In order to assess the effect of a new baby on social network contact and family support, 72 volunteer families were studied longitudinally from the last trimester of pregnancy through the ninth postpartum month.

Research

Emotional and material support received from families of origin was greater at three months postpartum than during the last trimester of pregnancy or at nine months postpartum, especially in the case of first-time parents. Even though the proximity of one's own family of origin predicts quantity of family contact and the extent to which it provides babysitting services, it does not relate to the degree of emotional and material support received or to the extent to which relatives are regarded as significant others.

Of interest to social workers, family counselors, and family physicians.

302.   BURKE, Ronald J., and Tamara Weir.   "Husband-wife helping-relationships: The 'mental hygiene' function in marriage." *Psychological Reports* 40 (1977): 911-925.

The relationships between several correlates and consequences of the husband-wife helping-relationship were examined.

Research

Effective husband-wife helping-relationships were significantly related to the quality of life of the marital partners.

Of interest to family therapists and marital counselors.

303.   HOWE, Anna L.   "Family support of the aged: Some evidence and interpretation." *Australian Journal of Social Issues* 14, no. 4 (1979): 259-273.

Presents a range of Australian material concerning family support for the aged.

Review

From a review of studies dealing with the family structure of the aged
and accounts of intergenerational contact and supportive exchanges
within families, including migrant families, considerable evidence of
family support is found. The implications of the absence of such
support are apparent from data on the use of services and admissions
to institutional care: the preventive effect of marriage and family is
clear, those aged without family being identified as most at risk.

Of interest to social and behavioral scientists.

304. HUSTON-HOBURG, Laura, and Carney Strange. "Spouse
support among male and female returning adult students."
Journal of College Student Personnel 27 (1986): 388-393.

This study examined whether male and female adults enrolled in a
two-year technical college differed in the degree and kind of spouse
support they received when they returned to formal education.

Research

Significant differences were found between male and female adult
students in the degree of attitudinal, emotional, and functional
support they received from their spouses after returning to school.

Of interest to mental health counselors, especially in college and
university settings.

305. International symposium· The family as a source of support for
the elderly." *Gerontologist* 23, no. 6 (1983): 573-656.

A symposium on family support of the aging containing cross-cultural,
cross-national, sociological, psychological, and economic
perspectives.

Symposium

An introduction and 14 research papers discuss family care of the
aging in Israel, Japan, China, Egypt, Poland, The United States,
Australia, and Norway from a variety of perspectives. Related studies
address the issues of caregivers who live with dependent elderly;
family support to the impaired elderly; a comparison of the helping
behavior of adult children with intact and disrupted marriages; racial
and cohort variations in filial responsibility norms; engaging
families as support resources in nursing home care; improving the
helping skills of family caregivers of older adults; and the family's
role in the use of public services for the aged.

Should interest sociologists, anthropologists, health professionals,
planners, and policymakers, and concerned lay persons; an excellent
overview for anyone interested in family care of the aged.

306. JOHNSON, Colleen Leahy. "Dyadic family relations and social
     support." *Gerontologist* 23 (1983): 377-383.

Examines the family support of 167 post-hospitalized elderly persons
to determine whether it is provided by the family as a functioning
unit or whether the major responsibility is assumed by one individual.

Research

The most comprehensive and unstressful support was found to be that
provided by a spouse. Among the widowed, the role of major caregiver
was assumed by a child. It was found that family members were
available in serial order rather than as a shared-functioning unit.
Impediments to family supports and the outcomes of care are also
reported.

Of interest to health professionals, especially geriatricians,
sociologists, and gerontologists.

307. KEMPLER, Hyman L. "Extended kinship ties and some modern
     alternatives." *The Family Coordinator* 25 (1976): 143-149.

Discusses some of the psychological advantages offered by extended kin
to the nuclear family, and examines some modern variants of the
traditional family in terms of their potential as substitutes for
kinship ties.

Descriptive

The author contends that close relationships with extended kin have
provided the nuclear family with psychological and instrumental
support, role models for the adult years, and a sense of historical
continuity and perspective. Family networks, communes, and the
affiliated family are critically evaluated with respect to their
potential utility as substitutes for kin ties.

Of interest to sociologists and anthropologists.

308. KITSON, Gay C., Robin N. Moir, Peyton R. Mason. "Family
     social support in crises: The special case of divorce."
     American Journal of Orthopsychiatry 52 (1982): 161-165.

Using data from a survey of divorced and separated men and women, this
study sought to identify the conditions under which families are
willing to give social support.

Research

When family members disapprove of the decision to divorce, they are
unlikely to help out if no other life events besides divorce are
considered. Families do extend a helping hand if other events besides
the divorce happen to the divorced person, regardless of their own
event-filled situation or their disapproval of the divorce.

Of interest to mental health practitioners, social workers, and family therapists.

309. KIVETT, Vira R. "Consanguinity and kin level: Their relative importance to the helping network of older adults." *Journal of Gerontology* 40 (1985): 228-234.

Help received by older adults living in a rural transitional area of the Piedmont area of North Carolina from family members related by blood or marriage or other associations was examined.

Research

Evidence is presented that suggests that little help is received from kin beyond the child or child-in-law level. These results support the "closeness" of relationships as crucial to social support.

Family sociologists and others interested in support theory will find this a useful paper.

310. KOBRIN, Frances E., and Gerry E. Hendershot. "Do family ties reduce mortality? Evidence for the United States, 1966-68." *Journal of Marriage and the Family* 39 (1977): 737-745.

Survey data are used to compute mortality rates for persons in different types of living arrangements.

Research

Mortality rates are lower for married persons, married persons with children, and non-married persons who are heads of households. Having the status of spouse, parent, or household head seems to protect one against risk of death.

Of interest to social scientists.

311. LADEWIG, Becky Heath, and Gail W. McGee. "Occupational commitment, a supportive family environment, and marital adjustment: Development and estimation of a model." *Journal of Marriage and the Family* 48 (1986): 821-829.

A multivariate model of marital adjustment among men and women in dual-earner marriages was developed and tested using structural equation analysis (LISREL VI).

Research

Higher levels of occupational commitment by wives adversely affected marital adjustment for both genders, yet both men and women perceived that the occupational commitment of husbands had no effect on marital adjustment. Higher levels of occupational commitment had a significant influence on perceptions of a supportive family environment for women, which, in turn, positively influenced marital adjustment. In the men's model, the path from occupational commitment to supportive family environment was not significant, yet greater perceived emphasis on a supportive family environment positively influenced the marital adjustment of men. The results of this study emphasize the importance of family system characteristics for understanding the impact of high work commitment on marital relationships.

Of interest to social and behavioral scientists.

312. PERELBERG, Rosine J. "Mental illness, family, and networks in a London borough: Two case studies by an anthropologist." *Social Science and Medicine* 17 (1983): 481-491.

This anthropological investigation explores how conjugal role relationships are related to patterns of coping during crises.

Research

Two families were studied following a period of acute mental illness. The results indicated that the family characterized by a more segregated role relationship and a more traditional/hierarchical family structure dealt in a different way with the crisis than the family with more joint role relationship between the spouses and a loose-knit network. The former sought help to cope with the crisis from within their network relations, whereas the latter tried to cope with it by themselves. They also differed in the way that each tried to understand the origin of the crisis.

This paper is helpful for anybody interested in family processes during times of crises, particularly social and cultural anthropologists, family sociologists, and social psychiatrists.

313. PERRAULT, Chantal, Allan L. Coates, Judith Collinge, Barry Pless, Eugene Outerbridge. "Family support system in newborn medicine: Does it work? Follow-up study of infants at risk." *Journal of Pediatrics* 108 (1986): 1025-1030.

Describes a family support system for a neonatal intensive care unit. The effectiveness was assessed by the evaluation of emergency room and inpatient hospital service utilization before and after the program was started.

Descriptive

There were no differences between the groups in the utilization of emergency services during the first year after discharge. However, during the second year, the control group used the emergency room twice as often as the study group. During the first two years, half of the control group was readmitted, compared to less than a third of the study group. The family support system was an effective way to reduce psychosocial sequelae of illness in newborn infants requiring intensive care.

Of special interest to neonatologists and nurses.

314. RAMSEY, Christian N., Jr., Troy D. Abell, Lisa C. Baker.
     "The relationship between family functioning, life events,
     family structure, and the outcome of pregnancy." *Journal of
     Family Practice* 22 (1986): 521-527.

A prospective study to evaluate the relationship of family
functioning, family structure, and life events with pregnancy outcome.

Research

The data from this study are congruent with the findings of other
studies with regard to the contribution of such factors as maternal
age, smoking, medical history, and parity. Taken together, these
factors account for approximately one-third of the total variance in
birth weight. Family structure and family functioning, both
significantly and independently, are related to birth weight. The
woman who lives alone is at risk for having a smaller baby; living
with her extended family improves her chances of having a heavier
baby, but not so much as does living with her husband.

Of interest to family physicians, obstetricians, and nurses.

315. SCOTT, Jean Pearson, Karen A. Roberto, J. Thomas Hutton.
     "Families of Alzheimer's victims. Family support to the
     caregivers." *Journal of the American Geriatrics Society*
     34 (1986): 348-354.

This study examined the instrumental and social-emotional support
provided by families to the primary caregivers of Alzheimer's
patients.

Research

While the major caregiving tasks were performed by the primary
caregiver, the types of assistance from family that seemed most
appreciated were visits and having persons stay with the parent so
that the caregiver could take a trip, rest, run errands, or get out of
the house for social activities. The majority of caregivers felt a
high degree of support from their families and reported low levels of
emotional upset resulting from family support efforts. The data
confirmed the hypothesis that family support was positively associated
with the caregiver's coping effectiveness.

Of interest to physicians, nurses, social workers, and families of
Alzheimer's patients.

316. SHANAS, Ethel. "The family as a social support system in old
     age." *Gerontologist* 19 (1979): 169-174.

Discusses research on two aspects of family social support.

Literature Review

The immediate family is the major source of social support for the
elderly, particularly in times of illness. Family visitation is the
primary tie of the elderly to the community.

Sociologists, gerontologists, and others working with the elderly will
find this a very useful summary.

317. SHAPIRO, Johanna. "Family reactions and coping strategies in
     response to the physically ill or handicapped child: A review."
     Social Science and Medicine 17, no. 14 (1983): 913-931.

Reviews a broad range of material that investigates coping processes
of individuals and families in response to serious illness.

Literature Review

Reviews the function of the family as a system, and emphasizes
feedback loops among all its members, which distribute responsibilities for dysfunction throughout the system. Concludes with a
discussion of the benefits for all health care professionals of
adopting a family-oriented treatment approach.

Of interest to all health care professionals.

318. SUCHET, Melanie, and Julian Barling. "Employed mothers:
     Interrole conflict, spouse support and marital functioning."
     Journal of Occupational Behavior 7 (1986): 167-178.

It was hypothesized that interrole conflict will have a direct effect
on marital functioning, while spouse support will exert both a direct
and moderating effect on the marital relationship.

Research

Interrole conflict and spouse support predicted marital satisfaction
and verbal communication. In addition, spouse support may moderate
negative effects of interrole conflict on marital satisfaction and
verbal communication. With regard to nonverbal communication, spouse
support was both a significant main effect and possibly a moderator of
interrole conflict.

Of interest to social workers, occupational therapists, and mental
health counselors.

319. Symposium: Aging and the family." *Gerontologist* 23, no. 1
     (1983): 24-50.

A symposium, originally presented at the 1980 meeting of the
Gerontological Society, presenting cross-cultural, sociological,
psychological, and economic perspectives on aging, families, and
family relations.

Symposium

The introduction and four papers address behavioral and social science perspectives on our knowledge, our myths, and our research on aging and family relations; family ties of the aged in cross-cultural perspective; a psychological perspective on autonomy and interdependence in the family of adulthood; research dilemmas and opportunities regarding the study of the frail elderly; and the role of the family in the economic well-being of the elderly.

An excellent overview for social and behavioral scientists and anyone else who is interested in aging and family relations.

c. Chapter

320. PILISUK, Marc, and Susan Hillier Parks. "Social support and family stress." *In* Hamilton I. McCubbin, Marvin B. Sussman, Joan M. Patterson (Eds.). *Social Stress and the Family.* New York: Haworth Press, 1983.

Reviews some of the evidence relating supporting ties of the type associated with family life to the maintenance of physical and emotional well-being.

Review and Analysis

Authors argue that some knowledge and consideration of personality dispositions is essential for students of family stress. Personality is an enduring and pervasive influence on the lives of family members, and it conditions the likelihood of stress and the individual's responses to it. How individuals with distinctive personalities interact over the life span is one of the least explored and most exciting topics for research in family studies.

Of interest to researchers of social support and stress.

d. Conference Proceedings

321. FOGEL, Robert W., Elaine Hatfield, Sara B. Kiesler, Ethel Shanas (Eds.). *Aging: Stability and Change in the Family.* New York: Academic Press, 1981.

The proceedings of a national conference on stability and change in the family as they are affected by aging.

Conference Proceedings

The last section of this book contains three chapters dealing with close relationships in the aging family. One chapter is particularly appropriate to the understanding of social support and deals specifically with love and its effects on mental and physical health.

An excellent resource for courses on the family and for better understanding of the family dynamics of aging.

B. FRIENDSHIP AND COMPANIONSHIP

a. Books

322. BECK, Alan, and Aaron Katcher. *Between Pets and People.* New York: G.P. Putnam, 1983.

Reports research on how people and companion animals interact.

Research

Interest in research on pets and people grew out of a study of patients with coronary heart disease. Patients with pets had increased survival rates during the first year of discharge. Other research reports the impact of pets on objective measures of health.

Of general interest to laymen and health professionals.

323. BELL, Robert R. *Worlds of Friendship.* Beverly Hills: Sage, 1981.

This book focuses on the blend of research using observational and theoretical sociology as it pertains to understanding friendship as a social institution.

Descriptive and Theoretical

Summarizes the literature on friendship and explores its meaning throughout the life span from adolescence to old age. A fresh perspective on friendship and supportive interactions is provided by the many insights this book provides.

Researchers, especially sociologists, will find this a very important book, dealing with a topic which has received little research attention.

324. BOISSEVAIN, Jeremy. *Friends of Friends.* Oxford: Basil Blackwell, 1974.

A model of social networks based on structural-functionalism, developed into a theoretical view of social interaction by the author.

Theoretical

Provides an important foundation in sociological theory for much of the current work on social support, clarifying the interaction and structure of networks, their basic link to values, and their vulnerability to manipulation.

Researchers and theorists alike will benefit from this book.

325. BRENTON, Myron. *Friendship*. New York: Stein and Day, 1975.

A study of American friendships.

Descriptive and Analytical

The author describes a wide range of friendship types and issues from childhood to old age. Describes same-sex and cross-sex friendships and how we take steps to turn strangers into friends and friends into strangers.

Of general interest.

326. DERLEGA, Valerian J., and Barbara A. Winstead. *Friendship and Social Interaction*. New York: Springer-Verlag, 1986.

A major goal of this volume is to develop theories and integrate research on the development and maintenance of friendships.

Book of Readings

The 13 chapters encompass a wide range of issues regarding friendship, including theoretical and methodological issues, strategies in developing friendships, same-sex friendships, loneliness, social support and stress, friendships in the work place, and friendship disorders.

Of particular interest to social psychologists and other social scientists.

327. FISCHER, Claude S. *To Dwell Among Friends. Personal Networks in Town and City*. Chicago: University of Chicago Press, 1982.

Shows how urban life changes personal relations and the ways people think and act socially. Discusses such matters as friendship, intimacy, involvement in the community, and life-style.

Theoretical and Research

Suggests public policy to improve the quality of people's personal networks. The global theoretical concerns stem from efforts to understand the personal consequences of urban life and, by extension, of modern life.

Of interest to social and behavioral scientists, especially sociologists, psychologists, anthropologists, and social workers.

328. LEYTON, Elliott (Ed.). *The Compact: Selected Dimensions of Friendship.* Newfoundland: University of Newfoundland Press, 1974.

An exploration of friendship from an anthropological view.

Book of Readings

This collection is divided into three parts, beginning with a survey of the literature, which covers the utilitarian and social functions of friendship and its major dimensions. The second part of the book presents ethnological perspectives, while the last part compares and contrasts friendships in five different cultural settings.

A must for theorists, researchers, and teachers who think, study, and instruct others about friendship.

329. SCHWARTZ, Gary, Don Merten, Fran Behan, Allyne Rosenthal. *Love and Commitment.* Beverly Hills: Sage, 1980.

This is a book about the meanings of love and intimacy in mainstream American culture.

Descriptive and Analytical

The body of the text is made up of a young girl's commentary on her dating and courtship relationships, which took place in the context of the youth culture of the mid 1960's. It gives the reader an "inside" look at the texture of lived experience and a feel for the meaning of growing up in middle-class culture. The text gives readers an opportunity to reflect on the significance of their own intimate relationships and to assess whether the author's analysis of the meaning of love in American culture sheds light on their own experiences.

Of interest to social scientists, as well as nonprofessional readers.

b. Articles

330. ATHANASIOU, Robert, and Gary A. Yoshioka. "The spatial character of friendship formation." *Environment and Behavior* 5 (March 1973): 43-65.

Several hypotheses related to choice of friends based on similarities in backgrounds, values, and interests and the effect of homogeneity of characteristics on friendship formation were tested.

Research

Similarities in leisure time interests were found to be a factor in friendship patterns, especially at small distances. Subjects' perceptions of their friends' political beliefs discriminated between friends and nonfriends better than did actual political affiliation.

Propinquity plays a part in friendship formation, but in order for friendships to be maintained over moderate or large distances, additional similarities in social class must be present.

Of particular interest to social and behavioral scientists.

331. BABCHUK, Nicholas. "Primary friends and kin: A study of the associations of middle class couples." *Social Forces* 43 (May 1965): 483-494.

This study describes the role of friendship in traditional dyadic relationships.

Research

In urban middle class couples, husbands were found to be more likely to initiate primary friendships for the couple at all stages of the family life cycle. The degree of family involvement, years of marriage, visitation patterns with friends, or children/spouse friendships appear not to affect the development of primary couple to couple friendships.

Family sociologists, students, and others interested in family dynamics and social support will find this an excellent study.

332. CAUCE, Ana Mari. "Social networks and social competence: Exploring the effects of early adolescent friendships." *American Journal of Community Psychology* 14 (1986): 607-628.

Explores the relationship between social network variables and social competence indices using a sample of 98 young black lower SES adolescents.

Research

Perceived emotional support from friends was positively related to the number of reciprocated best friends in an adolescent's social network. Perceived friend emotional support and number of reciprocated best friends contributed independently to school competence, peer competence, and perceived self-competence measures. The friendship network's school achievement orientation was related positively to school competence, but was unrelated to peer or perceived self-competence. Friendship network density did not add to the variance explained by the other network variables.

Of interest to researchers of social networks and social support.

333. FRIEDMANN, Erika, Aaron Honori Katcher, James J. Lynch, Sue Ann Thomas. "Animal companions and one-year survival of patients after discharge from a coronary care unit." *Public Health Reports* 95 (1980): 307-312.

A study of the effects of social isolation and social support on the survival of patients who had been hospitalized in a coronary care unit with a diagnosis of myocardial infarction or angina pectoris.

Research

The findings of this study confirm the independent importance of social factors in the determination of health status. Social data obtained during patients' hospitalization can be valuable in discriminating one-year survivors from nonsurvivors. Social affiliation and companionship have important health effects. Pet ownership can add significantly to survival following myocardial infarction.

Of interest to internists interested in coronary heart disease and social and behavioral scientists.

334. ROBB, Susanne S., and Charles E. Stegman. "Companion animals and elderly people: A challenge for evaluators of social support." *Gerontologist* 23 (1983): 277-282.

A comparative, retrospective study, which measured selected health-related effects of the association with companion-animals on humans.

Research

A sample of 56 predominantly elderly veterans, randomly selected from among clients of a home care program, who did (n=26) and did not (n=30) live with pets, were interviewed. No significant differences were found between the pet and non-pet groups with respect to health related variables. However, the failure to corroborate earlier findings may be partially attributable to methodological causes. The results provide some direction for future research.

Of interest to social science researchers.

335. TOKUNA, Kenneth A. "The early adult transition and friendships: Mechanisms of support." *Adolescence* 21, no. 83 (1986): 593-606.

Describes and categorizes the specific processes by which friends serve to influence the emerging life structures of early adulthood.

Research

Research indicates that friends are a primary choice of support for young adults faced with developmental tasks. In this study, open-ended interviews of 34 young adults ranging from 20 to 28 years of age were used to develop five categories describing friends in the roles of (1) models, (2) active agents for change, (3) reactors, (4) interactors, and (5) passive influences. Further specificity was gained through the descriptions of 13 subcategories. Implications of the preliminary findings using these categories are discussed.

Of interest to social and behavioral scientists.

c. Chapter

336. FLEMING, Raymond, and Andrew Baum. "Social support and stress--the buffering effects of friendship." *In* Valerian J. Derlega, and Barbara A. Winstead (Eds.). *Friendship and Social Interaction.* New York: Springer-Verlag, 1986.

Focuses upon the relationship between friendship, social support, and stress.

Review and Analysis

Although research generally indicates that a relationship between social support and stress exists, specifics of the relationship are not well-established. An over-reliance on life events measures as indicators of stress has tended to keep findings very general. Better techniques for measuring the stress response, including the use of multi-modal assessments, may allow greater freedom in the types of stressful situations studied with respect to social support.

Of interest to researchers of social support.

3. NETWORK INTERVENTIONS

a. Books

337. CAPLAN, Gerald. *Support Systems and Community Mental Health.* New York: Behavioral Publications, 1974.

A collection of selected lectures outlining concepts proposed by the author over a period of 20 years. Presents new ideas in their formative stages.

Theoretical

Discusses the nature of support systems, differentiates between types of support systems, and describes the process of organizing support systems and the use of naturally-occurring systems by mental health professionals.

Of interest to social and behavioral scientists and mental health professionals.

338. COLLINS, Alice H., and Diane L. Pancoast. *Natural Helping Networks: A Strategy for Prevention.* New York: National Association of Social Workers, 1976.

A how-to-do-it publication describing techniques used by the authors in making use of natural networks.

Manual

Contains an overview of networks (types and aspects), a review of pertinent literature, and a description of natural networks, as well as information regarding traditional approaches to networks, artificial networks organized to meet needs, consultation methods, modifications in techniques of consultation with natural neighbors, finding natural neighbors, and establishing a consultation service.

Of particular importance to social workers, but also to all types of helpers, e.g. psychologists, community health nurses.

339. HASSINGER, Edward W. *Rural Health Organization: Social Network and Regionalization.* Ames, IA: Iowa State University Press, 1982.

Deals with the effects of informal group networks and extralocal organizational relationships on the delivery of health services in rural areas.

Text

Rural health care delivery must be viewed within the context of the larger society, while attention is paid to the special characteristics of rural society that affect health care delivery. Chapters address rural society; health services and health status; primary groups and social networks related to use of health services; regionalization: concept, perimeters, and landmarks; control processes in regionalized interorganizational fields; unmanaged regionalization of health services; managed regionalization of health services; two case studies; and the organization of rural health delivery.

Should interest sociologists, health care planners, and policymakers.

340. McGUIRE, Lambert. *Understanding Social Networks.* Beverly Hills: Sage, 1983.

Deals with the development and evaluation of networking approaches in mental health and social services that maximize the use of natural helping networks.

Resource Book

Explains what networks are, which research supports their use, and how to organize supportive and helpful networks around individuals, self-help groups, communities, and organizations for the purposes of support, treatment, prevention, rehabilitation, advocacy, or improved communication and understanding. Establishes the foundation for network interventions in theory and practice, and examines network strategies applicable to individuals, self-help or mutual aid groups, organizations, and communities.

Useful to students and practitioners in the mental health or social service professions.

b. Articles

341. COHEN, Carl I., and Arlene Adler. "Assessing the role of social network interventions with an inner-city population." *American Journal of Orthopsychiatry* 56 (1986): 278-288.

Assesses an experimental network intervention program conducted in a single-room-occupancy hotel.

Research

The results reflect the desirability of refining the application of network interventions from nonspecific usages to a more strategic focus. Network interventions are not for every person or every problem. Situational factors, especially problems presented as crises, emerged as inappropriate for network intervention. Successful network intervention must be viewed as an unhurried, long-term effort.

Of interest to social workers and mental health professionals.

342. ENG, Eugenia, John Hatch, Anne Callan. "Institutionalizing social support through the church and into the community." *Health Education Quarterly* 12 (Spring 1985): 81-92.

Considers using the black church as an institutional framework for introducing and promoting health-related activities in rural black communities in North Carolina.

Literature Review

The uniqueness of the black church as both a unit of identity and of solution makes it a potentially effective unit of practice for health professionals. This framework is useful both as an analytical framework involving the complex networks of social support and influence, and as a foundation for eliciting participation and mobilizing resources.

Of interest to health professionals and social scientists.

343. ERIKSON, Gerald D. "The concept of personal network in clinical practice." *Family Process* 14 (1975): 487-498.

Discusses the impact of the expanding arena of practice of family therapists to include a variety of social networks.

Review and Analysis

Describes the social network as a curative resource in family therapy and explores its role in help-seeking and in mitigating the effects of diffusion from overinvolvement in multi-organizational linkages. Illustrates the importance to the therapist of personal networks as aids to intervention and action.

Family therapists, psychiatrists, psychologists, social workers, and other counselors will benefit from reading this thought-provoking article.

344. HOPPS, June Gary. "The catch in social support." *Social Work* 31 (1986): 419-420.

A plea for social workers to be aware, not only of the positive aspects of social support, but also of its constraints and areas in need of further exploration.

Editorial

The relationship between social welfare policies, social service programs, and informal support systems should be examined to determine how best they can complement each other. Natural helpers should be facilitated, rather than debilitated by overloading. Policies that advocate social support must examine the impact of demographics to be credible. Social support may not be universally positive. Social workers and allied professionals should, therefore, try to determine when, why, under what circumstances and conditions, and for whom various types and levels of support are effective and supportive.

Of interest to social workers and mental health professionals.

345. ISRAEL, Barbara A. "Social networks and health status: Linking theory, research and practice." *Patient Counselling and Health Education* 4 (1982): 65-79.

Attempts to link theory, research, and practice to social networks and their association with health status.

Literature Review

Evidence suggests there is a correlation between social networks and health status. The quality of these interactions seems to have a more significant relationship to well-being than the quantity. Health programs attempting to implement change should consider the influence of social networks.

Of interest to mental health professionals and health educators.

346. ———. "Social networks and social support: Implications for natural helper and community level interventions." *Health Education Quarterly* 12 (Spring 1985): 65-80.

Focuses on the link between social support and health education programs involving interventions at the network and community level.

Literature Review

Highlights several network characteristics that have been found to be related to physical and mental health and makes suggestions for their application to program strategies. Concludes with recommendations for research.

Of interest to health educators.

347. ————, and Kenneth R. McLeroy (Eds.). "Social networks and social support: Implications for health education." *Health Education Quarterly* 12 (Spring 1985): 1-106.

An entire issue of this journal, devoted to the effects of social networks and social support on health behavior and health status, and to the nature and extent of supportive relationships in which an individual is involved that may have health consequences.

Theoretical and Research

The seven articles focus on social network and social support interventions. Network therapy is one form of intervention designed to strengthen existing networks. Developing new social network linkages is a second form of network intervention. A third type of network intervention is making use of natural helpers to improve network functioning. The fourth type of network intervention involves strengthening overlapping networks to enhance their ability to identify, address, and solve community problems.

Of interest to health educators and to social and behavioral scientists.

348. McINTIRE, Eilene L.G. "Social networks: Potential for practice." *Social Work* 31 (1986); 421-426.

Examines social network concepts to explore their potential use for social work practice, particularly in regard to the provision of social support.

Theoretical

Discusses trends, strengths, and gaps in knowledge about social networks in relation to natural helping. Reviews current problems in the use of social network concepts in practice, and suggests directions for future research.

Of interest to social workers.

349. MORIN, Robert C., and Edward Seidman. "A social network approach and the revolving door patient." *Schizophrenia Bulletin* 12 (1986): 262-273.

A conceptual review and analysis of the literature reveals two Assessment methods, as well as strategies for balancing flexibility and stability are described. Enlarging the network, increasing multiplexity, and/or reducing the negative effects of attitudinal inflexibility encompass the strategies for increasing flexibility, while developing connections between individuals, generating spans between clusters of people in the network, and increasing multiplexity are recommended for increasing stability.

Of interest to mental health professionals.

350. SCOTT, Jean Pearson, and Karen A. Roberto. "Use of informal and formal support networks by rural elderly poor." *Gerontologist* 25 (1985): 624-630.

Results of a survey of a group of rural people at poverty level and a smaller group of rural adults with higher incomes, comparing their identification and use of social networks.

Survey Research

The poor sample tended to use formal networks only in situations of extreme need. All groups relied heavily on family support networks.

Social workers and others working with policy issues affecting the elderly may find this article useful.

351. SLATER, Mary A., and Lynn Wikler. "'Normalized' family resources for families with a developmentally disabled child." *Social Work* 31 (1986): 385-390.

Reviews stress-coping theories relevant to families with developmentally disabled children and recommends resources for helping them live in as normal a way as possible.

Theoretical

Social workers can assist families in living fuller, more normal lives by helping them to identify external informal sources of support, mobilizing informal network members to offer physical and emotional support, providing information and training for potential informal support members, and providing family therapy. Through this system, families are encouraged to obtain support from informal as well as formal networks, and function in a dynamic, relatively normal fashion while deriving support on a number of levels at the same time.

Of interest to social workers and other mental health professionals.

352. WEINBERG, Richard B., and Herbert A. Marlowe, Jr. "Recognizing the social in psychosocial competence: The importance of social network interventions." *Psychosocial Rehabilitation Journal* 6, no. 4 (1983): 25-34.

Reports on the use of network interventions as a tool for environmental modification by psychosocial rehabilitation practitioners.

Descriptive and Review

The importance and necessity of environmental modification are reviewed. Then the concepts of social networks and social support are defined and explicated. Empirical studies that examine the nature of the psychiatric client's social network are reviewed. Finally, several intervention strategies and current program efforts are presented.

Of interest to social and behavioral scientists and rehabilitation counselors.

353. WHITTAKER, James K. "Formal and informal helping in child welfare services: Implications for management and practice." *Child Welfare* 65, no. 1 (1986): 17-25.

Raises questions about whether and how informal and professional helping networks may work together to help children at risk of harm and families at risk of dissolution.

Theoretical

A systematic, thorough, critical review of informal helping strategies as a component of child welfare is warranted by the shift in preoccupation with formal helping to a growing recognition of the importance of informal helping for children and families. Preliminary evidence of the positive effects of social supports as a buffer to stress are encouraging, but not unequivocal. Many questions remain to be answered. Nevertheless, at some level, the multiple activities of skilled professionals and paraprofessionals must be buttressed by the socially supportive activities of preexisting or contrived networks of friends, kin, and acquaintances who can help clients sustain and consolidate gains made in professional helping.

Of interest to social workers, mental health professionals, and public policymakers.

c. Chapters

354. ATTNEAVE, Carolyn L. "Social networks as the unit of intervention." *In* Philip J. Guerin, Jr. (Ed.). *Family Therapy: Theory and Practice*. New York: Gardner Press, 1976.

Discusses social and family networks and the advantages for therapists of using them as the unit of intervention.

Review

Reviews the history of the concept of the social network, definitions and descriptions of social and family networks, clinical interpretations of networks, various models of network interventions, and preventive applications of network concepts.

Useful to students and practitioners in the mental health professions.

355. D'ANGELLI, Anthony R. "Social support networks in mental
     health." *In* J.K. Whittaker, and J. Garbarino (Eds.).
     *Social Support Networks: Informal Helping in the Human
     Services.* New York: Aldine, 1983.

A discussion of support networks and psychopathology, social network
correlates of mental health, social network interventions, and support
networks and the maintenance of mental health.

Essay

The social network model offers a framework to help the isolated and
to enrich the development of those embedded in social networks.
Professionals need to avoid interfering with social networks and,
instead, should strive to strengthen and expand them.

Of interest to mental health practitioners and researchers.

356. MacELVEEN, P.M. "Social networks." *In* Dianne C. Longo,
     and Reg Arthur Williams (Eds.). *Clinical Practice in
     Psychosocial Nursing: Assessment and Intervention.* New
     York: Appleton-Century-Crofts, 1978.

A consideration of the supportive nature of the social network.

Theoretical

Describes network structure, processes, functions, styles, and the use
of networks as resources for support by nurses seeking to initiate
interventions.

Of interest to social and behavioral scientists, nurses, and allied
health professionals.

357. SILVERSTONE, Barbara. "Informal social support systems for
     the frail elderly." *In* Committee on an Aging Society,
     Institute of Medicine and National Research Council (Ed.).
     America's Aging: Health in an Older Society. Washington,
     DC: National Academy Press, 1985.

Discusses the informal support systems of the chronically impaired
elderly, the nature and quality of informal support for the care of
frail elderly, and the still unmet needs of this population, and
presents future capabilities of the informal support system and of
public programs.

Literature Review

It was found that the chronically physically or mentally disabled
elderly generally have an extensive informal support system,
consisting primarily of next of kin, that provides a greater variety
of care than has usually been assumed, although wide variations do
exist among different subpopulations. However, many needs are still
unmet. Policy considerations to address these unmet needs in the next
two decades are offered. It is argued that future community services

should tie in with and complement the care provided by the informal support system.

Should interest gerontologists, as well as planners and policymakers of health care for the chronically disabled elderly.

4. HELP-SEEKING BEHAVIOR

a. Articles

358. BROWN, R. Bradford. "Social and psychological correlates of help-seeking behavior among urban adults." *American Journal of Community Psychology* 6 (1978): 425-431.

Investigates the differences between persons who seek help for major life changes from formal and informal support systems.

Research

Differences in terms of demographic background, personal resources, social networks, and psychological barriers to help-seeking were addressed. Generally, nonseekers who felt self-reliant and respondents who sought assistance seemed well prepared to handle major life events. Nonseekers, as well as help-seekers who contacted only professionals, were more at risk.

Of interest to behavioral scientists.

359. GOTTLIEB, Benjamin H. "Lay influences on the utilization and provision of health services: A review." *Canadian Psychological Review* 17 (1976): 126-136.

Documents the process and impact of the lay person in society on help-seeking behavior.

Literature Review

The lay referral and treatment networks are described, and future research directions are identified. The current state of knowledge of the impact of the lay community on health care, medical, and mental health services is discussed in light of professional practice.

Students and others interested in help-seeking behavior should read this article.

360. GOURNASH, Nancy. "Help-seeking: A review of the literature." *American Journal of Community Psychology* 6 (1978): 413-423.

Investigates help-seeking, examining those who seek help, the role of the social network in the help-seeking process, and possible outcomes of the helping interaction.

Literature Review

Help-seekers tend to be young, white, educated, middle class females
suffering from mild stress to severe emotional distress. Social
networks serve as a support system, and those who seek help are
generally satisfied, which results in a decrease in stress.

Will interest any professional dedicated to helping: social service
workers, counselors, and mental health professionals.

361. McKINLAY, John B. "Social networks, lay consultation and
     help-seeking behavior." *Social Forces* 51 (March 1973):
     275-292.

Considers the apparent role of the family, kin, and friendship
networks in the use of health and welfare services.

Research

Under-utilizers relied on an undifferentiated group of readily
available relatives and friends as lay consultants before using health
services, while utilizers appeared to both differentiate between
relatives and friends, and be independent of both of these sources of
social control.

Useful to family sociologists, researchers of health services
utilization, and social psychologists.

362. PILISUK, Marc, and Meredith Minkler. "Supportive ties: A
     political economy perspective." *Health Education Quarterly*
     12 (Spring 1985): 93-106.

Examines the interdependencies between supportive ties on individual
and community levels and the larger social and political environments
within which social networks operate.

Literature Review

Findings show that social isolation and disrupted personal ties may be
major risk factors in health breakdown. A central issue involves the
deficiencies in supportive environments for effective functioning of
social ties and natural helping networks on the individual, group, and
community levels. Health professionals have a role as advocates for a
less ruthless and more caring environment.

Of interest to health care professionals.

363. YOUNG, Carl E., Dwight E. Giles, Jr., Margaret C. Plantz.
     "Natural networks: Help-giving and help-seeking in two
     rural communities." *American Journal of Community Psy-
     chology* 10 (1982): 457-469.

A group of 213 respondents in rural communities were interviewed about their help-giving and help-seeking behavior related to 11 problems of living.

Research

Results indicate that over 80 percent of the respondents saw themselves as active help-givers and receivers in exchanges with spouses, friends, relatives, and others. A wide range of helping activities were reported, led by attempts to understand another person's situation and feelings and just listening. Respondents indicated a general willingness to tackle problems, a preference for help from people within their networks, and that this type of help is effective.

Of interest to teachers, administrators, and counselors.

c. Chapter

364. McKINLAY, John B. "Social network influences on morbid episodes and the career of help-seeking." *In* Leon Eisenberg, and Arthur Kleinman (Eds.). *The Relevance of Social Science for Medicine.* New York: Reidel, 1980.

Selectively reviews some studies that seek to explain the epidemiology of many different problems and the ways in which they are responded to, and discusses them in relation to the notion of a help-seeking career.

Review

Illustrates the potential of the concept of a social network for understanding the etiology of particular morbid episodes, how they are responded to, and recovery from them. Discusses the help-seeking career, the precise influence of social support systems, and their potential as a basis for effective interventions.

Should interest medical sociologists and epidemiologists.

d. Dissertation

365. RICHARDSON, John B. "Support systems and sense of well-being: A study of separated and divorced parents with physical custody of their children." D.S.W. dissertation, University of Southern California, 1981.

Examines the relationship between selected social, personal, and demographic factors; use of support systems, and sense of well-being; and the effect of differential use of support systems on a sense of well-being among separated and divorced parents.

Research

Parents primarily used informal support systems, especially for practical matters. Emotional problems were more likely to be handled by the use of personal resources than by support systems. Only social class correlated with use of support systems and sense of well-being; the main relationships in this study were strongest among middle-class people.

Of interest to social and behavioral scientists, and marital counselors.

CHAPTER 3

SOCIAL SUPPORT, PHYSICAL HEALTH
AND ILLNESS, AND REHABILITATION

a. Books

366. ANGERMEYER, Matthias C., and Otto Dohner (Eds.).
Chronische kranke kinder und jugendliche in der familie.
(German) Stuttgart: Ferdinand Enke Verlag, 1981.

Deals with psychosocial factors concerning the families of chronically
ill children.

Book of Readings

Starts with three general chapters, after which each chapter focuses
on a specific illness such as diabetes, hemophilia, cancer, and
schizophrenia. Each section contains a discussion of some aspect of
the psychosocial role of the family, particularly its adaptation to
the child's illness and it's involvement in treatment and
rehabilitation.

Of special interest to pediatricians, medical sociologists, and all
others interested in the psychosocial care and treatment of the
chronically ill child.

367. BADURA, Bernhard (Ed.).   *Soziale   Unterstützung   und*
      Chronische   Krankheit.   Zum   Stand   Sozialepidemiologischer
      Forschung. (German) Frankfurt am Main: Suhrkamp, 1981.

An overview of social epidemiological research on the influence of
social support on the development and treatment of chronic illness.

Theoretical and Research

Discusses theoretical models of the role of social support in chronic
illness; provides a review of the empirical findings in support of
these models; and describes the role of social support in the development, treatment, and rehabilitation of specific chronic diseases, such
as myocardial infarction, stroke, and cancer.

Useful to social epidemiologists, medical sociologists, stress researchers, and rehabilitation specialists.

368. BERKMAN, Lisa F., and Lester Breslow.   *Health and Ways of*
      Living: The Alameda County Study.   New York: Oxford
      University Press, 1983.

A presentation of the background, rationale, methods and results of
the Alameda County study, which examined the relationship between
social networks, daily behaviors, and health consequences.

Research

Analysis of the data revealed five common habits to be strongly, and
each one, independently, associated with mortality during the nine
years of follow-up. These habits, called high-risk health practices,
were 1) smoking cigarettes; 2) consuming excessive quantities of
alcohol; 3) being physically inactive; 4) being obese or overweight;
and 5) sleeping fewer than 7 or more than 8 hours per night. A Social
Network Index showed a gradient with mortality. Men constituting the
most isolated group had an age-adjusted mortality rate 2.3 times
higher than men with the strongest social connections; among women the
difference was 2.8 times.

Of interest to researchers concerned with social support and preventive medicine.

369. FRIEDMAN, Howard S., and M. Robin DiMatteo (Eds.).   *Inter-*
      personal Issues in Health Care. New York: Academic Press,
      1982.

Updated and expanded revision of Volume 35, no. 1, 1979 issue of the
Journal of Social Issues, titled "Interpersonal Relations in Health
Care."

Book of Readings

Presents current social psychological thinking on a number of basic
health care issues. Divided into four sections: perspectives on

social influence in health care; relations with others, social support, and the health care system; expectations, pain, and the nature of illness; patients' demands and the health care environment.

Directed at professionals and paraprofessionals involved in the social science aspects of health care. Also useful to graduate students in psychology and sociology and researchers new to the medical field.

370. WAN, Thomas, T.H. *Stressful Life Events, Social Support Networks, and Gerontological Health: A Prospective Study.* Lexington, MA: Lexington Books, 1982.

Presents findings from a ten year panel study of the impact of major life changes occurring in later life on health status and utilization of health services by persons of retirement age.

Research Monograph

Describes the major aspects of the Longitudinal Retirement History Study, conducted by the Social Security Administration. Presents the theoretical overview, research methodology, and findings pertaining to retirement and gerontological health, and determines the presumed effectiveness of social support systems or social resources in minimizing any adverse impact of life transitions on well-being of older people in the U.S.

Useful to gerontological researchers, social scientists, and others interested in life events, social support, and health.

371. WOLF, Stewart. *Social Environment and Health.* Seattle/ London: University of Washington Press, 1981.

An attempt to synthesize available data linking the quality of social relationships to physical health and disease.

Series of Lectures

Emphasizes the integrative functions of the central nervous system in regulating adaptive responses to environmental challenges of all sorts. Stresses the importance of intercommunication and interdependence in the process of social and biological homeostasis.

Of interest to students and practitioners of medicine, the biological sciences, and the social sciences, as well as interested laymen.

b. Articles

372. BERKMAN, Lisa F. "Assessing the physical health effects of social networks and social support." *Annual Review of Public Health* 5 (1984): 413-432.

Review of data relating social ties to physical health.

Review and Analytical

Issues regarding the definition and measurement of social networks and social support are addressed, and problems with particular study designs are discussed. The functions of social networks and social support, what they provide for people, and the potential biological pathways that link social networks to morbidity and mortality are discussed.

Of interest to social and behavioral scientists and health professionals in preventive medicine and public health.

373. BLAKE, Robert L., Jr., Carl Roberts, Thomas Mackey, Michael Hosokawa. "Social support and utilization of medical care." *Journal of Family Practice* 11 (1980): 810-812.

Tests the hypothesized association of weak social support with increased use of professional services in a rural primary care setting.

Research

When the respondents reported good health, social support did not affect utilization. When poor health status was reported, the subject with high social support showed a utilization rate of 1.5 compared to a rate of 2.2 for those with low support.

Of interest to health care professionals, especially those in rural settings.

374. BOSSE, R., D.J. Ekert, B.H. Vinick, J.K. Davis, C.M. Aldwin. "Retirement, social support, and self-reported health." *Gerontologist* 25, Supplement 1 (1985): 235.

The relationship between a variety of social support measures and changes in the self-reported health of 380 men, from the period in which they were working to three years after retirement, was examined.

Research Abstract

Changes in self-reported health following retirement were found to be significantly related to health before retirement, wife's happiness with retirement, retirement age, and social support measures, including contact with close friends.

Of interest to gerontologists, social workers, and social scientists.

375. BRODY, Stanley J., Walter Poulshock, Carla F. Masciocchi. "The family caring unit: A major consideration in the long-term support system." *Gerontologist* 18 (1978): 556-561.

Attempts to provide new data for long-term care planning which will identify the variables that govern the institutional or community placement of the functionally disabled elderly.

Research

The presence of caring units in terms of spouse, children, and other relatives is a critical factor in helping individuals to remain in the community despite serious physical impairment. It is suggested that planners be directed toward developing and providing support programs and services for families who provide home health care to their chronically ill or disabled relative if retention of the disabled in the community is a public goal. However, no one factor should be viewed as a sole solution for retaining the disabled in the community as long as possible.

Of special interest to health care planners and policymakers.

376. CHESNEY, Alan P., and W. Doyle Gentry. "Psychosocial factors mediating health risk: A balanced perspective." *Preventive Medicine* 11 (1982): 612-617.

Deals with the tendency in psychosocial and illness research to focus on susceptibility, while ignoring resistance factors.

Editorial

The authors propose a balanced model of health risks, and describe conditions of high and low health risk in which the balance would explain certain discrepancies in research findings. The model is important to health practitioners as it allows for a wide range of intervention to promote improved psychosocial functioning and thus, physical health.

Behavioral medicine researchers and practitioners will benefit from this thoughtful piece.

377. CORBIN, Juliet M., and Anselm L. Strauss. "Collaboration: Couples working together to manage chronic illness." *Image: The Journal of Nursing Scholarship* 16, no. 4 (1984): 109-115.

Deals with the management of chronic illness by couples.

Essay

Explores definitions of collaboration, its mechanisms of action, and the consequences of its demise. A three-step program for nursing intervention in cases where there is some problem with collaboration is presented.

Should interest nurses and other health care providers.

378. DIMSDALE, J.E., J. Eckenrode, R.J. Haggerty, B.H. Kaplan, Frances Cohen, S. Dornbusch. "The role of social supports in medical care." *Social Psychiatry* 14 (1979): 175-180.

Reviews the effect of social supports on health and the health care system.

Review

Social supports may positively affect an individual's coping resources, reducing the risk of morbidity and mortality. Medical care, itself, may serve a supportive function, and the medical care system may complement community support systems. Existing evidence regarding the relationship between social support systems and the utilization of health services is discussed.

Useful to health care professionals interested in social support.

379. FUSILIER, Marcelline R., Daniel C. Ganster, Bronston T. Mayes. "The social support and health relationship: Is there a gender difference?" *Journal of Occupational Psychology* 59 (1986): 145-153.

Investigates whether the benefits of social support are dependent upon the source of the support and the gender of the individual receiving it.

Research

Several health and satisfaction variables were investigated, controlling for variables which may be confounded with gender in the workforce, and the relationship between gender and amount of social support from various sources was explored. Findings suggest that social support has various beneficial effects on health outcomes, gender has little bearing on the amount of support received, and there are few gender differences in the effects of social support on health.

Of interest to social scientists.

380. GELEIN, Janet Larson. "The aged American female: Relationships between social support and health." *Journal of Gerontological Nursing* 6 (1980): 69-73.

Examines the concept of social support in relation to the health of older women.

Review and Analysis

The nature and characteristics of social support are described, the health conditioning effects of social support are examined, and the implications for health care providers regarding the mobilization of mechanisms of support for older women are detailed.

Of interest to social and behavioral scientists, nurses, social workers, and gerontologists.

381. HANNICH, H.J. "Psychological support of the patient during the operative period." *Acta Anaesthesiologica Belgica* 35, Supplement (1984): 436-439.

Provides a step-by-step procedure for the anesthesiologist's psychological preparation of the patient for surgery.

Descriptive

Details the important aspects of establishing rapport and conveying information to the patient preoperatively.

Of special interest to anesthesiologists, nurse anesthestists, surgeons, and other health professionals in the surgery suite.

382. HELLER, Kenneth, Ralph W. Swindle, Jr., Linda Dusenbury. "Component social support processes: Comments and integration." *Journal of Consulting and Clinical Psychology* 54 (1986): 466-470.

The lack of a good theory base has impeded the research on the health effects of social support, not advancing evidence from epidemiologic and public health studies.

Theoretical

Symbolic interactionism is suggested as one way to conceive of key components that might explain how social support protects one's health. Esteem-enhancing appraisals and stress-laden transactions are described, along with other significant issues raised in other research.

Of interest to theorists, researchers, and others seeking a framework for understanding social support.

383. HOUSE, James S., Cynthia Robbins, Helen L. Metzner. "The association of social relationships and activities with mortality: Prospective evidence from the Tecumseh Community Study." *American Journal of Epidemiology* 116 (1982): 123-140.

Social relationships and activities were reported by a cohort of men and women during a round of interviews and medical examinations in 1967-1969, and their prospective association with mortality during the succeeding nine to 12 years was examined in the Tecumseh Community Health Study.

Research

After adjustments were made for age and a variety of risk factors for mortality, men who reported a higher level of social relationships and activities in 1967-1969 were significantly less likely to die during the follow-up period. Trends for women were similar.

Of interest to researchers of stress and social support.

384. HUBBARD, Patricia, Ann F. Muhlenkamp, Nancy Brown. "The relationship between social support and self-care practices." *Nursing Research* 33 (1984): 266-270.

A study of the perceived level of social support and the performance of health practices.

Research

A strong positive association was found between perceived social support and a number of positive health practices. Implications for health professionals, particularly nurses, are discussed.

Of value to all health professionals and health behavior researchers.

385. HUNSBERGER, Mabel, Barbara Love, Carolyn Byrne. "A review of current approaches used to help children and parents cope with health care procedures." *Maternal and Child Nursing Journal* 13, no. 3 (1984): 145-165.

Reviews three approaches that are used to help children and parents cope with health care procedures.

Review

The provision of emotional support and the use of play to help children cope with procedures is strongly supported in the anecdotal and theoretical literature. However, few controlled studies have specifically analyzed the effects of play programs in pediatric settings.

Of interest to pediatricians and pediatric nurses.

386. KIECOLT-GLASER, Janice K., Warren Garner, Carl Speicher, Gerald M. Penn, Ronald Glaser. "Psychosocial modifiers of immunocompetence in medical students." *Psychosomatic Medicine* 46 (1984): 7-14.

Addresses the effects of stressful life events and loneliness on components of the immune response.

Research

Blood was drawn twice from 75 first year medical students, one month before final exams and on the first day of final exams. Median splits on scores from the Holmes-Rahe Social Readjustment Rating Scale and the UCLA Loneliness Scale produced a 2x2x2 repeated measures ANOVA when combined with the trials variable. Natural killer cell activity declined significantly from the first to the second sample. High scorers on stressful life events and loneliness had significantly lower levels of natural killer cell activity. Total plasma IgA increased significantly from the first to second sample, while plasma IgG and IgM, C-reactive protein, and salivary IgA did not change significantly.

Should interest researchers of stress, loneliness, and the immune system.

387. KIRITZ, Stewart, and Rudolf H. Moos. "Physiological effects of social environments." *Psychosomatic Medicine* 36 (1974): 96-114.

Surveys evidence supporting the link between social environments and their effects on physiological processes, presents a conceptual model of social environment, and discusses implications for person-environment interaction.

Theoretical--Literature Review

Social stimuli associated with the relationship dimensions of support, cohesion, and affiliation generally have been found to have a positive effect on health. Negative physiological effects, related to dimensions such as responsibility, work pressure, and change, have been reported.

Useful to teachers and researchers in the area of stress and its relationship to health.

388. KOBASA, Suzanne C., Salvatore R. Maddi, Stephen Kahn. "Hardiness and health: A prospective study." *Journal of Personality and Social Psychology* 42 (1982): 168-177.

Utilizing a prospective design, this study tested the hypothesis that hardiness--commitment, control, and challenge--functions to decrease the effect of stressful life events in producing illness symptoms.

Research

Hardiness functions as a resistance resource in buffering the effects of stressful events. It is suggested that social supports might be effective in preserving health when hardiness is high.

Of interest to researchers of stress and social support.

389. KOBASA, Suzanne, C.O., Salvatore R. Maddi, Mark C. Puccetti, Marc A. Zola. "Effectiveness of hardiness, exercise and social support as resources against illness." *Journal of Psychosomatic Research* 29 (1985): 525-533.

The effects of the resistance resources of personality, hardiness, exercise, and social support, taken singly and in combination on concurrent and prospective levels, and the probability of illness were studied.

Research

Suggests that passive implications of social support have only a modest buffering effect, and provokes curiosity about how many resistance resources it is useful to have in the attempt to remain healthy despite stressful circumstances. It appears that the more resources one possesses, the less likely one is to be at risk for serious illness.

Of interest to researchers of social support and stress.

390. LEVY, Rona L. "Social support and compliance: A selective review and critique of treatment integrity and outcome measurement." *Social Science and Medicine* 17 (1983): 1329-1338.

A selective review and critique of the literature on social support as a factor in the enhancement of patient compliance and medical regimens.

Review and Analysis

Highlights several studies that measure the correlation between social support and compliance. The manner in which studies operationalize social support is discussed. Several research recommendations suggest ways social support could be studied as a clear and strong independent variable.

Of interest to teachers and researchers interested in social support and compliance behavior.

391. LILJA, Paula. "Recognizing the effect of social support on compliance to medical regimen in the elderly chronically ill." *Home Healthcare Nurse* 2, no. 5 (November-December 1984): 17-22.

A study of the role of social support in compliance to medical regimen in elderly patients.

Theoretical

Compliance to medical regimen is related to an individual's competence and perceived strains. A model is offered demonstrating how supportive behaviors and attitudes by health care professionals, especially nurses, may affect competence and strains, resulting in improved compliance. The model is extended to similar issues in community health nursing.

Primarily useful to nurses and other health professionals working with the elderly.

392. McKAY, David A., Robert L. Blake, Jr., Jack M. Colwil, Edward E. Brent, Jimmy McCauley, Robert Umlauf, Gail W. Stearman, Daniel Kivlahan. "Social supports and stress as predictors of illness." *Journal of Family Practice* 20 (1985): 575-581.

The incidence and pattern of self-reported illness was studied over a six-month period in panels of 292 women and 188 men, categorized by their experience of stressful life changes and their perceived supportive relationships.

Research

Analysis of the interaction of stressful changes with social supports showed that women with a combination of high changes and low supports experienced 2.5 times the rate of illness of those with low changes and high supports. This interaction was not found for men.

Of interest to researchers of stress and social support.

393. MONROE, Scott M. "Social support and disorder--toward an untangling of cause and effect." *American Journal of Community Psychology* 11 (1983): 81-97.

This statistical study, using a historical approach, examines the relationship of social support to psychological and physical symptoms with and without controlling for previous symptoms or interaction effects.

Research

Results demonstrate that the relationship of support to disorders varies as a function of the research design, the control of mistakes, and the types of disorders under study.

Will be very useful to researchers attempting to evaluate the existing literature on social support.

394. MOOS, Rudolf H., and Bernice Van Dort. "Student physical symptoms and the social climate of college living groups." *American Journal of Community Psychology* 7 (1979): 31-43.

Student physical symptoms were related to the social climates of university living groups. A Physical Symptom Risk Scale was developed.

Research

Living groups characterized by high student physical symptoms were perceived by students as low in involvement and support, high in competition, and low in student influence. The results indicate that certain types of social environments may be "high risk" settings in that they support and possibly facilitate complaints of physical symptoms. These settings may be amenable to early "environmental diagnosis," preventive counseling, and change-oriented social systems intervention.

Of interest to school psychologists, counselors, and physicians in university health services.

395. MUHLENKAMP, Ann F., and Judy A. Sayles. "Self-esteem, social support, and positive health practices." *Nursing Research* 35 (1986): 334-338.

A study to identify relationships among perceived social support, self-esteem, and positive health practices in adults living in a southwestern metropolitan area.

Research

Using a sample of 98 persons selected from the population of an adult apartment complex, three self-report questionnaires (Personal Resources Questionnaire, Coopersmith Self-Esteem Inventory, and Personal Lifestyle Activities Questionnaire) were used to measure the variables of perceived social support, self-esteem, and positive health practices; a theoretical causal model was developed and tested; and both the direct and indirect effects of various independent variables on life style were determined. The results indicated a positive association among the variables and suggested that both self-esteem and social support are positive indicators of life style. Furthermore, social support was found to exert influence indirectly through its direct effect on self-esteem.

Of interest to social scientists and health care providers.

396. NORRISBAKER, C. "Changes over time in informal social supports and health of the elderly in rural communities." *Gerontologist* 25, Supplement 1 (1985): 96-97.

Explores the relationship between instrumental, expressive, and structural aspects of support systems and the health status of the elderly.

Research Abstract

Data show a single linear relationship between changes in aspects of health and changes in social support, with the number of close friends and the hospitalizations highest of the variants. Implications for the relationship between health and support of the elderly in rural communities are discussed.

Of interest to gerontologists.

397. PESZNECKER, Betty L., and Jo McNeil. "Relationship among health habits, social assets, psychologic well-being, life change, and alterations in health status." *Nursing Research* 24 (1975): 442-447.

This community survey examined variables that may temper life change and enable persons to withstand high degrees of change without developing illness.

Research

The study found no evidence for the buffering effects of social support on illness after significant life changes. Health habits, psychological well-being, and social assets (supports) were only weakly associated with health maintenance.

Nurses and others interested in community health assessments may find this an interesting article.

398. PILISUK, Marc. "Delivery of social support: The social innoculation." *American Journal of Orthopsychiatry* 52 (January 1982): 20-31.

A review of the literature on health breakdown and susceptibility to mental and physical illness.

Review and Analysis

Social marginality and loss are commonly associated with a high incidence of breakdown in diverse forms. The mechanism by which relationships may affect the immunological system and the social mechanisms that promote continued social ties are examined. The emergence of supportive networks and the preventive role of mental health workers are considered.

Of interest to mental health practitioners and researchers of social support.

399. RADELET, Michael L. "Health beliefs, social networks, and tranquilizer use." *Journal of Health and Social Behavior* 22 (1981): 165-173.

Identifies health beliefs and social networks that distinguish tranquilizer users from nonusers.

Research

Major differences between the two groups indicate that those who use tranquilizers are more reluctant to admit unpleasurable feelings, are more likely to define anxiety as a biophysical problem, are less critical of over-the-counter-drug advertisements, use more over-the-counter medications, and are more likely to have friends and family members who also use tranquilizers than are nonusers.

Of interest to medical sociologists and pharmacy educators.

400. RAHE, Richard H., Merle Meyer, Michael Smith, George Kjaer, Thomas H. Holmes. "Social stress and illness onset." *Journal of Psychosomatic Research* 8 (1964): 35-44.

Examines the effect of environmental variables on time of illness onset.

Research

A major deterioration of health status was often preceded by an accumulation of social stress during the two years preceding the change in health. Interpersonal stresses seemed to play the most significant role among the psychosocial life crises.

Of particular relevance to stress researchers and other scientists interested in psychosomatic medicine.

401. SCHAEFER, Catherine, James C. Coyne, Richard S. Lazarus. "The health-related functions of social support." *Journal of Behavioral Medicine* 4 (1981): 381-406.

Compared social network size and three types of perceived social support--tangible, emotional, and informational--in relation to stressful life events with psychological symptoms, morale, and physical health status in a sample of 100 persons, 45-64 years of age.

Research

Social network size was empirically separable from, though correlated with, perceived social support and had a weaker overall relationship to outcomes. Low tangible support and emotional support, in addition to certain life events, were independently related to depression and negative morale. Informational support was associated with positive morale. Neither social support nor stressful life events were associated with physical health.

Of interest to researchers of stress.

402. SOMERS, Anne R. "Marital status, health and use of health services: An old relationship revisited." *Journal of the American Medical Association* 241 (1979): 1818-1822.

A review of the premise that married persons live longer on the average than unmarried persons and generally make less use of health care services.

Research

The complex cause and effect relationship between marriage and better health has long been recognized, but there is now some indication that the relationship is less strong than before. Perceptions of health, illness, and "need" for health care are constantly changing and, as the family's role in health has declined, there has been a concurrent rise in the "need" for, and cost of, the external health care system. The future of these trends depends, on part, on the future of the American family.

Of general interest to laymen and health professionals.

403. THOMAS, P.D., W.C. Hunt, J.M. Goodwin, J.S. Goodwin.
    "Stress, social support, and biochemical indicators of health
    status--a preliminary investigation." *Clinical Research* 31,
    no. 1 (1983): 38A.

Examined the relationship of social support, stress associated with
aging, and biochemical indicators of uric acid, blood cholesterol and
immunologic functions of lymphocyte count and mitogen response.

Research Abstract

Negative correlations were found between degree of social support and
blood cholesterol level and uric acid, while positive correlations
were found between social support and lymphocyte counts. Mitogen
responses were not affected by social support. These data indicate
that social support is related to lower levels of stress and greater
immunologic activity, all of which may be protective of health.

Social and behavioral scientists will benefit from this study, which
offers social biological parameters that strengthen the otherwise
subjective measures of stress and support.

404. THOMAS, Paula D., Jean M. Goodwin, James S. Goodwin.
    "Effect of social support on stress-related changes in choles-
    terol level, uric acid level, and immune function in an elderly
    sample." *American Journal of Psychiatry* 142 (June 1985):
    735-740.

Hypothesized that individuals with confidant relationships would have
lower cholesterol and uric acid levels and higher immune response than
those with poorer social support systems.

Research

The authors found that, among 256 healthy elderly adults, individuals
with good social support systems tended to have lower serum cholesterol and uric acid levels and higher indices of immune function;
these correlations were independent of age, body mass, tobacco use,
alcohol intake, and degree of perceived psychological stress.

Of interest to mental health professionals, physicians in general,
nurses, and social workers.

405. VAN EŸK, J. "De verwerking van enkele levensgebeurtenissen
    en steun uit sociale netwerken." (Dutch) *Gezondheid en
    Samenleving* 1 (1980): 83-101.

Investigates the influence of life events and social network support
on morbidity.

Research

It was found that hospitalization of a family member resulted in an increase of minor complaints, whereas the occurrence of an acute illness led to an increase of serious complaints among family members. Low or superficial network support was positively associated with the number of complaints presented to a general practitioner during stressful conditions.

Of interest to social scientists, in particular, stress researchers, and also to general practitioners and family physicians.

406. WALLSTON, Barbara S., Sheryle W. Alagna, Brenda M. DeVellis, Robert F. DeVellis. "Social support and physical health." *Health Psychology* 2 (1983): 367-391.

Delineates stages at which social support can mediate health outcome.

Theoretical

The authors suggest a new course for social research by emphasizing the need for differentiating between specific components of social support, delineating the physical health outcome stage at which support is provided, making use of extant theory to relate social support causally to other variables, matching measurement procedures to theoretical conceptualizations of support, and considering, where appropriate, individual as well as situational factors that might influence psychological processes related to social support.

Useful to researchers of social support.

c. Chapters

407. LAESSLE, R., and R. Ellmann. "Effects of the social situation on health and utilization of medical care services: Results from the Munich Follow-up Study" *In* Ulrich Laaser, Raoul Senault, Herbert Viefhues (Eds.). *Primary Health Care in the Making.* Berlin: Spring-Verlag, 1985.

An analysis of the data from a seven year follow-up study of a representative sample of the adult population of the Federal Republic of Germany regarding the influence of working and housing conditions, the place of residence, and social support as intervening variables in health and utilization behavior.

Research

People of lower socioeconomic status tend to give poorer health ratings, but some status differences in health ratings can be explained by other variables. Objective material conditions do relate to health; however, individual dissatisfaction seems to play an important intervening role. When social support and degree of satisfaction were added in the regression equation, there was no change in the social class effect.

Of interest to health administrators and health professionals interested in utilization behavior.

408. MADDOCKS, Ian. "The impoverishment of community life and the need for community health." *In* N.F. Stanley, and R.A. Joske (Eds.). *Changing Disease Patterns and Human Behavior.* London: Academic Press, 1980.

Attempts to show how the structure of the modern city can deprive people of natural supports and promote unease and sickness.

Theoretical

Suggests that crowding limits what people can offer one another, cities are diverse and destructive to the sense of community, city life is demanding and stressful, and the disruption of the coherence that simpler societies possess leads to unease and sickness. Community health depends upon a sense of community, and health professionals must redefine their role accordingly.

Should interest social and behavioral scientists.

409. OAKLEY, Ann. "The family, marriage, and its relationship to illness." *In* David Tuckett (Ed.). *An Introduction to Medical Sociology.* London: Tavistock, 1976.

Deals with the family as a unit of analysis in the study of illness.

Literature Review

Discusses the family context of illness, including a curative agent, recuperative agent, and mediator of health services. Gender roles and role strain are described as they relate to their association in the literature of family and illness.

Sociology students, social workers, and others interested in the sociology of illness will find this a thorough and analytic review.

d. Dissertations

410. BOHM, Lori C. "Social support and well-being in older adults: The impact of perceived control." Ph.D. dissertation, Yale University, 1983.

Examines whether feelings of control and efficacy affect the supportiveness of social relationships and, consequently, health outcomes.

Research

Feelings of control and efficacy were found to affect the social support/health outcome relationship. Differences in feelings of efficacy explained the association between social support and well-being. Persons with less control overall and in their relationships were less likely to deal adaptively with illness.

Useful for gerontologists, social scientists, and health care utilization researchers.

411. BREITENSTEIN, Donna L. "Health behaviors of women relative to marital status and social support." Ed.D. dissertation, University of Tennessee, 1984.

Never married women were compared with married women in regard to preventive health behaviors and how these are influenced by supportive social relationships.

Research

The two groups were similar in preventive health behavior. There were some differences in sources of support for choosing or maintaining these health behaviors. Married women received most support from their direct families, while unmarried women relied more on friends and others.

Useful for health educators and promoters, and researchers of health behavior.

412. JOHNSON, Robert J. "The impact of chronic illness on social supports." Ph.D. dissertation, University of Utah, 1983.

A study of the influence of chronic illness on several dimensions of social support, using a symbolic interaction framework.

Research

Although chronic illness tended to have a negative impact on social support resources, even reduced levels of support were effective for coping with the stressful condition of a chronic illness.

Of interest to social and behavioral scientists and rehabilitation specialists.

413. RIPORTELLA-MULLER, Roberta. "Social network influences on health perception and medical care utilization in a low income elderly population." Ph.D. dissertation, University of Wisconsin-Madison, 1985.

A study of the effect of social network contacts on health perception and health care utilization among low income elderly people.

Research

The results indicate that social contacts have a positive influence on both perception of health and utilization of health care. This is of particular importance, since this population is generally in high need of medical care.

Should interest health professionals, planners and providers, and gerontologists.

414. UHL, Joan E.H. "Health related outcomes of marital status and social support among the elderly." Ph.D. dissertation, University of Utah, 1985.

A study of the association of marital status, sex, and age with social support, household size, health status, and need for assistance.

Research

The major finding was that the inability to drive an automobile was an important social support risk indicator for elderly persons. This risk indicator is positively associated with age, being female, and having fewer social outings and friends. It was also associated with physical limitations and solitariness.

Of interest to social workers, health care providers, community planners, and gerontologists.

1. PREGNANCY, CHILDBIRTH, AND GYNECOLOGICAL PROBLEMS

a. Articles

415. KLAUS, Marshall H., John H. Kennell, Steven S. Robertson, Roberto Sosa. "Effects of social support during parturition on maternal and infant morbidity." *British Medical Journal* 293 (September 6, 1986): 585-587.

Investigates the clinical effect of support during labor on maternal and neonatal morbidity.

Research

Two hundred and forty-nine healthy primagravidous women undergoing labor were compared to 168 who had supportive female companions throughout their labor. The women with companions had significantly fewer perinatal complications, including caesarean sections and oxytocin augmentation, and fewer infants admitted to neonatal intensive care. Among those women who had an uncomplicated labor and delivery requiring no interventions, those with a companion had a significantly shorter duration of labor. Results suggest that constant human support may be of great benefit to women during labor.

Of interest to obstetricians, nurse midwives, and researchers of social support.

416. OAKLEY, Ann. "Social support in pregnancy: The 'soft' way
      to increase birthweight?"   *Social Science and Medicine*
      11 (1985): 1259-1268.

Examines the thesis that social support in pregnancy is capable of
affecting birthweight, as one easily measurable aspect of pregnancy
outcome.

Review

Reviews the published literature on social support in pregnancy,
including simple observational and nonrandomized intervention studies
and randomized controlled trials of social interventions. Methodological problems associated with some of these studies are discussed.

Of interest to social and behavioral scientists and obstetricians and
gynecologists.

417. PASCOE, John M., John Chessare, Evelyn Baugh.   "Which
      elements of prenatal social support improve neonatal morbidi-
      ty?" *Pediatric Research* 19, no. 4 (1985): 206A.

This study sought to define those elements of social support which
alter neonatal morbidity.

Research Abstract

This study of 201 mothers identified as important support factors,
"help with daily chores," a communicative male, and emergency child
care. The data suggest that prenatal help with daily tasks and the
support of a communicative male improve neonatal morbidity for infants
of indigent, urban, and multigravida mothers.

May be helpful to social workers, obstetricians, and others working
with high risk populations of pregnant women.

418. ROBBINS, James M., and John D. DeLamater. "Support from
      significant others and loneliness following induced abortion."
      Social Psychiatry 20 (1985): 92-99.

The relationship between support from significant others and feelings
of loneliness one week after induced abortion was investigated.

Research

Support from the male partner before, during, and after the procedure
was shown to be related to less frequent feelings of loneliness among
228 abortion recipients. Involvement or support of parents before and
during the procedure had no effect on loneliness.

Of interest to obstetricians, gynecologists, nurses, and social
workers.

419. WEBB, Christine.   "Professional and lay social support for
      hysterectomy patients."   *Journal of Advanced Nursing*   11
      (1986): 167-177.

Description of a study of social support for women undergoing
hysterectomy.

Descriptive

Post-hysterectomy follow-up at three months showed the "information
group" was less hostile, but more critical of their hospital treatment. The study also confirms previous findings by the same author of
generally high levels of satisfaction, health, and resumption of
activities after hysterectomy.

Of interest to nurses and obstetricians/gynecologists.

420. ————, and Jenifer Wilson-Barnett.   "Self-concept, social
      support and hysterectomy."   *International Journal of Nursing
      Studies*   20 (1983): 97-107.

Reports on part of a larger study concerned with describing recovery
from hysterectomy and evaluating an experimental counseling session
aimed at helping women to plan and manage their own recovery.

Research

Women in this study showed no evidence of adverse changes in self-
concept. Depression levels were reduced after operation, and the
majority of women were glad to have had a hysterectomy. Low levels of
support from partner, family, and friends were associated with poorer
outcome on some of the indicators used.

Of interest to gynecologists, family physicians, nurses, and social
workers.

b. Dissertations

421. BROWN, Marie A.   "Social support and symptomatology: A
      study of first time expectant parents."   Ph.D. dissertation,
      University of Washington, 1983.

A study of the effects of stress and social support on health during
pregnancy.

Research

Social network support, in particular, partner support, and stress
were the most important predictors of experienced symptoms during
pregnancy for both the future mother and father. The data provided
some evidence that supportive behavior between partners tends to be
reciprocal, not unidirectional from the future father to a pregnant
wife.

Should interest researchers and providers of prenatal care.

422. KELLER, Nancy A.   "Relationship between social support and mothers' perceptions of the birth experience in the early postpartum period."   D.S.N.   dissertation, University of Alabama in Birmingham, 1985.

The effect of social support on the birth experience among 105 new mothers who had normally delivered term infants in satisfactory condition was studied.

Descriptive Research

Birth experience was generally perceived as positive, but was not affected by the amount of available social support.   Only duration of labor was correlated with perceptions of the birth experience.

Should interest nurses, obstetricians, and other health professionals working with pregnant women.

423. PASS, Cleo Massicotte.   "Relationship between social support and premenstrual syndrome."   D.S.N. dissertation, University of Alabama in Birmingham, 1983.

Examines the relationship between social support and premenstrual syndrome (PMS), and social support and selected personal characteristics.

Research

Evidence was found that an increase in the severity of PMS is accompanied by a decrease in the social support network.   A number of personal characteristics, like marital status, educational level, and religious participation, were related to support variables.

Of interest to women with PMS, gynecologists, and social scientists.

2. CARDIOVASCULAR DISEASES

a. Books

424. BRUHN, John G., and Stewart Wolf.   *The Roseto Story: An Anatomy of Health*.   Norman, OK: University of Oklahoma Press, 1979.

A summary of a 15 year study of an Italian-American community in Pennsylvania, which was found to have a lower death rate from heart attacks than neighboring communities of different ethnic compositions.

Research

The importance of social support as a buffer against stress was noted. As the community began to change and assume values of the larger American culture, the rate of heart attacks began to rise.

Of interest to social and behavioral scientists, community workers, and mental health professionals.

425. CAPLAN, Robert D., R. Van Harrison, Retha V. Wellons, John R.P. French, Jr. *Social Support and Patient Adherence: Experimental and Survey Findings.* Ann Arbor: The University of Michigan, 1980.

This study focuses on patients who are in treatment for high blood pressure to uncover the social-psychological differences between those who do and those who do not have their blood pressure under adequate control.

Research

Higher levels of affective support from someone at home led to higher levels of perceived support from both the physician and the nurse. When physician support was high, somatic complaints and depression were low. Support from the nurse was also perceived to be high when somatic complaints were low. The findings relating to partner variables suggest that involvement at the clinic may be beneficial for the patient. The partner accurately perceives the support the nurse attempts to provide the patient, which increases the partner's motivation to support the patient and, in turn, the support the partner actually attempts to provide the patient. Finally, the patient accurately perceives the support offered by the partner.

Of interest to social and behavioral scientists, health educators and specialists in hypertension.

426. CAPLAN, Robert D., Elizabeth A.R. Robinson, John R.P. French, John R. Caldwell, Marybeth Shinn. *Adhering to Medical Regimens: Pilot Experiments in Patient Education and Social Support.* Ann Arbor: Institute for Social Research, 1976.

Describes a pilot effort to identify factors that determine why hypertensive patients do or do not adhere to their regimens.

Research

The role of social support was a major focus of this study. Social support from the spouse was associated with low levels of depression, while social support from other sources had no such effect. On the other hand, social support from the spouse and physician tended to be highest for patients who were highly motivated to adhere, and social support from the physician was an important correlate of perceived consequences of nonadherence. Social support from one source was not always substitutable for social support from other sources.

Of interest to researchers of social support, especially physicians specializing in hypertension, health educators, and social and behavioral scientists.

427.   CROOG, Sydney H., and Sol Levine. *The Heart Patient Recovers.* New York: Human Sciences Press, 1977.

Follows the history of a group of men after a first heart attack. Presents data for a period of one year following admission to the hospital, which describes and analyzes life patterns or careers, examines the relationship between psychosocial and medical variables to morbidity and mortality, and examines variables associated with "outcome."

Research

The primary role of the family as a support and resource was manifest in this study. A type of surrogate family--friends and neighbors--also provided considerable assistance. Individuals who received support from one source were likely to receive it from other sources. Thus, the more socially integrated the individuals, the more support they were likely to receive. Religion also provided support. While religion may have provided support for a considerable segment of the patients, for men who did not value it before the illness, it was not a support to which they turned in time of stress.

Of interest to cardiologists and rehabilitation counselors, as well as social and behavioral scientists.

428.   LYNCH, James J. *The Broken Heart.   The Medical Consequences of Loneliness.* New York: Basic Books, 1977.

The lack of human companionship--chronic loneliness and social isolation, as well as the sudden loss of loved ones--is one of the leading causes of premature death. While the lack of human companionship is related to virtually every major disease from cancer to tuberculosis to mental illness, the link is particularly marked in the case of heart disease.

Research

The most simple forms of human contact have proven dramatic effects on the body, and especially the heart. In a society in which the divorce rate is rising, the family is fragmenting, social and community bonds are fleeting, and children and the aged are neglected, our physical survival is threatened.

Of interest to social and behavioral scientists, health professionals, and the lay public.

429. OSTFELD, Adrian, and Elaine D. Eaker (Eds.). *Measuring Psychosocial Variables in Epidemiologic Studies of Cardiovascular Disease.* Proceedings of a Workshop. U.S. Department of Health and Human Services, Public Health Service, National Institutes of Health. NIH Publication No. 85-2270, March 1985.

Proceedings of a workshop on the measurement of psychosocial variables associated with cardiovascular disease.

Workshop Proceedings

Session 2 is composed of four presentations on social support and social networks, discussions of each paper, and a group summary. Suggestions for research of the role of social support in cardiovascular disease are presented.

Of interest to social and behavioral scientists, epidemiologists, and researchers of coronary heart disease.

b. Articles

430. ALLEN, Jerilyn, and Diane Becker. "Determinants of early physical activity following coronary bypass surgery. *Circulation* 74, Supplement II (October 1986): 291.

This study attempted to determine the relative influence of both physical and social factors on self-reported physical activity levels one month following coronary bypass surgery.

Research Abstract

A panel of 70 men undergoing coronary bypass surgery at less than 65 years of age were interviewed before hospital discharge and four to six weeks later. Analysis revealed age, number of bypass grafts, postoperative spouse encouragement, length of preoperative disability, and physician encouragement each made a significant and independent contribution to physical activity level. The findings suggest that spouse support is influential in determining early physical activity level and that wives should be given specific information to enhance their supportive roles.

Should interest cardiologists, cardiac care nurses, and rehabilitation specialists.

431. ALONZO, Angelo A. "The impact of the family and lay others on care-seeking during life-threatening episodes of suspected coronary artery disease." *Social Science and Medicine* 22 (1986): 1297-1311.

Focuses on the impact of the spouse, other family members, and lay others on life-threatening illness behavior surrounding acute episodes of coronary heart disease.

Research

Analyzing the care-seeking behavior of those individuals within life threatening illness behavior and situational perspectives, analyses revealed that family members, especially a spouse, had both positive and negative influences on the duration of time between acute symptom onset and arrival at a hospital emergency room.

Of interest to social and behavioral scientists.

432. BADURA, Bernhard, and Millard Waltz. "Social support and the quality of life following myocardial infarction." *Social Indicators Research* 14 (1984): 295-311.

A longitudinal investigation of the influence of the social environment on successful adaptation and well-being among 980 male, German cardiac patients.

Research

The quality of interpersonal relationships and of experienced socioemotional support were found to affect both the positive and negative dimensions of psychological well-being. Perceived health status and physical disability mainly influenced the negative dimension.

Should interest social scientists and health care professionals.

433. BERKMAN, Lisa F. "Social network analysis and coronary heart disease." *Advances in Cardiology* 29 (1982): 37-49.

A review of the importance of social and community ties and resources to the risk of coronary heart disease.

Review

Social networks influence the prevalence and mortality of coronary heart disease. However, there are still no data on the relationship of networks to the incidence of myocardial infarction or any other disease. Such data are necessary to our further understanding of how social networks influence disease processes.

Of interest to researchers of coronary heart disease and social support.

434. BRUHN, John G., Betty Chandler, M. Clinton Miller, Stewart Wolf, Thomas N. Lynn. "Social aspects of coronary heart disease in two adjacent, ethnically different communities." *American Journal of Public Health* 56 (September 1966): 1493-1506.

A community study of coronary heart disease was carried out in Bangor, Pennsylvania, and the death rate from myocardial infarction was found to be higher there than in its adjacent neighbor, Roseto, a predominantly Italian-American community.

Research

Individuals who had experienced a myocardial infarction in the two communities shared more similarities than differences in regard to the psychosocial variables examined; however, the two communities differed notably in their culture and group dynamics. The more homogeneous and stable of the two communities was found to have a lower incidence of deaths from myocardial infarction and a lower incidence of treated mental illness.

Of interest to social and behavioral scientists, epidemiologists, community mental health, and public health professionals.

435. BRUHN, John G., Billy U. Philips, Stewart Wolf. "Lessons from Roseto 20 years later: A community study of heart disease." *Southern Medical Journal* 75 (May 1982): 575-580.

Findings of a community study of coronary artery disease were reviewed, retrospectively, to highlight applications to current research and clinical practice.

Review

Social support and close family ties were found to be important buffers of the deleterious effects of stress and life change, factors which have been implicated in the occurrence of myocardial infarction and sudden death.

Of interest to health professionals in general, to epidemiologists, and to community health workers.

436. CHAMBERS, William N., and Morton F. Reiser. "Emotional stress in the precipitation of congestive heart failure." *Psychosomatic Medicine* 15 (1953): 38-60.

An investigation of the role of emotional factors in the development of congestive heart failure in a representative group of patients.

Research

The life histories of these patients were characterized by a realistic lack of material and social security and stability. At the time of the study, most were functioning in an environment and social milieu which had a very limited capability of affording material and emotional support. Dependence upon tenuous relationships with relatively few key figures, upon symbols (such as familiar living quarters), and even upon illusions, is understandably exaggerated in such a setting.

Of interest to internists and to social and behavioral scientists.

437. COOPER, C.L., E.B. Faragher, C.L. Bray, D.R. Ramsdale. "The significance of psychosocial factors in predicting coronary disease in patients with valvular heart disease." *Social Science and Medicine* 20 (1985): 315-318.

A retrospective survey of patients with valvular disease who had undergone routine coronary angiography followed by valve replacement.

Research

Psychosocial factors improved the preoperative predictive power of significant coronary artery disease on four criteria: previous history of hypertension, previous history of myocardial infarction, signs of peripheral vascular disease, and ECG evidence of myocardial infarction. All psychosocial factors except work stress enhance the predictive power of regression equations, particularly the cumulative effect of a number of adverse life events occurring in a short period of time and the lack of social support from family and friends to help to overcome them.

Of interest to cardiologists, rehabilitation specialists, and social and behavioral scientists.

438. DHOOPER, Surjit Singh. "Social networks and support during the crisis of heart attack." *Health in Social Work* 9 (1984): 294-303.

The type, source, and extent of support received by the families of heart attack victims were investigated.

Research

Although grown children, friends, and neighbors were found to be the families' greatest source of emotional support, professional intervention is needed to mobilize and supplement informal networks.

Of interest to social workers and mental health professionals.

439. DOHERTY, W.J., H.G. Schrott, L. Metcalf, L. Iasiello-Vailas. "Effect of spouse support and health beliefs on patient adherence." *Controlled Clinical Trials* 3 (1982): 137.

Support and health beliefs of wives were assessed by structured interviews of participants, wives, and medical staff of the Coronary Primary Prevention Trial.

Research Abstract

The correlation of spouses' health beliefs with their perceived support was significant for their scores on susceptibility, severity, and benefits, but not for costs. The high support participants had spouses with higher scores on perceived benefits. Thus, men with higher wife support adhered better to medication, and wives with strong belief in the benefits, as opposed to costs of the program, were most supportive.

Of interest to health educators and professionals in preventive medicine and community health.

440. DRESSLER, William W., Alfonso Mata, Adolfo Chavez, Fernando E. Viteri, Philip Gallagher. "Social support and arterial pressure in a central Mexican community." *Psychosomatic Medicine* 48 (1986): 338-350.

Research on the relationship of social support and arterial blood pressure, conducted in a town in central Mexico.

Research

A culturally appropriate measure of social support was developed assessing perceived support from relatives, friends, neighbors, and compadres. For males, more support from all four sources was related to lower arterial pressure, whereas amount of social contact was related to higher diastolic blood pressure; support from compadres had the largest inverse correlation with blood pressure. For females, the pattern of correlations was dependent on age: support from relatives and friends was related to higher blood pressure for younger females, whereas support from relatives was related to lower blood pressure in older females.

Of interest to physicians and social and behavioral scientists.

441. EAKER, Elaine D., Suzanne G. Haynes, Manning Feinleib. "Spouse behavior and coronary heart disease in men: Prospective results from the Framingham Heart Study II: Modification of risk in Type A husbands according to the social and psychological status of their wives." *American Journal of Epidemiology* 118 (1983): 23-41.

Describes the results of a prospective study of heart disease and the etiological significance of the wives' behavior or social status.

Research

Confirms what is generally known about the Type A/B personality regarding heart disease, and lists the education of the spouse and her personality as a risk factor in the etiology of the disease. This finding is apparent regardless of the husband's coronary risk profile.

An important study for researchers interested in heart disease, which offers much promise for additional research.

442. EARP, Jo Anne L., Marcia G. Ory, David S. Strogatz. "The effects of family involvement and practitioner home visits on the control of hypertension." *American Journal of Public Health* 72 (October 1982): 1146-1154.

Two groups of hypertensive patients, subjected to different social support strategies designed to lower their blood pressure, were compared to each other and to a control group receiving routine care in a randomized clinical trial extending over two years.

Research

Neither support strategy was clearly shown to be more effective than the other over time. The efficacy of the interventions is discussed with respect to cost and feasibility of implementation.

Of interest to nurses and physicians, especially those interested in behavior change.

443. GARRITY, Thomas F. "Social involvement and activeness as predictors of morale six months after first myocardial infarction." *Social Science and Medicine* 7 (1973): 199-207.

A theory relating social involvement to morale is tentatively used to predict the morale of 62 first myocardial infarction patients.

Research

Although an association is found between social involvement and morale, it appears to be explained by the patient's perception of his health. The findings call for a modification of social gerontology's theory of morale.

Of interest to researchers of social support and to gerontologists.

444. HILBERT, Gail A. "Spouse support and myocardial infarction patient compliance." *Nursing Research* 34 (1985): 217-220.

An investigation of the relationship between spouse support and compliance of myocardial infarction patients.

Research

Data were obtained from a sample of 60 couples during home interviews with the husband at least three months following his infarction. Husband's self-reported compliance was obtained for each of 10 aspects of the regimen. Wives completed a spouse support questionnaire that estimated the degree to which they engaged in theoretically supportive behaviors. Demographic and illness variables were also obtained. The hypothesis that there is a positive relationship between spouse support and compliance was not supported and compliance was not related to demographic or illness variables. However, those subjects engaged in a cardiac rehabilitation program had significantly higher compliance than those who had stopped attending.

Of interest to health professionals involved with myocardial infarction patients.

445. KNOX, Sarah S., Töres Theorell, Jan Ch. Svensson, Dick Waller. "The relation of social support and working environment to medical variables associated with elevated blood pressure in young males: A structural model." *Social Science and Medicine* 21 (1985): 525-531.

An examination of the interaction of working environment factors and individual social support networks with medical variables related to blood pressure elevations in young hypertensives.

Research

The medical variables, which explained a significant amount of the variation in systolic blood pressure, were found to be blood hemoglobin, plasma adrenaline, and relative weight. High relative weight was associated with a low level of employment security and high plasma adrenaline with a poor self-reported social network as well as a job that provided few possibilities for learning new things.

Of interest to researchers studying stress and social support.

446. LEVY, Rona L. "Social support and compliance--update." *Journal of Hypertension* 3, Supplement 1 (1985): 45-49.

An update of a selective review and critique of the literature on social support as a factor in the enhancement of patient compliance with medical regimens, with hypertension and hypertension risk factors as a particular focus.

Literature Review and Critique

Three problem areas in using the social support variable are cited: inconsistent and/or low levels of specificity in using the social support variable, inconsistent and/or inadequate outcome measures, and inattention as to whether independent variables are carried out as planned in an experiment. It is suggested that social support research utilize compliance enhancement strategies as a measure of social support behaviors and to ensure greater compliance with experimental manipulations.

Of interest to social and behavioral scientists, especially researchers interested in social support and compliance behavior.

447. LYNCH, James J., and William H. Convey. "Loneliness, disease, and death: Alternative approaches." *Psychosomatics* 20 (1979): 702-708.

Illustrates a psychosomatic approach that takes stress-producing factors into consideration and is proving effective in treating a selected number of patients with drug-resistant hypertension.

Descriptive

A psychosomatic treatment approach that combines insight therapy, especially regarding interpersonal relationships, and behavioral techniques in treating hypertension is illustrated by case histories. Useful to physicians and health professionals interested in psychosomatic medicine.

448. LYNCH, James J., Sue A. Thomas, David A. Paskewitz, Aaron H. Katcher, Lourdes O. Weir. "Human contact and cardiac arrhythmia in a coronary care unit." *Psychosomatic Medicine* 39 (1977): 188-192.

An extension of studies on the cardiac effects of pulse palpation among patients in a coronary care unit.

Research

Significant reduction in ventricular arrhythmias occurred following pulse palpation. These data suggest that significant changes in ventricular arrhythmia can occur as a result of even minimally arousing psychosocial interactions.

Of interest to cardiologists, nurses, and other health care professionals providing direct patient care.

449. O'REILLY, Patrick. "Social support networks and maintenance of improved cardiovascular risk status." *Circulation* 74, Supplement II (October 1986): 320.

Reports on a study undertaken to clarify the relationship between social support networks and maintaining an improved cardiovascular status.

Research Abstract

Three years after the completion of the Multiple Risk Factor Intervention Trial (MRFIT), 290 participants were rescreened to identify who had improved risk status at the end of MRFIT and who had maintained improvement. Although no significant relationship was found between maintenance and general social support or in the sociodemographic patterns of maintainers versus non-maintainers, significant associations were found for four types of support specific to risk reduction--information/advice, encouragement, caring, and availability--and for three network components--size, density, and relational content. The data suggest a relationship between long-term maintenance of risk-reducing behaviors and the provision of specific supportive behaviors by close, primarily family, network members.

Of interest to cardiologists, rehabilitation specialists, and social and behavioral scientists.

450. REED, Dwayne, Daniel McGee, Katsuhiko Yano, Manning
Feinleib. "Social networks and coronary heart disease among
Japanese men in Hawaii." *American Journal of Epidemiology*
117 (1983): 384-396.

A group of 4,653 men of Japanese ancestry living in Hawaii was studied
for the association of measures of social networks with both the
prevalence and incidence rates of coronary heart disease.

Research

There was little evidence of reduced risk of incidental coronary heart
disease associated with the social network scale for men in high risk
categories relating to serum cholesterol, blood pressure, and cigarette smoking. With prevalence data, social network scores were
inversely related to total coronary heart disease and, to some extent,
with angina and myocardial infarction.

Useful to epidemiologists and social and behavioral scientists studying coronary heart disease.

451. SIEGRIST, J., K. Dittmann, H. Weidemann. "The role of
psychosocial risks in patients with early myocardial infarction." *Acta Nervosa Superior* (Praha) 24 (1982): 14-24.

Results of a retrospective case-control study on 380 male patients
with clinically documented first myocardial infarction (age 30-55) as
well as findings of a follow-up over 18 months are presented.

Research

Workload, lack of social support, and/or life changes are significantly related to the recurrence of cardiac symptoms in an 18 month
follow-up of cardiac patients.

Of interest to family physicians, internists, rehabilitation counselors, and social and behavioral scientists.

452. SOMMERS, Marilyn Sawyer. "Creating a therapeutic environment during cardiopulmonary resuscitation." *Focus on Critical Care* 12, no. 3 (1985): 22-29.

A description of the aspects of maintaining a supportive emotional
atmosphere in a critical care unit.

Descriptive

The life and death situation of a cardiopulmonary arrest is extremely
stressful for patients, families, other patients, and the critical
care staff. The staff must meet the needs of patients and their
families, as well as provide emotional support and ongoing information. The population of the critical care unit also needs support.

Of particular interest to health professionals working in critical care units of hospitals.

453. WALTZ, Millard. "Marital context and post-infarction quality of life. Is it social support or something more?" *Social Science and Medicine* 22 (1986): 791-805.

Concerned with intimacy attachment, social role strains, and the self-concept in relation to well-being after myocardial infarction.

Research

Marital status, the emotional quality of the spouse relationship, and longstanding marital stressors were found to have direct and indirect effects on the two dimensions of the Bradburn Affect Balance Scale. The same is true of continuing problems associated with the heart attack, relative to perceptions of having coped effectively with the after effects of illness.

Of interest to social and behavioral scientists.

454. WILLIAMS, Carolyn A., Shirley A. Beresford, Sherman A. James, Andrea Z. La Croix, David S. Strogatz, Edward H. Wagner, David G. Kleinbaum, Lawrence M. Cutchin, Michel A. Ibrahim. "The Edgecombe County High Blood Pressure Control Program. III. Social support, social stressors, and treatment dropout." *American Journal of Public Health* 75 (1985): 483-486.

In a hypertension prevalence survey of a stratified random sample of 1,000 households, 2,030 adults were interviewed and information on psychosocial variables collected.

Research

Among 359 hypertensives, there was a consistent relationship, in women, between indicators of difficulty in the social environment and dropout from treatment. Compared to those who remained in treatment, women who dropped out had less social support on the job, had less perceived spouse approval (if married), had a lower level of perceived access to supportive resources, and, if they were homemakers, were more likely to report feeling pushed most or all of the time.

Of interest to social and behavioral scientists, health educators, family physicians, and cardiologists.

c. Dissertations

455. FLOWERS, Retha Vivian Wellons. "Effects of social support on adherence to therapeutic regimens." Ph.D. dissertation, University of Michigan, Ann Arbor, 1978.

A quasi-experimental study of the effects of social support on adherence to therapeutic regimens and consequent goal attainment among a group of hypertensive patients.

Research

It was found that objective social support, as provided to the patient by a nurse, positively affected regimen adherence and goal attainment, primarily through perceived social support and objective knowledge of the therapeutic regimen. The group of patients who had a partner and received support from a nurse showed a significantly larger increase in the proportion of controlled blood pressure than either the group that received support only from a nurse or the control group.

Of interest to researchers of the utilization of health services and primary health care professionals.

456. GENERAL, Dale A.   "Type A behavior and social support in coronary heart patients."   Ph.D. dissertation, North Texas State University, 1983.

Investigates the relationship between Type A behavior and perceived quality of social support among patients with symptomatic coronary disease.

Research

As expected, a negative correlation was found between Type A and perceived quality of social support.   Type A was also significantly associated with interpersonal stress, but not with a number of other measures of support used.

Of interest to social and behavioral scientists, in particular stress researchers.

457. JOSEPH, Jill G.   "Social affiliation, risk factor status, and coronary heart disease: A cross-sectional study of Japanese-American men."   Ph.D. dissertation, University of California, Berkeley, 1980.

Investigates the effects of social affiliation and social disconnection on the risk of coronary heart disease.

Research

Social affiliation was, in addition to age, physical inactivity, and family history of heart infarcts, found to be significantly associated with prevalence of coronary heart disease in the expected direction. This association was stronger in the presence of lower levels of the other risk factors of coronary heart disease.

Useful to social scientists, social epidemiologists, and physicians interested in psychosomatic medicine.

458. PATTERSON, Judith P. "Family structure, social support, and
cardiovascular risk factors." Ph.D. dissertation, University
of Texas at Austin, 1984.

The effects of social support, provided by living in extended families, on the levels of a number of cardiovascular risk factors were
studied in a Mexican-American and an Anglo-American sample.

Research

Mexican-Americans were more likely to live in extended families, but
did not show significantly different levels of cardiovascular risk
factors. However, household structure and visiting patterns were
found to be associated with levels of cardiovascular risk factors.

Of interest to social scientists and other researchers in the prevention of cardiovascular disease.

3. EPILEPSY, STROKE, AND MULTIPLE SCLEROSIS

a. Articles

459. EVANS, Ron L., and Lawrence K. Northwood. "Social support
needs in adjustment to stroke." *Archives of Physical Medicine and Rehabilitation* 64, no. 2 (1983): 61-64.

Examines the relationship of interpersonal social contact to adjustment after rehabilitation for stroke.

Research

The adjustment of stroke patients to rehabilitation and their chronic
physical limitations was related to their ability to recognize sources
of social support and express their personal need for it. Those
patients not recognizing direct social support resources were alienated and entered cycles of isolation.

Physical and occupational therapists and other health professionals
interested in the rehabilitation of stroke victims will benefit from
this article.

460. GRANT, Igor. "The social environment and neurological disease." *Advances in Psychosomatic Medicine* 13 (1985):
26-48.

Reviews the literature on research concerned with psychosocial influences on epilepsy, stroke, and multiple sclerosis.

Literature Review

Reviews some methodological and theoretical issues in research linking
the social environment to illness, and then focuses on three specific

neurological entities to examine evidence for a possible association between neurological illness and life stress.   The role of social support as a moderator variable for stress is discussed.

Of interest to health professionals concerned with psychosocial factors in neurological and cardiovascular diseases.

461. McIVOR, Geraldine P., Manuel Riklan, Marvin Reznikoff. "Depression in multiple sclerosis as a function of length and severity of illness, age, remissions, and perceived social support."   *Journal of Clinical Psychology*   40 (1984): 1028-1033.

Describes a study of social support, conditional parameters of multiple sclerosis, demographic factors, and depression.

Research

More depressed individuals were found to be more likely to be disabled, to be older, and to perceive less social support from family and friends.   Those subjects who had experienced remission in their disease were less depressed.

Psychologists, social workers, and others interested in rehabilitation research will benefit from this study.

462. McLEROY, Kenneth R., Robert De Vellis, Brenda De Vellis, Berton Kaplan, James Toole. "Social support and physical recovery in a stroke population." *Journal of Social and Personal Relationships* 1 (1984): 395-413.

A longitudinal study of 393 stroke cases, examining several aspects of social support.

Research

Different types of social support had different effects on physical recovery.   Instrumental assistance had a significantly negative effect, compared to the positive effects of informational and affective support.   Instrumental support was a better predictor of functioning than was social network structure.

Of importance to physicians, especially internists and family physicians, rehabilitation specialists, and physical and occupational therapists.

b. Dissertations

463. McIVOR, Geraldine P.   "Depression in multiple sclerosis as a function of length and severity of illness, age, remissions, and perceived social support."   Ph.D. dissertation, Fordham University, 1981.

Investigates the effect of a number of illness, demographic, and

Depression was significantly associated with degree of disability, age, absence of remissions, and lack of perceived social support, but not with length of illness. Perceived social support, severity of disability, and course of illness were the best predictors of depression in this group of patients.

Of interest to social scientists and health professionals, in particular, those who work with MS patients.

4. CANCER

a. Books

464. GOLDBERG, Jane G. (Ed.). *Psychotherapeutic Treatment of Cancer Patients.* New York: Free Press, 1981.

Provides a thorough overview of key components of adjunctive psychotherapy as well as insights into its importance during orthodox medical treatment for cancer.

Book of Readings

Edited in five parts to represent the important social support components of adjunctive psychotherapy in cancer. These include theoretical considerations, psychosomatic components of cancer treatment, the role of the therapist, the role of group therapy, and the family.

Essential reading for those providing supportive care for cancer victims and their families.

b. Articles

465. BLOOM, Joan R. "Social support, accommodation to stress and adjustment to breast cancer." *Social Science and Medicine* 16 (1982): 1329-1338.

Develops a model specifying the interrelationships between social support, coping response, and adjustment to illness.

Research

Social support was the strongest predictor of coping response, and had indirect effects on all three measures of adjustment: self-concept, sense of power, and psychological distress. Of the social background factors, only social status and employment had direct effects on adjustment, as measured by sense of power and self-concept. These relationships were not predicted. The results suggest that women who have more support use fewer modes of accommodation to the stress of breast cancer.

Useful to physicians, nurses, and allied health professionals working
with patients rehabilitating from breast cancer.

466. ————, and David Spiegel. "The relationship of two dimensions
      of social support to the psychological well being and social
      functioning of women with advanced breast cancer." *Social
      Science and Medicine* 19 (1984): 831-837.

Discusses the mechanism through which social support provides protection for individuals enduring stressful life circumstances.

Research

Women with advanced breast cancer were interviewed to assess the
relationship of their outlook and social functioning to the social
support they were receiving. Emotional support was found to be
strongly related to outlook, and opportunities for social exchange,
affected functioning, outlook, and interactive processes.

Of interest to social workers and health professionals.

467. COBB, Sidney, and Christine Erbe. "Social support for the
      cancer patient." *Forum on Medicine* 1 (November 1978):
      24-29.

Identifies the function of the support network for the cancer patient
in relation to the function of the treatment team.

Theoretical

Explains the importance of social support to the cancer patient
experiencing the loss of role and identity and reduced social activity. Defines the need for support counselors whose responsibility is
to the patient's family and whose work will benefit the patient
indirectly.

Of interest to health professionals caring for cancer patients.

468. FUNCH, Donna P., and James Marshall. "The role of stress,
      social support, and age in survival from breast cancer."
      Journal of Psychosomatic Research 27 (1983): 77-83.

A study focused on the relationship of objective and subjective stress
to survival from breast cancer.

Research

Objective stress was related to survival for the oldest group, while
subjective stress was related to survival for the youngest group.
Neither stress was related to survival for women aged 40-60. Using
the entire sample, the stage of cancer at the time of diagnosis was
the best predictor of survival.

Of interest to oncologists and social and behavioral scientists.

469. FUNCH, Donna P., and Curtis Mettlin. "The role of support
     in relation to recovery from breast surgery." *Social
     Science and Medicine* 16 (1982): 91-98.

The relationship between support and short-term recovery from breast
surgery was examined retrospectively in 151 female breast cancer
patients, 3-12 months postoperative.

Research

Social and professional support had a significant positive relationship to psychological adjustment, and financial support was positively
related to physical recovery.

Of interest to oncologists and other health professionals concerned
with the rehabilitation of cancer patients.

470. LEV, Elise L. "Community support for oncology patient and
     family." *Topics in Clinical Nursing* 7 (April 1985): 71-78.

Explores community resources available to families and patients
dealing with life-threatening illness.

Literature Review

Discusses various social networks involved in family support during
crisis, including community support, hospice programs, cancer support
teams, and self-help groups. Points out that the literature regarding
management of these situations is much more abundant than the actual
helping process, and offers recommendations for improvement of
implementation.

Of interest to all who deal with the terminally ill.

471. LINDSEY, Ada M., Jane S. Norbeck, Virginia L. Carrieri,
     Elizabeth Perry. "Social support and health outcomes in
     postmastectomy women: A review." *Cancer Nursing*
     4 (October 1981): 377-384.

Compares major conceptualizations of social support, and summarizes
studies in which some component characteristics of social support in
adjustment to a mastectomy have been examined.

Review

Weaknesses were found in the conceptualization of social support. The
instruments used to measure social support or components of social
support were varied and inadequate. The work, to date, on social
support as a moderator variable in coping with mastectomy is scattered
and essentially noncumulative in nature.

Of interest to researchers of social support.

472. MAISIAK, Richard, Richard Gams, Esta Lee, Bobbie Jones.
      "The psychosocial support status of elderly cancer outpa-
      tients." *Progress in Clinical and Biological Research*
      120 (1983): 395-403.

A study to identify the psychosocial problems of elderly cancer
outpatients, which differ from those of younger cancer patients, and
from those of the general elderly population.

Research

The results suggest that psychosocial support for cancer patients
should be directed differently for older and younger adult patients.

Of interest to oncologists, gerontologists, and social and behavioral
scientists.

473. MONACO, Grace Powers. "Resources available to the family of
      the child with cancer." *Cancer* 58 (1986): 516-521.

Focuses on the societal, professional, and peer resources needed for
survival and coping from the point of diagnosis through treatment,
relapse, and death.

Review and Analysis

Families require access to a firm, unfragmented foundation of support,
incorporating a multidisciplinary network of resources, involving the
combined efforts of the primary health care team and the community.
Medical and emotional counseling, peer support, spiritual guidance,
and special community services contribute to the optimal care of both
patient and family.

Of particular interest to pediatric oncologists and social workers.

474. MORROW, Gary R., Paul J. Carpenter, Alice C. Hoagland.
      "The role of social support in parental adjustment to pediatric
      cancer." *Journal of Pediatric Psychology* 9 (1984): 317-329.

The effects of treatment stage, parental sex, age, and perceived
social support network on psychological adjustment for parents of
pediatric cancer patients were examined.

Research

In the case of parents of a child who was not undergoing active
medical treatment, only support from relatives appeared to temper
adjustment difficulties. Parents of a child who had died did not
appear to benefit from any source of social support.

Of interest to pediatric oncologists, pediatric nurses, and social workers.

475. MORROW, Gary R., Alice Hoagland, Charles L. Carnrike. "Social support and parental adjustment to pediatric cancer." *Journal of Consulting and Clinical Psychology* 49 (1981): 763-765.

Assesses the psychosocial adjustment of 107 parents whose children had cancer.

Research

Parents whose children were still in treatment and parents over 30 years of age showed better adjustment than those parents whose children had died. Results suggest that attention should be focused on the psychosocial adjustment of young bereaved parents.

Should interest researchers of the psychosocial aspects of cancer and bereavement.

476. RAY, Colette, Janet Grover, Tom Wisniewski. "Nurses' perceptions of early breast cancer and mastectomy, and their psychological implications, and of the role of health professionals in providing support." *International Journal of Nursing Studies* 21 (1984): 101-111.

This study focused on the nurse's role in the psychological management of breast cancer.

Research

A survey found a mixed attitude regarding the efficacy of treatment outcomes, and a general enthusiasm for health education as a means of enhancing support for women experiencing mastectomy. Nurses reported their preference for a support giving role, but did not see themselves as counselors.

Nurses and others providing psychological support to mastectomy patients will find this article helpful.

477. REVENSON, Tracey A., Carol A. Wollman, Barbara J. Felton. "Social supports as stress buffers for adult cancer patients." *Psychosomatic Medicine* 45 (August 1983): 321-331.

Examines the relationship between naturally occurring, supportive behaviors and psychological adjustment to the illness of 32 nonhospitalized adult cancer patients, and includes follow-up data collected seven months after the initial interview.

Research

Although support appeared to have few effects on adjustment at either point in time for the sample as a whole, social support was related to poorer adjustment for patients not undergoing chemotherapy or radiation treatments or with many limitations on physical functioning.

Of interest to physicians and other health professionals treating cancer patients.

478. SATARIANO, William A., and Dorothy Eckert. "Social ties and functional adjustment following mastectomy: Criteria for research. *Progress in Clinical and Biological Research* 120 (1983): 387-394.

Presents a research strategy to investigate the extent to which social ties with others affect functional adjustment following mastectomy.

Theoretical

Contains a discussion of methodological and design issues in measuring and assessing social support in mastectomy patients.

Of interest to social and behavioral scientists.

479. TEBBI, Cameron K., Marilyn Stern, Michele Boyle, Curtis J. Mettlin, Eugene R. Mindell. "The role of social support systems in adolescent cancer amputees." *Cancer* 56 (1985): 965-971.

To examine the role of social support systems, 27 adolescents who had undergone amputations for cancer were interviewed. Inquiries were made regarding patients' perceived social support providers and the impact of amputation upon their lives and independence.

Research

Parents, especially mothers, were perceived as realistic and most helpful at the time of surgery, followed by professional hospital staff and siblings. Friends of patients were less helpful, as many reported their friends felt sorry for them, avoided them, or drifted away. Only 7.4 percent of the patients expressed a clear preference to be associated with other amputees.

Of interest to mental health professionals, especially social workers and rehabilitation counselors.

480. WEISMAN, Avery D., and J. William Worden. "Psychosocial analysis of cancer deaths." *Omega* 6 (1975): 61-75.

The investigators used information from psychological autopsies of cancer deaths and correlated observed survival with psychosocial findings.

Research

Patients who lived significantly longer tended to maintain cooperative and mutually responsive relationships, especially towards the end of their lives. Patients with death wishes, depression, apathy, and long-standing mutually destructive relationships survived for shorter periods than expected.

Of interest to oncologists and social and behavioral scientists.

481. WELLISCH, David K. "The psychologic impact of breast cancer on relationships." *Seminars in Oncology Nursing* 1 (1985): 195-199.

Assesses four areas of interaction of breast cancer and the patient's personal relationships.

Theoretical

An excellent discussion of general interactional themes of the patient's personal relationships; the impact of social support, in general, and the support of the marital partner on patient adjustment; the impact of breast cancer on the marital and parent-child relationship.

Of interest to oncologists and all other health professionals relating to cancer patients.

482. WORTMAN, Camille B. "Social support and the cancer patient. Conceptual and methodologic issues." *Cancer* 53, Supplement (May 15, 1984): 2339-2360.

Highlights some of the issues that potential cancer researchers face in deciding how to conceptualize and measure social support.

Literature Review and Theoretical

Highlights the importance of designing research that will shed light on the precise mechanisms by which support influences health outcomes. Hopefully, such research will clarify how social support interacts with other important psychosocial variables, such as coping strategies and self-esteem.

Of interest to social and behavioral scientists and cancer researchers.

c. Chapters

483. BLOOM, Joan R. "Social support systems and cancer: A conceptual view." *In* Jerome Cohen, Joseph W. Cullen, L. Robert Martin (Eds.). *Psychosocial Aspects of Cancer.* New York: Raven Press, 1982.

Reviews the literature on the nature and use of social support and its role in disease prevention, health maintenance, and the alleviation of the impact of illness on the stricken individual and those close to him.

Literature Review

Understanding what social support is and the process by which it operates will facilitate the development of methods for defining individuals and groups at risk, ways to mobilize resources for such individuals and groups, alternative sources of social support, and cost-effective ways to provide such support to both cancer victim and family.

Should be of particular interest to planners and providers of health care.

484. JOSEPH, Jill Gregory, and S. Leonard Syme. "Social connection and the etiology of cancer: An epidemiological review and discussion." *In* Jerome Cohen, Joseph W. Cullen, L. Robert Martin (Eds.). *Psychosocial Aspects of Cancer.* New York: Raven Press, 1982.

Examines the relationship between social connection and cancer etiology.

Literature Review

Existing studies suggest an association between social connection and cancer etiology. Research methods need to be improved so that sharper, more informed inferences can be drawn.

Should interest social scientists involved in research on the association of social networks, social support, and disease etiology.

d. Dissertation

485. CLARK, Elizabeth J. "The role of social support in adaptation to cancer." Ph.D. dissertation, University of North Carolina at Chapel Hill, 1981.

Examines the relationship between social support and adaptation to cancer.

Research

Results indicated that social support was an important factor with respect to adaptation to cancer. It was shown to have a mediating effect on adaptation, so that persons with decreased support were at increased risk of poor adaptation.

Of interest to rehabilitation specialists and all health care professionals concerned with the treatment of cancer patients.

5. RENAL DISEASE

a. Articles

486. BURTON, H.J., R.M. Lindsay, S.A. Kline. "Social support as
      a mediator of psychological dysfunctioning and a determinant
      of renal failure outcomes." *Clinical and Experimental Dialysis
      and Apheresis* 7 (1983): 371-389.

A study of end stage renal disease and social support to determine
whether social support directly influenced successful continuation of
home dialysis, was related to certain psychological traits, and
affected the mediation of stress associated with the disease.

Research

Social support was not found to be related to the successful continuation of home care, but was related to less introversion, hypochondria-
sis, and anxiety. The role of social support in mediating the
stresses of living with end stage renal disease was unequivocal.

Researchers interested in how psychological adjustment to chronic,
life-threatening diseases is influenced by social support will benefit
from this work.

487. SMITH, Marc D., Barry A. Hong, Michael A. Province, Alan M.
      Robson. "Does social support determine the treatment setting
      for hemodialysis patients?" *American Journal of Kidney
      Diseases* 5 (1985): 27-31.

A study of the effect of social support on the quality and location of
treatment for end-stage renal disease.

Research

The selection of home versus center dialysis was unrelated to the
level of social support available to the patient and appeared to be a
function of the attitudes and actions of clinical staff favoring one
or the other setting.

Health administrators, health services researchers, and others interested in decision theory pertaining to treatment for chronic disease
will benefit from this paper.

6. DIABETES MELLITUS

a. Articles

488. EDELSTEIN, Jacqueline, and Margaret W. Linn. "The influence
      of the family on control of diabetes." *Social Science and
      Medicine* 21 (1985): 541-545.

Evidence suggests that family members can influence the control of adult onset diabetes.

Research

Patients in better control of their disease perceived their families
to be low in conflict and organization and oriented toward achievement. Families with high achievement orientation appeared to stimulate self-responsibility, which is related to better disease control.

Health care providers may find this a useful summary of factors
affecting the control of diabetes.

489. HEITZMANN, Carma A., and Robert M. Kaplan. "Interaction
     between sex and social support in the control of Type II
     diabetes mellitus." *Journal of Consulting and Clinical Psy-
     chology* 52 (1984): 1087-1089.

A study investigating the role of social support in the control of
Type II diabetes mellitus.

Research

In women, satisfaction with supportive relationships was found to be
associated with control of the diabetic state, while, in men, the
converse was found to be true. These results suggest that social
support may operate differently for men than women, and that wives may
have a greater impact on the health behavior of their husbands than
vice versa.

Psychologists, health educators, and others interested in patient
compliance research will benefit from reading this study.

490. PEYROT, Mark, and James F. McMurray, Jr. "Psychosocial
     factors in diabetes control: Adjustment of insulin-treated
     adults." *Psychosomatic Medicine* 47 (1985): 542-557.

Two groups of 10 insulin-treated diabetic adults were studied to
identify psychosocial factors important in blood glucose control. The
groups were similar in composition and sexually balanced, but one was
in "poor" control and the other in "good" control.

Research

Behavioral variables investigated included predisposing, enabling, and
conditioning factors. Psychophysiologic variables were stress-
response factors, including social support and psychologic coping
responses. A strong relationship was found between psychosocial
adjustment and diabetic control, suggesting that adjustment affects
control through both behavioral and psychophysiological mechanisms.
One major implication of the findings is that psychosocial factors
affecting diabetic control cannot be fully understood when studied
separately, as complex relationships among factors would be missed.
Recommendations are made for further studies.

Should interest physicians, clinical researchers, and social scientists.

491. SCHLENK, Elizabeth A., and Laura K. Hart. "Relationship between health locus of control, health value, and social support and compliance of persons with diabetes mellitus." *Diabetes Care* 7 (1984): 566-574.

This study was undertaken to identify the relationship between patient compliance with the diabetes therapeutic regimen and the social learning theory variables of health locus of control, health value, and perceived social support.

Research

A statistically significant relationship was found between compliance and social support, powerful others health locus of control, and internal health locus of control.

Of interest to nurses, physicians, and health educators.

492. SCHWARTZ, Lee S., Joy Springer, Joseph A. Flaherty, Reza Kiani. "The role of recent life events and social support in the control of diabetes mellitus. A pilot study." *General Hospital Psychiatry* 8 (1986): 212-216.

This study evaluated the relationship between recent life events, social support systems, and blood glucose control in diabetic patients.

Research

A higher number of life events was associated with a higher percentage of abnormal fasting blood glucose and glycosylated hemoglobin results, and improved social support was associated with a smaller percentage of abnormal glycosylated hemoglobin scores.

Of interest to physicians and other health care providers working with diabetic patients.

493. SHENKEL, Randee Jae, Joseph P. Rogers, Greg Perfetto, Robert A. Levin. "Importance of 'significant others' in predicting compliance with diabetic regimen." *International Journal of Psychiatry in Medicine* 15 (1985-1986): 149-155.

A psychosocial model of behavioral prediction developed by Fishbein was used to examine compliance interventions among diabetic patients.

Research

How important following the regimen was to "significant others" in a patient's life was a stronger predictor of behavioral intention than were the patient's own beliefs.

Of interest to physicians, nurses, and health educators.

b. Dissertation

494. WIERENGA, Mary E. "The interrelationship between multidimensional health locus of control, knowledge of diabetes, perceived social support, self-reported compliance and therapeutic outcomes six weeks after the adult patient has been diagnosed with diabetes mellitus." Ph.D. dissertation, Michigan State University, 1979.

Examined the relationships of health locus of control, knowledge, social support, and compliance on therapeutic outcomes of adult patients with newly diagnosed diabetes.

Research

Significant associations were found between internal locus of control and social support, compliance and therapeutic outcomes, powerful others' orientation and knowledge, social support and outcomes. Knowledge was positively related to compliance and outcomes, and there was a negative association between compliance and therapeutic outcomes.

Should interest health educators and health providers.

7. ASTHMA

a. Article

495. DE ARANJO, Gilberto, Donald L. Dudley, Paul P. Van Arsdel, Jr. "Psychosocial assets and severity of chronic asthma." *Journal of Allergy and Clinical Immunology* 50 (1972): 257-263.

Examines the effect of psychosocial assets on steroid treatment needs among asthma patients.

Research

Patients with lower psychosocial assets required significantly higher dosages of steroids for their treatment than did patients with more psychosocial assets.

Of interest to psychosomatic researchers, particularly those concerned with the treatment of asthma patients.

b. Dissertation

496. McCARTNEY, Christine M.   "Coping with asthma in adulthood:
      Relationship to severity of asthma and life satisfaction."
      Ph.D. dissertation, Purdue University, 1984.

A study of the impact of chronic asthma on life satisfaction, as
modified by coping strategies, locus of control, and social support.

Research

General findings include a positive association between physical
condition and use of active coping strategies and a significant
correlation between life satisfaction and the number and quality of
social relationships.

Of interest to social and behavioral scientists, in particular,
researchers interested in psychosomatic diseases.

8. RHEUMATOID ARTHRITIS

a. Article

497. LAMBERT, Vickie A.   "Relationships among the factors psycho-
      logical well-being, social support, functional status, and
      demographic characteristics of rheumatoid arthritic women."
      Nursing Research 33 (1984): 50-51.

This study investigated selected factors related to the psychological
well-being of women afflicted with rheumatoid arthritis.

Research

Older women who had had rheumatoid arthritis for a long time were
found to be more dependent on others and tended to have more external
support. Psychological well-being was related to pain and difficulty
in performing tasks.

Nurses and others who care for rheumatoid arthritics will benefit from
this study.

b. Dissertation

498. HEACOCK, Patsy R.   "An analysis of coping strategies and
      social supports of rheumatoid arthritics." Ph.D. dissertation,
      University of Texas at Austin, 1983.

A study of coping strategies, social support systems, and anxiety and
depression among rheumatoid arthritics.

Research

Results indicated that acceptance was the main coping strategy arthritics used to deal with their illness, although other strategies
were also present. Primary groups, in particular, were sources of
social support, community ties were more restricted.

Helpful for rheumatologists, rehabilitation specialists, and others
interested in or involved with rheumatoid arthritics.

9. ACQUIRED IMMUNODEFICIENCY SYNDROME (AIDS)

a. Articles

499. ABRAMS, Donald I., James W. Dilley, Linda M. Maxey, Paul A.
      Volberding. "Routine care and psychosocial support of the
      patient with the acquired immundeficiency syndrome." *Medical
      Clinics of North America* 70, no. 3 (1986): 707-720.

Focuses on routine medical care and psychosocial support of the
patient with AIDS.

Descriptive

A description of the cooperative AIDS program of San Francisco General
Hospital in cooperation with the City of San Francisco and University
of California. A comprehensive, community-based organization for
providing support is described.

Of interest to urologists, oncologists, psychiatrists, nurses, social
workers, allied health professionals, and counselors.

500. WOLCOTT, Deane L. "Psychosocial aspects of acquired immune
      deficiency syndrome and the primary care physician." *Annals
      of Allergy* 57 (1986): 95-102.

Reviews the basic psychosocial principles useful in understanding and
treating individuals with life-threatening illness, the psychosocial
aspects of AIDS, the functional psychiatric and organic mental disorders seen in patients with AIDS-related complex (ARC) and AIDS, the
psychosocial stresses on social network members of AIDS and ARC
patients and on health professionals caring for them, and the primary
physician's role in the care of AIDS and ARC patients.

Review

While the needs and problems of AIDS patients are similar to those of
other young adults with chronic life-threatening illness, multiple
factors create unique patterns of stress for AIDS patients, members of
their social network, and health care personnel. The primary care
physician needs to concern himself with understanding the psychosocial

stresses of AIDS and working with a multidisciplinary team to provide support for the patient and his family.

Of interest to primary care physicians.

501. ――――, Fawzy I. Fawzy, Robert O. Pasnau. "Acquired immune deficiency syndrome (AIDS) and consultation-liaison psychiatry." *General Hospital Psychiatry* 7 (1985): 280-292.

The psychosocial effects of AIDS for patients, family and friends, and health care professionals are discussed.

Descriptive

An integrated multidisciplinary team providing coordinated medical and psychiatric care to patients during inpatient and outpatient phases of treatment should be developed by each institution that treats a significant number of AIDS patients. This approach would greatly facilitate optimal clinical patient care, as well as longitudinal research that is needed to characterize the psychiatric and psychosocial problems of AIDS patients more fully.

Of interest to virologists, consultation and liaison psychiatrists, social workers, nurses, and other health professionals caring for AIDS patients.

502. WOLCOTT, Deane L., Sheila Namir, Fawzy I. Fawzy, Michael S. Gottlieb, Ronald T. Mitsuyasu. "Illness concerns, attitudes towards homosexuality and social support in gay men with AIDS." *General Hospital Psychiatry* 8 (1986): 395-403.

A study of 50 gay men, recently diagnosed with AIDS, to document health status, psychologic status, and aspects of social support in patients with life-threatening illness.

Research

Subjects reported levels of illness-related concerns comparable to those of previously studied cancer patients, attitudes towards homosexuality similar to those of previously studied healthy homosexual males, variable social support needs, variable satisfaction with specific types of social support, and moderately small social networks. Illness concerns, attitudes toward homosexuality, and social support satisfaction were significantly correlated with each other, with previously reported levels of psychologic distress, and with subjective (but not objective) measures of health status.

Of interest to social scientists, especially researchers of social support, and physicians working with AIDS patients.

b. Dissertation

503. BECHTEL, Gregory A. "Purpose-in-life and social support in gay men with the Acquired Immunodeficiency Syndrome." Ph.D. dissertation, Texas Woman's University, Denton, Texas, 1986.

An investigation of the relationship between purpose-in-life and social support in gay men with AIDS and gay men who may be at risk for developing AIDS.

Research

Results demonstrated a significant difference between purpose-in-life scores in the two groups of gay men, although there was no significant difference in their social support scores. Income was found to be the only variable consistently related to social support.

Of interest to AIDS researchers, public health professionals, health educators, nurses, social workers, and gay organizations.

10. HERPESVIRUS

a. Articles

504. GLASER, Ronald, Janice K. Kiecolt-Glaser, Carl E. Speicher, Jane E. Holliday. "Stress, loneliness, and changes in herpesvirus latency." *Journal of Behavioral Medicine* 8 (1985): 249-260.

A prospective design was used to examine the influence of examination stress and loneliness on herpesvirus latency.

Research

High-loneliness subjects had significantly higher Epstein-Barr virus antibody titers than low-loneliness subjects. Data suggest that stress-related immunosuppression can significantly modulate herpesvirus latency.

Of interest to social and behavioral scientists and physicians.

505. MANNE, Sharon, Irwin Sandler, Alex Zautra. "Coping and adjustment to genital herpes: The effects of time and social support." *Journal of Behavioral Medicine* 9 (1986): 163-177.

This study investigated the effects of the passage of time and of membership in a self-help group on coping behaviors and distress among people with genital herpes.

Research

Results indicated that people employed fewer coping strategies with increasing time since the onset of the stressor. This pattern was particularly clear in non-support-group subjects. Support-group members did not exhibit as significant a decrease in the use of coping strategies or as great an improvement in the level of depression and the degree bothered by herpes over time.

Of interest to physicians, psychologists, preventive medicine specialists, and social workers.

506. SILVER, Paul S., Stephen M. Auerbach, Nahum Vishneavsky, Lisa G. Kaplowitz. "Psychological factors in recurrent genital herpes infection: Stress, coping style, social support, emotional dysfunction, and symptom recurrence." *Journal of Psychosomatic Research* 30 (1986): 163-171.

The relationship among stress, coping style, emotional dysfunction, social support, and severity of symptoms was investigated in females and males suffering from severe cases of genital herpes.

Research

Negative life stress was unrelated to psychopathology, and was associated only with duration among the symptom measures. Regression analyses indicated that higher frequencies of recurrence and greater symptom discomfort were associated with an external locus of control, a tendency to use emotion-focused wishful thinking, and avoiding the use of cognitive strategies to cope with the stress of herpes.

Of interest to internists and family physicians.

11. OTHER MEDICAL PROBLEMS

a. Articles

507. GIERSZEWSKI, Susan Abbott. "The relationship of weight-loss, locus of control, and social support." *Nursing Research* 32 (1983): 43-47.

A study investigating the relationship between weight loss, locus of control, and social support.

Research

A negative relationship between social support and weight reduction was found in women with internal locus of control. The results are discussed and recommendations given for health professionals planning weight reduction programs.

Will interest general audiences, health professionals, and others working in weight loss programs.

508. LEIMKÜHLER, Anne M. "Familie und chronische krankheit.
     Ein überblick über die neuere familien-und medi-
     zinsociologische forschung unter besonderer berück-
     sichtigung der chorea Huntington." (German) *Fortschritte
     in Neurologie und Psychiatrie* 53 (1985): 105-116.

Discusses the importance of social support and social networks for the
care and rehabilitation of chronically ill patients. Includes a
special section on Huntington's chorea patients.

Review

Offers a sociological analysis of concepts commonly used in research
on the social relationships of chronically ill patients. Problems
with concepts like family structure, family dynamics, and family
systems are discussed. A note on methodological issues concludes this
paper.

Should be very useful to social scientists interested in social
support research, and helpful to rehabilitation specialists, particularly those working with Huntington's chorea patients.

509. MAGILVY, Joan K. "Quality of life of hearing-impaired older
     women." *Nursing Research* 34 (1985): 140-144.

An examination of the major influences on the quality of life experienced by older hearing-impaired women, and a comparison of those who
were prevocationally deaf and those who had a later onset of significant hearing loss.

Research

Sixty-six hearing impaired women, aged 54 to 96, including 27
prevocationally deaf and 39 later onset subjects, were interviewed.
Predictors of quality of life included age, age at onset of hearing
loss, financial adequacy, social hearing handicap, perceived health,
and functional social support. A causal model was specified that
proposed that health, social support, hearing handicap, and financial
adequacy would directly affect quality of life as well as mediate the
effect of the demographic variables, age, and age at onset of loss on
this outcome. Results of the path analysis showed the best predictors
of quality of life to be social hearing handicap, functional social
support, and perceived health. The later onset group had an overall
lower perception of quality of life, this relationship being mediated
as predicted.

Should interest health professionals and social scientists.

510. MORGAN, M., D. Patrick, J. Charlton. "Social support and
     the course of disability." *Journal of Epidemiology and Com-
     munity Health* 37 (1983): 161-162.

The relationship between social support and the course of disability was examined in a sample of 585 people, age 45-75, living at home and having some functional limitation or activity restriction.

Research Abstract

A low level of social contact was significantly associated with deterioration in psychosocial disability over a two year period and, in both psychosocial and emotional disability, over a 12 month period, with the effect of the level of support being greatest in the presence of adverse life events. There was no significant relationship between the level of emotional support and the course of disability.

Of interest to rehabilitation counselors.

511. ORY, Marcia G., T. Franklin Williams, Marian Emr, et al. "Families, informal supports, and Alzheimer's disease. Current research and future agendas." *Research on Aging* 7 (1985): 623-644.

Reviews the current state of knowledge regarding how families and other social supports affect and are affected by Alzheimer's disease (AD) and related disorders, and suggests future directions for research.

Literature Review

Background knowledge of the epidemiology, diagnosis, classification, etiology, and treatment of Alzheimer's disease, and of systems of care is important for understanding how familial and other informal support factors relate to Alzheimer's disease. Current knowledge about AD patients and their families is based on small nonrepresentative samples and should not be considered definitive. Future research on families, informal supports, and AD should include studies on: a) the availability of family members to care for AD patients; b) caregivers' perception of and response to symptoms of AD; c) the influence of familial factors on the onset and/or exacerbation of AD symptoms; d) the burden of AD on caregivers; and e) informal and formal resources.

Of interest to health professionals, particularly geriatricians and social science researchers.

512. PATRICK, Donald L., Myfanwy Morgan, John R.H. Charlton. "Psychosocial support and change in the health status of physically disabled people." *Social Science and Medicine* 22 (1986): 1347-1354.

An exploration of the influence of different types of psychosocial support on different types of disability experienced by community residents with a physically disabling illness.

Research

A high level of social contact had a more protective effect on the physical functioning of respondents with arthritis or heart trouble who also reported depression. The level of emotional intimacy was not a significant influence on reported health status change. Confiding relationships do not appear to be important for adults with pre-existing illness who are not at significant risk of developing stress-related conditions.

Of interest to social and behavioral scientists.

513. STOTTS, R. Craig, and Beverly A. Hall. "Formal and informal bases of support for families of persons with Alzheimer's: A position paper." *Archives of the Foundation of Thanatology* 12 (1986): 23-.

Analyzes the societal trends that have particular relevance to the situation in which families of Alzheimer's victims find themselves.

Analytical

Attention is given to both the informal and formal support systems available to the families of Alzheimer's victims. The responsibilities of communities and societies in providing access to support services and promoting the overall health of the affected individuals and families are juxtaposed against the families' responsibilities. Recommendations are made for changes in health policies and decision making processes.

Of interest to health professionals, social workers, and public policymakers.

514. WEINBERGER, Morris, Sharon L. Hiner, William M. Tierney. "Improving functional status in arthritis: The effect of social support. *Social Science and Medicine* 23 (1986): 899-904.

Data from a longitudinal study of patients with symptomatic osteoarthritis testing the hypothesis that social support, provided by telephone interviewers, may improve the patients' functional status.

Research

After six months of receiving bi-weekly telephone calls from interviewers inquiring about stressors they had experienced and their self-assessment of their health, the patients' functional status (physical disability, psychological disability, and pain) improved significantly. In addition, the patients reported more social support at six months than at baseline, suggesting that the telephone interviews were viewed as a source of support by elderly persons who may have a support deficit. Suggestions are made for future studies involving telephone interviewers to further enhance social support and provide greater potential for improving patients' health status.

Should interest geriatricians, gerontologists, and social workers.

515. WILLIAMS, K., V. Bahlinger, B. Heroman, D. Madrigal, P. Brantley. "The relationship between perceived social support and illness reports in Hansen's disease patients." *International Journal of Leprosy* 53 (1985): 162-163.

Examines the relationship of social support to patients' reports of physical symptoms in Hansen's disease patients.

Research Abstract

Results indicated that perceptions regarding the quality of social relationships were significantly related to the number of physical symptoms they endorsed on the physical symptom checklist. The actual number of social contacts appeared to be a far less important determinant of illness reports.

Should interest physicians as well as researchers in the social and behavioral sciences.

b. Dissertations

516. BROWNE, Susan E. "Social networks, social support, and general well-being of lesbians with chronic illness or hidden disabilities." D.N.Sc. dissertation, University of California, San Francisco, 1985.

A study of the relationships of lesbian and chronic illness identities, social networks, and social support to general well-being.

Research

Results indicated complex relationships between lesbian identity, chronic illness identity, network structure, nature of relationships with network members, and general well-being. Availability of network support and knowledge of lesbian identity were important determinants of support for chronic illness.

Should interest nurses, social workers, and social scientists.

517. SUNDE, Carol R. "Social support and adaptation to an ostomy: An examination of members and nonmembers of a medical mutual aid group." Ph.D. dissertation, University of Southern California, 1985.

Examines the influence of formal and informal sources of social support on mental health and functional status indices following an ostomy.

Research

Social support and stress had direct effects on the health and functional status measures, but no interactive effect was found. Members of the mutual aid group experienced relatively better adaptation than nonmembers.

Of interest to social and behavioral scientists, and to rehabilitation specialists, particularly those working with ostomy patients.

12. REHABILITATION

a. Books

518. ANGERMEYER, Matthias C., and Hellmuth Freyberger (Eds.). *Chronisch kranke erwachsene in der familie.* (German) Stuttgart: Ferdinand Euke, 1982.

An overview of research on the role of the family in the treatment and/or rehabilitation of chronically ill patients.

Book of Readings

Each chapter focuses on a particular chronic condition (e.g., arthritis or cancer) or treatment (e.g., dialysis), and provides information on research that has been conducted on the family situation of chronically ill patients. Most chapters concentrate on how the family can contribute to the post-hospitalization care and rehabilitation of these patients. A variety of physical illnesses are discussed.

Of special interest to physicians, rehabilitation specialists, medical psychologists, and medical sociologists.

b. Articles

519. CLUFF, Claudia B., and Leighton E. Cluff. "Informal support for disabled persons: A role for religious and community organizations." *Journal of Chronic Diseases* 36 (1983): 815–820.

Discusses the need for informal support systems for the disabled.

Theoretical

The treatment and care provided by the formal health care system are not sufficient to meet all the needs of the disabled; therefore, a better organized informal, volunteer support system should be developed. Religious and community organizations, in particular, are suggested as appropriate providers of that type of informal support.

For all those interested in rehabilitation, community health care planning, and health care delivery.

520. DAVIDSON, Terrence N., M. Leora Bowden, Daniel Tholen, Michael H. James, Irving Feller. "Social support and post-burn adjustment." *Archives of Physical Medicine and Rehabilitation* 62 (1981): 274-278.

Interviews were conducted with 314 persons who had sustained burns and were treated at a major burn center between 1956 and 1976.

Research

The data indicate that social support is both directly and indirectly related to patient's post-burn adjustment. Measures of social support from family, friends, and peers were significantly related to several subjectively assessed outcomes, such as life satisfaction, self-esteem, and participation in social and recreational activities.

Of interest to rehabilitation specialists, nurses, surgeons specializing in the treatment of burns, and social workers.

521. EL-ISLAM, M.F. "Rehabilitation of schizophrenics by the extended family." *Acta Psychiatrica Scandinavia* 65 (1982): 112-119.

Describes the patterns of care of extended and nuclear families for their members.

Research

A study of 540 Arab schizophrenic outpatients found the extended family to be more tolerant than the nuclear family of patients' minor behavioral abnormalities and temporary withdrawals, and more helpful in the supervision of medication taking, social adjustment and leisure activities. Nuclear family members were more likely to tax the patients' emotional resources and limited repertoire of social skills.

Psychiatrists, psychologists, and social workers interested in cross-national research will find this a very interesting and enlighting study.

522. LIFCHEZ, Raymond. "The environment as a support system for independent living." *Archives of Physical Medicine and Rehabilitation* 60 (1979): 467-476.

This study of the support provided by the environment to physically disabled young adults presents a very new way of conceptualizing social support, reviewing issues of the relationships between physical form and social support in the physical environment.

Research

One hundred and fifty physically disabled young adults living independently were interviewed to determine the psychosocial accommodation of their physical environment to supporting the behavioral needs of the whole person. Mayer Spivak's construct of "archetypal place" is used to describe the behaviors supported there, such as shelter supports, emotional recuperation, and social contact.

Should interest social scientists and rehabilitation specialists.

523. NEW, Peter Kong-Ming, Anthony T. Ruscio, Rhea Pendergrass Priest, Dora Petritsi, Linda A. George. "The social structure of heart and stroke patients: A study of the role of significant others in patient rehabilitation." *Social Science and Medicine* 2 (1968): 185-200.

Concerned with the 'presentation of the self' by 48 heart and stroke patients subsequent to their discharge from a rehabilitation institute.

Research

Even though patients can identify those whom they felt have helped them most, and presumably this would mean some degree of consensus between the patients and their helpers, those significant others are not all in agreement with the patients' capabilities. Lacking this degree of consensus, the significant others may attribute to the patient more or less independence. When this occurs, one can anticipate adjustment problems for the patient.

Of interest to health professionals working with heart and stroke patients.

524. PALMER, Sally, Lino Canzona, John Conley, George Wells. "Vocational adaptation of patients on home dialysis: Its rela tionship to personality, activities and support received." *Journal of Psychosomatic Research* 27 (1983): 201-207.

A study of psychosocial characteristics associated with the vocational adaptation of home dialysis patients.

Research

Only support received from household members was associated with good adaptation. Support from the dialysis team seemed to have the opposite effect. Social introversion was found to be the best predictor of vocational adaptation.

Of interest to health professionals working in home dialysis teams, and to rehabilitation specialists in general.

525. ROBERTSON, El Dora K., and Richard M. Suinn. "Determination of the rate of progress of stroke victims through empathy measures of patients and family." *Journal of Psychosomatic Research* 12 (1968): 189-191.

This study was concerned with the role of empathy in rehabilitation progress.

Research

Improved rates of progress were associated with higher ability of the subjects in predicting the attitudes of others. The results point to the necessity of attending to the psychosocial aspects of the patient and his family.

Of interest to physical and occupational therapists and other health professionals working with rehabilitating patients.

526. SCHULZ, Richard, and Susan Decker. "Long term adjustment to physical disability--the role of social support, perceived control, and self-blame." *Journal of Personality and Social Psychology* 48 (1985): 1162-1172.

Interviews of 100 middle-aged and elderly spinal-cord-injured persons, conducted an average of 20 years after the disability occurred, collected data on perceived control attributions of blame and the nature of social comparisons made by the respondents.

Research

Respondents reported levels of well-being only slightly lower than the population means of nondisabled persons of similar age for all three outcome measures. After controlling for health status and current income, it was found that persons who have high levels of social support, are satisfied with their social contacts, and feel they have high levels of perceived control report high levels of well-being. Self-blame and the perceived avoidability of the cause of the disability correlated only moderately with the three measures of adjustment, suggesting that there are important differences between coping successfully immediately following a traumatic event and coping successfully many years later.

Of interest to social and behavioral scientists, social workers, and mental health professionals.

527. SMITH, Richard T. "Rehabilitation of the disabled: The roles of social networks in the recovery process." *International Rehabilitation Medicine* 1 (1979): 63-72.

This study examines the role of informal and formal intervention systems utilized by the chronically disabled in the process of rehabilitation and recovery.

Research

In addition to formal community resources (agents and agencies), the disabled tend to rely on informal social networks (family and peers) as sources of support in the recovery process. The findings focus on the extent to which formal interventions and informal resources are supportive of the disabled and the effect of these support systems on outcome.

Of interest to rehabilitation specialists.

c. Chapters

528. BADURA, Bernhard, Josef Bauer, Gary Kaufhold, Harald Lehmann, Millard Waltz. "Herzinfarctrehabilitation und soziale unterstützung. Erste ergebnisse der oldenburger longitudinalstudie." (German) *In* Christian von Ferber, and Bernhard Bandura (Eds.). *Laienpotential, Patientenaktivierung und Gesundheitsselbsthilfe.* Munchen: R. Oldenbourg Verlag, 1983.

A study of the effects of psychosocial stressors and supports during rehabilitation from myocardial infarction.

Research

Patients who reported a good marriage were much less depressed and anxious after an MI than patients who were unmarried or reported a bad marriage. Social support from the patient's spouse and adult children was found to be positively associated with general well-being immediately following an MI and after 6 months of rehabilitation. Lack of support from family members was positively related to a negative emotional state after MI.

Of particular interest to social scientists interested in psychosomatic medicine, rehabilitation specialists, and cardiologists.

529. BRODY, Elaine M. "Informal supports systems in the rehabilitation of the disabled elderly." *In* Stanley J. Brody, and George E. Ruff (Eds.). *Aging and Rehabilitation: Advances in the State of the Art.* New York: Springer, 1986.

Discusses the impact on the family of a disabled elderly family member, and the family's role in his/her rehabilitation.

Review

Families provide 80 to 90 percent of medically related care and home nursing, personal care, household maintenance, transportation, and shopping for elderly disabled relatives, as well as the "expressive" support that is the form of help most wanted by the elderly, with little help from the formal support system. The rehabilitation team needs to recognize that family members are at risk of mental and physical problems if their caring roles become unduly stressful and provide counseling or referral to community agencies that provide family-focused services, such as respite care, day hospitals, and day care centers, which offer "formal" patient and family support.

Of interest to rehabilitation specialists, gerontologists, geriatricians, social workers, and mental health professionals.

530. BRODY, Stanley J. "Impact of the formal support system on rehabilitation of the elderly." *In* Stanley J. Brody, and George E. Ruff (Eds.). *Aging and Rehabilitation: Advances in the State of the Art.* New York: Springer, 1986.

Discusses the formal support system for the physically and mentally

disabled elderly, the scarcity of social support programs for these
people, and the needs that must be met to improve the quality of their
lives.

Review

Public programs provide for acute care medical and income maintenance
needs of the physically and mentally disabled elderly, but there are
few social support programs: rehabilitation services that go beyond
medical treatment are sparse. Public policy needs to recognize and
support the psychosocial needs of the elderly and the elderly disabled
and their families and build upon the accomplishments that have been
achieved in lengthening life by improving the quality of the lives
that have been lengthened.

Of interest to rehabilitation specialists and public policymakers.

531. SMITH, Richard T. "Disability and the recovery process: Role
      of social networks." *In* E. Gartly Jaco (Ed.). *Patients,
      Physicians and Illness.* Third edition. New York: Free
      Press, 1979.

This study is both a replication and an extension of studies relating
socially supportive networks to rehabilitation and recovery of the
disabled in society.

Research

Results include an analysis of the extent to which social networks
affect the recovery of disabled adults with chronic conditions, and
the role of informal networks in this process. Other findings relate
to the role of the formal intervention system, specifically vocational
rehabilitation services, in improving outcome.

Of interest to rehabilitation counselors, physical and occupational
therapists, and social and behavioral scientists.

d. Dissertations

532. ALTMAN, Barbara H. "Examination of the effects of individual,
      primary and secondary resources on the outcomes of impair-
      ment." Ph.D. dissertation, University of Maryland, 1984.

Identifies supportive resources available to impaired individuals and
examines their effect on physical, social, and psychological outcomes.

Research

Individual resources, such as age and race, were significantly predictive of impairment outcomes. Some evidence was found that primary
resources, such as family social support, moderated disability, but
the effects of rehabilitation and financial assistance were less
clear.

Particularly useful for rehabilitation specialists.

533. BRUGGE, Patricia A.   "The relationship between family as a social support system, health status, and exercise of self-care agency in the adult with a chronic illness." Ph.D. dissertation, Wayne State University, 1981.

Descriptive study of the influence of family support and health status on the exercise of self-care agency among the chronically ill.

Research

Family as a support system showed a moderate, but significant, positive (linear) relationship with the exercise of self-care agency. Health-related dysfunction was moderately inversely associated with exercise of self-care agency.

Interesting for health care professionals working with chronically ill patients, the patients' families and friends, and rehabilitation specialists.

534. DECKER, Susan D.   "Social support and well-being in middle-aged and elderly spinal cord injured persons: A social-psychological analysis." Ph.D. dissertation, Portland State University, 1982.

A study of factors contributing to the well-being of middle-aged and elderly community-residing spinal cord injured persons.

Research

Severity of injury was not significantly associated with subjective well-being. High levels of well-being were correlated with favorable social conditions, amount of perceived control over one's life, self-reported health status, and social support.

Valuable to rehabilitation specialists and to patients with spinal cord injuries and their families.

535. McLEROY, Kenneth R.   "The effects of social support on physical functioning at six months in a hospitalized stroke population." Ph.D. dissertation, University of North Carolina at Chapel Hill, 1982.

Examines the influence of social support on rehabilitation from stroke.

Research

Results indicated complex relationships between social support/network variables and rehabilitation outcomes.

Of special interest to rehabilitation specialists and professionals concerned with the treatment of stroke patients.

536. SMITH, Patricia A. "Adjustment to spinal cord injury: Social
      support, locus of control, time since onset of injury."
      Ph.D. dissertation, Ohio State University, 1984.

Investigates the effect of social support, health locus of control,
and time since onset of injury on adjustment to injury.

Research

Social support was a significant, positive predictor of successful
adjustment and "Powerful Others Health Locus of Control" was a significant negative predictor.

Should interest rehabilitation specialists and social scientists.

CHAPTER 4

SOCIAL SUPPORT, MENTAL HEALTH,
AND MENTAL ILLNESS

1. MENTAL HEALTH AND PSYCHOLOGICAL WELL-BEING

a. Book

537. CAPLAN, Ruth, in collaboration with Gerald Caplan, David E.
Richards, Anson Phelps Stokes, Jr. *Helping the Helpers to
Help: Mental Health Consultation to Aid Clergymen in Pastoral
Work*. New York: The Seabury Press, 1972.

Describes a mental health consultation program designed to support
clergy in the management of cases within their congregations in which
mental health issues arise that are beyond their usual expertise.

Text

Describes the development of a collaborative program of the Episcopal
Diocese of Massachusetts and the Harvard Laboratory of Community
Psychiatry, beginning with a brief history; discusses the theory and
techniques of mental health consultation, using case presentations as
illustrations; and describes the impact of the program and its continuing evolution.

Very important to clergy and others working in the community mental
health movement.

b. Articles

538. ANDERSON, Donna and Rita Braito. "The mental health of the
never-married: Social protection, social reaction, and social
selection models." *Alternative Lifestyles* 4 (1981): 108-124.

Reviews research relevant to mental health and marital status as it pertains to never-marrieds.

Review and Analytical

The mental health of never-marrieds is examined from the perspective of three popular models of mental health--the social protection, social reaction, and social selection models--each of which offers competing explanations for differences in rates between married and unmarried people and between unmarried men and women. Recent data have questioned the long-held belief that never-marrieds are less mentally healthy than married people. The authors of this article conclude that the mental health of the never-married is a very complex and superficially charted area. Methodological problems and current gaps in research are pointed out, and suggestions are offered for improving research on the mental health of the never-married.

Should interest social scientists and mental health professionals.

539. BANKOFF, Elizabeth A. "Effects of friendship support on the psychological well-being of widows." *Research in the Interweave of Social Roles* 2 (1981): 109-139.

Deals with the importance of friendship and other interpersonal support on the psychological well-being of widows.

Literature Review and Research

Describes the role of the social network in the adaptation to widowhood, and presents the results of a study of the indicators of psychological distress in the crisis and transition stages of loss.

Useful to sociologists and others working with the widowed and the elderly.

540. BILLINGS, Andrew G., and Rudolf H. Moos. "Social support and functioning among community and clinical groups: A panel model." *Journal of Behavioral Medicine* 5 (1982): 295-311.

An examination of the relationship between social support and personal functioning in a longitudinal assessment of a representative sample of community men and women.

Research

Although there was considerable temporal stability in several indices of support and personal functioning, changes in levels of support during the follow-up period were associated with changes in functioning. These relationships varied according to the individual's gender and source of support.

Useful to researchers in the area of stress and social support.

541. BOWERS, Clint A., and Ellis L. Gesten. "Social support as a buffer of anxiety." *American Journal of Community Psychology* 14 (1986): 447-451.

The anxiety-buffering role of social support was investigated using an experimental analogue.

Research

Subjects accompanied by a friend showed a smaller increase in state anxiety than those in the other two groups. There was no group difference on the Palmar Sweat Measure. No significant relationship between perceived social support and changes in state anxiety was found.

Of interest to psychologists.

542. CHAPMAN, Nancy J., and Marie Beaudet. "Environmental predictors of well-being for at-risk older adults in a mid-sized city." *Journal of Gerontology* 38 (1983): 237-244.

Examines the influence of the physical and social environment on well-being.

Research

Several environmental factors were associated with general well-being in this study sample, in particular, living in quiet, well-maintained residential neighborhoods outside the center of the city. This type of neighborhood appeared to stimulate interaction with neighbors, family, and friends.

Should be useful to social epidemiologists and health care planners.

543. D'ARCY, Carl, and C.M. Siddique. "Social support and mental health among mothers of preschool and school-age children." *Social Psychiatry* 19 (1984): 155-162.

Examines the mental health functions of spouse and community support in a sample of mothers with preschool and school age children.

Research

The results indicate that mothers with strong spouse support have better mental health than those without spouse support. Community support is protective and moderately correlated only in the absence of spouse support.

Useful to mental health researchers and community psychologists.

544. ECKENRODE, John. "The mobilization of social supports: Some individual constraints." *American Journal of Community Psychology* 1 (1983): 509-528.

Examines the relationship of locus of control and help-seeking beliefs, along with sociodemographic variables, on the mobilization of social support.

Research

Supports the importance of internal locus of control, higher income and education, and membership in the dominant culture as critical in the mobilization of social support and help-seeking behavior in general.

Community psychiatrists and others working with neighborhood health centers or disadvantaged groups will benefit from this paper.

545.   FISCHER, Pamela J., Sam Shapiro, William R. Breakey, James C. Anthony, Morton Kramer. "Mental health and social characteristics of the homeless: A survey of mission users." *American Journal of Public Health* 76 (1986): 519-524.

Selected mental health and social characteristics of 51 homeless persons drawn as a probability sample from missions are compared to those of 1,338 men, aged 18-64 years, living in households.

Research

Differences between the two groups were small with respect to age, race, education, and military service, but the differences in mental health status, utilization patterns, and social dysfunction were large. Social dysfunction among the homeless was indicated by fewer social contacts and higher rates of arrests as adults than among domiciled men.

Of interest to social and behavioral scientists, mental health professionals and public health professionals.

546.   FRANKEL, B. Gail, and R. Jay Turner. "Psychological adjustment in chronic disabilities--the role of social support in the case of the hearing impaired." *Canadian Journal of Sociology* 8 (1983): 273-291.

Concerned with psychological adjustment among a group of individuals with hearing impairment acquired in adulthood.

Research

Social support, measured in a variety of ways, is the most important predictor of psychological adjustment. Another predictor is the experience of handicap or social disruption related to hearing loss.

Of interest to rehabilitation counselors and health professionals working with the hearing impaired.

547. GILHOOLY, Mary L.M.   "The impact of caregiving and care-
     givers: Factors associated with the psychological well-being of
     people supporting a dementing relative in the community."
     British Journal of Medical Psychology 57 (1984): 35-44.

This paper presents findings concerning a variety of factors expected
to influence, either directly or indirectly as mediators, the psychological well-being of persons caring for a dementing relative in the
community.

Research

Sex of dependent, sex of supporter, satisfaction with help from
relatives, blood/role relationship, duration of care, frequency of
visits from a home help and community nurse were significantly correlated with supporters' morale and mental health. The directions of
these correlations were not as expected, e.g. the longer the duration
of caregiving the higher the supporters' morale and the better the
supporters' mental health.

Of interest to mental health professionals.

548. HIRSH, Barton J., and Bruce D. Rapkin.   "Multiple roles,
     social networks, and women's well-being." *Journal of Person-
     ality and Social Psychology*. 51 (1986): 1237-1247.

Concerned with the frequency and conditions under which both positive
and negative outcomes of multiple roles occur.

Research

Using data from a random sample of 235 married female nurses, this
study focused on marital and job satisfaction as important criteria in
managing multiple roles. Cluster analysis identified five different
profiles of marital and job satisfaction, which were found to be
meaningfully associated with measures of psychological symptomatology
and overall life satisfaction. When linkages were considered between
the profiles and measures of social support and social rejection
provided by five key network·members, the strongest univariate profile
discriminator was found to be the level of work rejection from the
spouse, which was even more powerful when compared to that received
from the next closest family member.

Of interest to social scientists.

549. HUGHES, Michael, and Walter R. Gove.   "Living alone, social
     integration and mental health." *American Journal of Sociology*
     87 (1981): 48-74.

Examines the impact of living alone on mental health, mental well-being, and maladaptive behaviors.

Research

Living alone was not found to result from previous psychological problems or other adverse factors, and was not necessarily associated with an increase in mental health problems, but unmarried persons living alone were more likely to use drugs and alcohol than other unmarried persons. A framework is provided for the effects of social integration on mental health.

Useful to sociologists interested in social networks and mental health.

550. HUNTER, Kathleen, Margaret W. Linn, Rachel Harris, Theodore C. Pratt. "Living arrangements and well-being in elderly women." *Experimental Aging Research* 5 (1979): 523-535.

The present study examined the relationship between three types of living situations and various measures of functioning.

Research

Women living alone were found to have lower life satisfaction, lower self-esteem, and higher social dysfunction than those living with a spouse or others. No differences were found with respect to depression, somatization, diet, or activity level. There was a significant interaction effect between race and living arrangement with respect to anxiety, with blacks less anxious than whites when living with others and more anxious when living alone or with only a spouse.

Of interest to gerontologists and social and behavioral scientists.

551. INSEL, Paul M. "Task force report: The social climate of mental health." *Community Mental Health Journal* 16 (1980): 62-78.

Focuses on the contributions the field of social ecology can make to understanding and assessing the social environment, with special reference to the prevention of mental illness.

Theoretical

Intervention in the social environment for the prevention of mental illness calls for an adequate concept of the environmental effects of mental health; a classification method for measuring and comparing different environments; a knowledge of the relationships between environmental variables and behavioral or psychological outcomes; and a way of determining the most effective interventions.

Of interest to social and behavioral scientists.

552. MITCHELL, Roger E., and Christine A. Hudson. "Coping with domestic violence: Social support and psychological health among battered women." *American Journal of Community Psychology* 11, no. 6 (1983): 629-654.

Examines the impact of stress, personal resources, social support, institutional responsiveness, and coping upon the psychological health of battered women.

Research

Increased levels of violence, minimal personal resources, lack of institutional or other social support, and avoidant coping styles were related to low self-esteem and continued fear.

Psychologists, social workers, and counselors will benefit from this paper.

553. O'CONNOR, Gail. "Presidential address 1983--Social support of mentally retarded persons." *Mental Retardation* 21 (1983): 187-196.

This presidential address focuses on the concept of social support and its importance for the adequate functioning of both the individual and the family.

Review

The quality of social relationships and interactions are vital to a real community of spirit. The author stresses that individuals working with the mentally retarded gain a better understanding of social support and social networks.

Of particular interest to persons working with the mentally retarded.

554. ROOK, Karen A. "The negative side of social interaction: Impact on psychological well-being." *Journal of Personality and Social Psychology* 46 (1984): 1097-1108.

Evidence is provided suggesting that social interaction can have a negative impact on well-being.

Research

This study of 120 widowed women found that negative social outcomes of interaction were more consistently and strongly related to well-being than were positive social outcomes. The degree of social involvement, background characteristics, and the quality of social ties were unrelated to this main effect or finding.

Those involved in designing social network interventions will benefit from this article.

555. SCHULTZ, B.J., and D.H. Saklofske. "Relationship between social support and selected measures of psychological well-being." *Psychological Reports* 53 (1983): 847-850.

A study of social support and loneliness, stress, locus of control, and psychological impairment.

Research

Social support as a general construct was not found to correlate with
any of the psychological variables, although helpfulness was a distinguishing factor in high and low levels of loneliness.

Psychologists and others interested in the psychological effects of
social support will find this an interesting study.

556. SYROTUIK, John, and Carl D'Arcy. "Social support and mental
      health: Direct, protective and compensatory effects." *Social
      Science and Medicine* 18 (1984): 229-236.

This study deals with the relationship between social support and
mental health.

Research

Results indicated that spousal support generally had more important
implications for psychological well-being than did community support.
However, the relative impact of these different sources of support
appeared to be related to the degree to which the mental health
symptomology reported was defined. Spousal support was found to
moderate the relationship between certain job strains (pressure) and
mental health. No protective effects were found for community
support.

Of interest to social and behavioral scientists and mental health
professionals.

557. TRAN, Thanh Van, and Roosevelt Wright, Jr. "Social support
      and subjective well-being among Vietnamese refugees." *Social
      Service Review* 60 (1986): 449-459.

This study attempts to identify the causal predictors of subjective
well-being among Vietnamese refugees in the United States.

Research

Social support, social interaction anxiety, family income, and mental
status were found to have significant direct effects on Vietnamese
refugees' sense of well-being.

Of interest to sociologists, anthropologists, and psychologists.

558. TURNBULL, C. "Work status preference and social support--
      effects on well-being in women." *Bulletin of the British
      Psychological Society* 37 (November 1984): 141.

An investigation of the possible protective affects of work on
self-reported well-being in married women.

Research Abstract

The mediating effect of social support and of preferred work status was explored. Emotional support was found to have a significant effect on self-esteem and tension.

Should interest mental health professionals.

559. TURNER, R. Jay. "Social support as a contingency in psychological well-being." *Journal of Health and Social Behavior* 22 (1981): 357-367.

A study of the relationship between social support and psychological well-being in diverse populations.

Research

A modest, but reliable association, found to exist between social support and well-being, was found to be reciprocal. Social support had an important direct effect on well-being, independent of levels of stress, but these relationships were not the same in all populations.

Should interest social and behavioral scientists.

560. WILLER, Barry, and James Intagliata. "Social-environmental factors as predictors of adjustment of deinstitutionalized mentally retarded adults." *American Journal of Mental Deficiency* 86 (1981): 252-259.

Mentally retarded adults from five state institutions were studied two to four years after they were placed in either foster family care or community residences.

Research

Multiple regression analysis revealed that social-environmental factors and other characteristics of community settings played an important role in individuals' adjustment. Individual level of functioning had little or no bearing on social support. Larger family care homes were more likely to encourage social support. In community residential facilities, younger residents were more likely to have social support from outside the home.

Of interest to mental health professionals, social workers, and personnel working with state mental health/mental retardation organizations.

c. Dissertations

561. BURRELL, Deanna L. "General well-being and use of social support." Dr.P.H. dissertation, University of Texas Health Science Center, School of Public Health, 1983.

A study of levels of self-perceived well-being and the use of formal or informal sources of social support.

Research

The data showed some evidence that perceived well-being is related to use of social support. Persons with low perceived well-being were more likely to use formal and/or informal sources of social support.

Of interest to social and behavioral scientists. ·

562. FRIESEN, Marilyn R.   "Unemployment and the relationship between social support and individual and family health." Ph.D. dissertation, California School of Professional Psychology, Fresno, 1983.

Investigates the mediating effect of social support on the relationship between unemployment and physical and psychological health.

Research

One component of social support, directive guidance, was related to lowered anxiety and depression among unemployed men and their wives. Support satisfaction led to lower symptom levels.

Should be of particular interest to stress researchers.

563. JONES, Betty B.   "Mental health and the structure of support." Ph.D. dissertation, University of Michigan, 1981.

Examined the structural dimensions of social support and the way in which these dimensions affected mental health in a national sample of 652 women, following the loss of an important relationship.

Research

Utilization of large informal networks resulted in superior outcomes on all measures of mental health. Utilization of only one support was associated with the poorest mental health outcome. Larger professional networks were associated with greater self-esteem and zest.

Of interest to social scientists and mental health professionals.

564. LEVIN, Deborah Marcia.   "Psychological adjustment among the physically disabled: The role of social support and coping strategies."   Ph.D. dissertation, University of Western Ontario (Canada), 1982.

A study of the influence of social support and coping on psychological adjustment among the disabled.

Research

Disability related variables were not particularly associated with psychological adjustment. Evidence was reported that social support

was an important factor in adjustment of the disabled, when controlling for relevant variables.   Coping proved to have a much weaker
relationship with psychological adjustment.

Of interest to rehabilitation specialists.

565. MALLET, Lydia G.   "The effects of social support and the
      source of social support on motivation to respond to losing a
      job due to a plant closing and psychological adjustment."
      Ph.D. dissertation, Michigan State University, 1982.

Evaluates associations between social support and motivation to
respond to job loss and psychological adjustment.

Research

The data indicated that subjective psychological support had a positive influence on affect, especially among married subjects.   An
economically poor situation resulting from a plant closing was related
to feelings of depression, low self-esteem, and anomie. Subjects with
negative tangible support were more likely to ask for job information.

Primarily of interest to policy workers/planners, but also useful to
social scientists.

566. PUGLIESI, Karen L.   "The well-being of women: The effects of
      marital status, employment and social support resources."
      Ph.D. dissertation, Washington State University, 1985.

Examined the influence of social status on social support and self-esteem and, subsequently, on well-being.

Research

Results indicated that married women have more social support resources, with the social support being positively related to self-esteem
and well-being.   Employed women showed similar relationships, but
marriage had a negative effect on the self-esteem of employed women.

Should interest social and behavioral scientists, particularly social
psychologists.

567. RAVEIS, Victoria H.   "Psychological well-being in women: A
      social structural analysis."   Ph.D. dissertation, Columbia
      University, 1984.

A study of the relationship between work stressors, several social
roles, and psychological functioning among women.

Research

The results focused on the associations between the stressors encountered in work; marital, homemaker, and parental roles; and levels of

distress, with social and personal resources of support as buffering variables. Personal resources had more consistent mediating effects on role stressors than did social resources of support.

Should interest social scientists, particularly those involved in women's studies.

568. ROWLEDGE, Lorinda R.   "Stress, social support and mental health: The moderating effects of personal characteristics." Ph.D. dissertation, University of Oregon, 1984.

A study of the direct and interactive effects of social support and other social and personal variables on depression in a sample of college students.

Research

Negative life events or perceived stress, social support, and several personal characteristics contributed to the presence of depression. A number of personal characteristics, such as interpersonal dependency and personal orientation toward support, moderated the effects of social support on depression.

Of interest to social and behavioral scientists, in particular, stress researchers.

2. PSYCHOLOGICAL DISTRESS AND DISORDERS

a. Book

569. HENDERSON, Scott.   *Neurosis and the Social Environment.* Sydney: Academic Press, 1981.

An extensive study of individual vulnerability to adversity, which would be an excellent text for a basic course in psychopathology and health.

Monograph

Contains an extensive review of the epidemiology of neurosis, which concludes with an elaboration of the social bond hypothesis. A detailed review of the literature on measuring social relationships is presented, as well as the description of an extensive study of personality, social relationships, and illness.

Research oriented psychiatrists, clinical psychologists, and social workers will find this a thorough review of literature, methods, and classical studies of neurosis.

b. Articles

570. ARNETZ, Bengt B., Bengt Edgren, Lennart Levi, Ulf Otto.
     "Behavioral and endocrine reactions in boys scoring high on
     sensation neurotic scale viewing an exciting and partly violent
     movie and the importance of social support." *Social Science
     and Medicine* 20 (1985): 731-736.

Describes a study of the effect of social support on the
psychobiologic reactions of neurotic boys.

Research

Deals with the behavioral and endocrine changes in three groups of
boys classified neurotic by the Sennton Neurosis Scale. Two groups
were from a normal school population, the third included boys who had
been treated for psychoneurosis. The study demonstrates both the
psychological and endocrine effects of being amongst friends during
stressful situations.

Psychologists and others interested in the effects of social support
on youth will benefit from this study.

571. BRAMWELL, Lillian, and Ann L. Whall. "Effect of role clarity
     and empathy on support role performance and anxiety."
     Nursing Research 35 (1986): 282-287.

This study focused on wives' perceptions as they attempted to develop
a support role during the rehabilitation phase following a first
myocardial infarction of their husbands.

Research

The findings indicate that support role performance has a direct
negative effect on anxiety, and trait anxiety has a direct positive
effect on anxiety. Descriptive data also provided documentation of
uncertainty as another source of anxiety.

Of interest to social and behavioral scientists, nurses, internists
and family physicians and rehabilitation counselors.

572. CAMASSO, Michael J., and Anne E. Camasso. "Social sup-
     ports, undesirable life events, and psychological distress in a
     disadvantaged population." *Social Service Review* 60 1986):
     378-394.

Examines two processes that are believed to account for the inverse
relationship between socioeconomic status and psychological distress.

Research

The findings indicate that undesirable life events contribute positively to levels of anxiety and depression, whereas social supports
protect against these illnesses.

Of interest to researchers of stress and social support.

573. COMPAS, Bruce E., Leslie A. Slavin, Barry M. Wagner, Kathryn Vannatta. "Relationship of life events and social support with psychological dysfunction among adolescents." *Journal of Youth and Adolescence* 15 (1986): 205-221.

Relationships among major life events, perceived social support, and psychological disorder were assessed in a sample of older adolescents.

Research

Negative life events and satisfaction with social support were significantly and independently related to a range of psychological symptoms. The relationship between negative events and disorder was moderated by gender, the types of events experienced, and anticipated change in the psychosocial environment.

Of interest to psychologists, psychiatrists, and social workers.

574. DUCKITT, John. "Social support, personality and the prediction of psychological distress: An interactionist approach." *Journal of Clinical Psychology* 40 (1984): 1199-1205.

Examines the influence of six personality factors, derived by a principal component analysis of the 16 PF, on the relationship between social support and symptoms of psychological distress in a student sample.

Research

Results indicate a significant interaction between extroversion and social support; extroverts showed a substantially heightened sensitivity to social support variations.

Of interest to social and behavioral scientists.

575. FLAHERTY, Joseph A., Robert Kohn, Alexander Golbin, F. Moises Gaviria, Susan Birz. "Demoralization and social support in Soviet-Jewish immigrants to the United States." *Comprehensive Psychiatry* 27 (1986): 149-158.

Two hundred seventy-four recent Soviet-Jewish immigrants to the Chicago area were interviewed and completed psychosocial questionnaires on migration history, social support, and demoralization.

Research

Older individuals, women, and those with weak social support systems had higher demoralization scores.

Of interest to social and behavioral scientists.

576. HENDERSON, A.S. (Ed.). "Social support and neurosis." *Social Psychiatry* 19, no. 2 (1984): 49-91.

The six articles in this special issue describe the current state of the science regarding social support and mental health.

Special Journal Issue

A good overview of social support and the principal hypotheses of most current research.

Will be of interest to a general audience.

577. ————, and P.A.P. Moran. "Social relationships during the onset and remission of neurotic symptoms: A prospective community study." *British Journal of Psychiatry* 143 (1983): 467-472.

In a prospective study of a community sample, the authors examined changes in social relationships accompanying the onset and remission of neurotic symptoms.

Research

For those who developed symptoms in the course of 12 months, no decrease was found in the availability or reported adequacy of either close or diffuse ties, compared to those who remained symptom-free. For those having a remission, an increase in the adequacy of social relationships and a decrease in rows was observed only in those who improved later on, at the 12 month interview.

Of interest to mental health professionals.

578. HENDERSON, Scott. "Social relationships, adversity and neurosis: An analysis of prospective observations." *British Journal of Psychiatry* 138 (1981): 391-398.

A four month follow-up of respondents reporting adversity in a point prevalence survey of 756 Canberra residents provides evidence of continuing neurosis among those reporting neurotic symptomatology in the initial interview and continued relationship problems.

Research

This study suggests that the lack of supportive relationships during adversity is less predictive of neurosis than the perception of these as being inadequate. This result is interpreted to reflect the importance of intrapsychic and personality factors in neurosis.

Mental health professionals should benefit from this study.

579. ———, D.G. Byrne, P. Duncan-Jones, Ruth Scott, Sylvia
      Adcock. "Social relationships, adversity and neurosis: A
      study of associations in a general population sample." *British
      Journal of Psychiatry* 136 (1980): 574-583.

Evidence is presented showing that attachment and social integration
are negatively associated with neurosis, even in the face of
adversity.

Research

This point prevalence study of nonpsychotic disorder was based on a
systematic sample of 756 Canberra residents. The work demonstrates an
association between neurosis and lack of social ties.

Mental health professionals and social epidemiologists will find this
an interesting study.

580. ———, Donald G. Byrne, Paul Duncan-Jones, Sylvia Adcock,
      Ruth Scott, Greg P. Steele. "Social bonds in the epi-
      demiology of neurosis." *British Journal of Psychiatry* 132
      (1978): 463-466.

A preliminary study, which looks at the association between social
bonds and neurosis, examines a range of social bonds.

Research

In a random sample of the general population, a strong inverse relationship was found between social bonds and the presence of neurotic
symptoms. This association was strongest in the case of close
affectional ties. Together, measures of social bonds accounted for 47
percent of the variance in neurotic symptoms.

Of interest to mental health professionals.

581. ———, P. Duncan-Jones, D.G. Byrne, Sylvia Adcock, Ruth
      Scott. "Neurosis and social bonds in an urban population."
      Australian and New Zealand Journal of Psychiatry 13 (1979):
      121-125.

The hypothesis that a deficiency in social bonds is a significant
causal factor in neurosis was examined in a sample of an urban
population.

Research

An association was found between neurosis and a deficiency, particularly a perceived deficiency, in social bonds.

Of interest to mental health professionals.

582. HOBFOLL, Stevan E., and Perry London. "The relationship of
     self-concept and social support to emotional distress among
     women during war." *Journal of Social and Clinical Psychology*
     4 (1986): 189-203.

This study examined the relationship of self-concept, the existence of
intimate relationships, and the receipt of support during the crisis
period to women's psychological distress reactions in an extreme
crisis.

Research

Coping traits (self-esteem and mastery) were negatively related to
psychological distress (state anxiety and state depression). Contrary
to predictions, social support was related to greater psychological
distress.

Of interest to social and behavioral scientists.

583. HOBFOLL, Stevan E., and Shlomo Walfisch. "Coping with a
     threat to life: A longitudinal study of self-concept, social
     support, and psychological distress." *American Journal of
     Community Psychology* 12 (1984): 87-100.

A study of the relationship of self-concept and social support to
psychological distress among women about to experience biopsy for
suspected cancer and three months later in those found benign.

Research

Women with stronger self-concepts and more social support experienced
less depression and anxiety, even though social support was found to
be less important than self-concept in the relationship of the
variables.

Social scientists and others interested in social/behavioral factors
in disease will benefit from this study.

584. HOLAHAN, Charles J., and Rudolf H. Moos. "Social support
     and psychological distress: A longitudinal analysis." *Journal
     of Abnormal Psychology* 90 (1981): 365-370.

Examines the relationship between changes in social support and
psychological maladjustment.

Research

Findings show a negative relationship between social support and
maladjustment with decrease in family social support during the year
of study, usually leading to an increase in psychological
maladjustment.

Of interest to social and behavioral scientists, especially researchers studying stress.

585. LEAVY, Richard L. "Social support and psychological disorder: A review." *Journal of Community Psychology* 11 (January 1983): 3-21.

Describes current conceptualizations of social support, and presents a distillation of empirical evidence on the relationships between stress, social support, and psychological disorder.

Review

The structure of support links and the quality of the relationships they provide appear to be associated with a range of mental health issues. Methodological problems with current research are assessed, and suggestions for appropriate design and conceptualization are offered.

Of use to teachers and researchers interested in social support and mental health.

586. LINDENTHAL, Jacob J., S. Thomas Claudewell, Jerome K. Myers. "Psychological status and the perception of primary and secondary supports from the social milieu." *Journal of Nervous and Mental Diseases* 153 (1971): 92-98.

Examines the sources of help for psychologically impaired persons in times of crisis.

Research

The impaired perceived formal resources of support as more helpful for a much greater number of crises than did their healthy peers. The impaired were less likely to seek support from primary-group relationships, which may be an indication of their poor fit in their immediate psychosocial environment.

Useful for mental health professionals, psychotherapists, and psychiatric epidemiologists.

587. MAGNI, Guido, Allesandra Silvestro, Modesto Carli, Diego De Leo. "Social support and psychological distress of parents of children with acute lymphocytic leukaemia." *British Journal of Medical Psychology* 59 (1986): 383-385.

A study of the relationship between psychological distress and social support.

Research

The Symptom Distress Checklist and the Social Support Questionnaire were completed by 26 parents of children with acute lymphocytic leukemia during the diagnostic phase. A high percentage of subjects reported a score of moderate psychological distress in four subscales of the Symptom Checklist: Obsessiveness-Compulsiveness, Depression, Anxiety, and Sleep Disturbances. The data indicated social support to have a "buffering" effect on the impact of the stress occasioned by the diagnosis of acute lymphocytic leukemia in a child. However, the results should be interpreted with caution, given the lack of a control group and the use of questionnaires only.

Of interest to social scientists and members of the helping professions.

`588. MILLER, P., and G. Ingham. "Friends, confidants, and symptoms." *Social Psychiatry* 11 (1976): 51-58.

A study of social support and symptom reporting of psychological and physical illnesses among 337 female patients from one general practice.

Research

Women without an intimate confidant had psychological symptoms of significantly greater severity than those with adequate supports.

Family physicians and other health providers interested in symptom reporting will find this article useful.

589. SOLOMON, Zahava, Mario Mikulincer, Stevan E. Hobfoll. "Effects of social support and battle intensity on loneliness and breakdown during combat." *Journal of Personality and Social Psychology* 51 (1986): 1269-1276.

A comparison of 382 Israeli soldiers who developed combat stress reactions (CSR) during the 1982 Israel-Lebanon War with groups of carefully matched controls who did not develop CSR.

Research

Lack of social support from officers and intensity of battle were both related to greater feelings of loneliness and greater likelihood of CSR in soldiers. Lack of social support from buddies was related to greater loneliness. A path model that suggests that battle intensity and officer support lead to CSR directly and indirectly by causing increased feelings of loneliness was tested and supported. Possible cognitive and psychodynamic explanations for the findings are offered, and the the limitations of making causal statements from retrospective perceptions are discussed.

Of interest to social and behavioral scientists and mental health professionals.

590. TURNER, R. Jay, and Samuel Noh. "Class and psychological vulnerability among women--the significance of social support and personal control." *Journal of Health and Social Behavior* 24 (1983): 2-15.

Focuses on social support and personal control as variables in the relationship between class position and psychological distress.

Research

Findings show that the role and importance of both social support and personal control is conditional and complex, varying according to both class grouping and stress level. When social support and personal control are both high, these variables may explain the relationship.

Of special interest to social and behavioral scientists.

c. Chapter

591. HENDERSON, Scott, Donald G. Byrne, Paul Duncan-Jones. "Neurosis and the social environment." *In* David T. Lyhken (Ed.). *Personality and Psychopathology, A Series of Monographs, Texts, and Treatises*, No. 27. Sydney: Academic Press, 1981.

Examines the extent to which factors in the social environment contribute to the etiology of neurosis.

Monograph

The main findings suggest that the actual availability of social relationships has no apparent effect on the development of neurosis. However, a perceived inadequacy of social contacts, especially under adversity, seems to be linked to the subsequent onset of neurotic symptoms; persons who perceive their relationships to be inadequate for their needs are more likely to develop neurotic symptoms than others.

Of particular interest to social scientists doing research in life events, social support, and health outcome relationships.

d. Dissertations

592. LECKLITER, Ingrid N. "Social support, coping, and psychological distress: An interactional and transactional analysis." Ph.D. dissertation, Virginia Polytechnic Institute and State University, 1984.

A study of the buffering effects of coping skills and social support on depression and physiological arousal using a transactional model.

Research

Social support moderated the effects of stress on depression and coping moderated the effects of stress on physiological arousal.

Of interest to social scientists, particularly, stress researchers and health psychologists.

593. PETERS, Larry. "The relationship between the structure and function of social support and psychological distress among the widowed elderly." Ph.D. dissertation, University of Saskatchewan, Canada, 1983.

Identifies the structural and functional dimensions of social support associated with psychological adjustment to widowhood among elderly women.

Research

Results indicated that larger support networks were associated with greater availability of social support. At the functional level, all types of support were related to an absence of psychological distress, particularly when friends provided emotional support.

Should interest gerontologists.

3. PSYCHIATRIC DISORDERS

a. Books

594. BROWN, George, and Tirril Harris. *Social Origins of Depression: A Study of Psychiatric Disorder in Women.* New York: The Free Press, 1978.

Seeks to explain the etiology of depression, and attempts to interpret it theoretically.

Research and Theory

Several samples of depressed women were studied in an attempt to determine the impact of the social environment on psychiatric disorder. A model was developed in which provoking agents, such as life events, vulnerability factors, and symptom-formation factors, were examined. Severe life events involving long-term threats such as loss and, to a lesser extent, major difficulties were found to contribute to the onset of all types of depression. Women who lacked intimate ties, had three or more children under age 14, or had lost their mother before age 11 were much more likely to break down in the presence of these provoking agents. Working class women were found to be more vulnerable than more affluent women because they experienced more severe life events and major difficulties.

Should interest social and behavioral scientists.

595. DEAN, Alfred (Ed.). *Depression in Multidisciplinary Perspective.* Brunner/Mazel: New York, 1985.

A multidisciplinary set of contemporary papers on depression, representing the state-of-the-art and future issues in epidemiologic findings, clinical diagnosis, pharmacological approaches, and psychological treatments, which reflect the approaches of psychiatrists, psychologists, and sociologists.

Text

The ten chapters are divided into three major sections: 1) psychosocial epidemiology and etiology; 2) special diagnostic and treatment issues and neglected areas; and 3) therapeutic innovations. Chapter 1 discusses the definition and measurement of social support and stressors, social supports, and personal resources in the age structure.

Useful to practitioners, students, faculty, and researchers.

596. LIN, Nan, Alfred Dean, Walter M. Ensel (Eds.). *Social Support, Life Events, and Depression*. New York: Academic Press, 1986.

Describes the research experiences and results of a team that have been working together since 1977 to look into the social process of mental health.

Book of Readings

A single theme continues throughout the book: How does social support, along with life events, affect depressive symptoms?

Intended for researchers, scientists, professionals, and instructors who are interested in examining both conceptual and methodological issues regarding social factors in mental health.

597. WEISSMAN, Myrna M., and Eugene S. Raykel. *The Depressed Woman: A Study of Social Relations*. Chicago: University of Chicago, 1974.

Deals with an aspect of depression--social adjustment. The social and family life of women when they are acutely depressed and when they recover are described.

Research

Depressed patients show disengagement and withdrawal. Marital relationships become an arena for the depression and are characterized by friction, poor communication, dependency, and diminished sexual satisfaction. The depressed woman feels a lack of affection towards her husband, together with guilt and resentment; communication is poor and hostility overt. Although much of the social disturbance subsides with recovery from symptomatic illness, the relationship between symptoms and social disturbance is not close. Many of the social disturbances of depression are a consequence of acute illness; about three-quarters subside with recovery, and many return with relapse. Social disturbances correlate poorly with symptom severity at the height of the illness.

Of interest to mental health professionals and social and behavioral scientists.

b. Articles

598. ANDREWS, Gavin, Christopher Tennant, Daphne Hewson, Malcolm Schonell. "The relation of social factors to physical and psychiatric illness." *American Journal of Epidemiology* 108 (1978): 27-35.

A study in social status associated with illness status was conducted in an Australian suburban community.

Research

Life event stress, adverse childhood experience, and poor social support were related to both physical and psychiatric illness. Twenty percent of the physical illness and 37 percent of the psychiatric impairment could be attributed to the presence of social factors.

Of interest to mental health professionals, epidemiologists, and social and behavioral scientists.

599. AYUSO-GUTIERREZ, J.L., F. Fuentenebro de Diego, I. Mateo Martin. "Psychosocial factors in later life depression." *International Journal of Social Psychiatry* 28 (1982): 137-140.

A study of the psychosocial precipitants of depression in late life.

Research

The onset of depression is preceded by disturbing life changes significantly more often among the aged than among younger subjects. Death of a spouse and changes in residence or family structure are the most frequent events precipitating depression among the elderly. Any therapeutic approach should include supportive psychotherapy.

Of interest to gerontologists and psychiatrists.

600. BEISER, Morton. "Personal and social factors associated with the remission of psychiatric symptoms." *Archives of General Psychiatry* 33 (1976): 941-945.

A community sample of 50 people with neurotic disorders were followed for up to five years, using both clinical and quantitative techniques.

Research

Ability to obtain emotional support from significant others was an attribute found to improve the chances of recovering from an episode of illness. The following were found to be important in predicting the remission of symptoms: a basic sense of self-worth, the ability to use others in the environment for emotional support, and a sense of long-term satisfaction.

Of interest to mental health professionals.

601.   BELL, Roger A., Joseph B. LeRoy, Judith J. Stephenson. "Evaluating the mediating effects of social support upon life events and depressive symptoms." *Journal of Community Psychology* 10 (October 1982): 325-340.

Using data gathered as part of a major epidemiological study, the authors examine the relationships between depressive symptoms, social support, stressful life events, and socioeconomic status.

Research

Direct effects were found for social support, stressful life events, and socioeconomic status upon depressive symptoms. However, there were no interactive effects. Findings demonstrate direct effects of social support and stressful life events upon depressive symptoms.

Of interest to researchers of stress and social support.

602.   BILLINGS, Andrew G., and Rudolf H. Moos. "Chronic and nonchronic unipolar depression. The differential role of environmental stressors and resources." *Journal of Nervous and Mental Diseases* 172, no. 2 (1984): 65-75.

Investigates the effect of psychosocial factors on the onset and course of depressive disorders.

Research

Chronic and nonchronic depressed patients did not differ in experience of stressors or amount of social resources. Stressors and social resources were of importance to functioning of nondepressed controls and nonchronic depressed, but not of the chronically depressed. It was suggested that severity of depression may be related to psychosocial factors for only specific subgroups of patients.

Helpful for psychiatrists, psychiatric epidemiologists, stress researchers.

603.   ———.   "Coping, stress, and social resources among adults with unipolar depression." *Journal of Personality and Social Psychology* 46 (1984): 877-891.

A study of the roles of stress, social resources, and coping among subjects entering treatment for depression.

Research

The results indicated that chronic role status was more strongly related to the dysfunction of depressed persons than particular negative life events. Furthermore, some forms of coping were associated with better functioning, and strength and quality of support were the most protective aspects of social resources with respect to the patients' functioning.

Helpful for stress researchers and mental health professionals.

604. —————— "Life stressors and social resources affect posttreatment outcomes among depressed patients." *Journal of Abnormal Psychology* 94 (1985): 140-153.

Explores the role of life stressors and social resources in the course of depressive disorders after treatment.

Research

Examines pre- to post-treatment changes in life stressors and social resources and their association with treatment outcomes in a 12 month follow-up of 424 adults with unipolar depression. While there were increases in patients' social resources and improvements in functioning, no overall decrease in stress was observed.

Psychologists and others interested in the recovery factors in depression will benefit from this article.

605. BLAZER, Dan. "Impact of late-life depression on the social network." *American Journal of Psychiatry* 140 (February 1983): 162-166.

Tests the hypothesis that a major depressive disorder contributes to a decline in social support by studying data from 331 subjects, 65 years of age and older.

Research

Impaired social support was associated with the presence of a major depressive disorder. Thirty months later, however, the surviving subjects whose social support had improved were 2.62 times more likely to have been depressed earlier than those whose social support did not improve. Major depressive disorder was a significant predictor of improvement in social support at follow-up.

Of interest to mental health professionals.

606. BROWN, G.W., B. Andrews, T. Harris, Z. Adler, L. Bridge. "Social support, self-esteem and depression." *Psychological Medicine* 16 (1986): 813-831.

Reviews a prospective study of 400 largely working-class women with children living at home to predict the risk of depression in the year following the occurrence of a stressor.

Research and Analysis

Low self-esteem and emotional support were associated with a greatly increased risk of depression following the occurrence of a stressor. Lack of support from a significant other at the time of a crisis was particularly predictive of an increased risk of depression. The authors conclude that it is essential for prospective enquiries to take account of the actual mobilization of support in the follow-up period.

Of interest to social and behavioral scientists and mental health professionals.

607. CHANCE, N.A. "A cross-cultural study of social cohesion and depression." *Transcultural Psychiatric Research Review* 1 (1964): 19-21.

Describes a test of the hypothesis that psychotic depression and membership in highly cohesive groups are associated.

Research

Describes a study, using the Depression Questionnaire, of several samples classified according to cohesion of the cultural groups to which they belonged. Those in more cohesive groups had higher psychotic depression scores. This result is described in light of social control theory.

Sociologists and cultural anthropologists will benefit from this interesting comparative study.

608. COHEN, Carl I., and Jay Sokolovsky. "Schizophrenia and social networks: Ex-patients in the inner city." *Schizophrenia Bulletin* 4 (1978): 546-560.

A study of the social interactions of schizophrenics, examining the notion of isolation among them.

Research

Findings indicate that schizophrenics have significantly fewer linkages than nonpsychotics, but even the most impaired schizophrenics are not totally isolated. Within the schizophrenic spectrum, there are differences with respect to network size, complexity, directionality, and interconnectedness. Rehospitalization is dependent upon degree of psychopathology and social network size.

Of interest to psychiatrists, psychologists, and social workers.

609. COSTELLO, Charles G. "Social factors associated with depression: A retrospective community study." *Psychological Medicine* 12 (1982): 329-339.

This study seeks to determine factors associated with depression and to test a hypothesis regarding social vulnerability and affective disorders.

Research

A lack of intimacy with spouse, cohabitants, and/or boyfriend increased the risk of depression, consistent with previous work on the vulnerability model.   Severe life events and other difficulties exacerbated affective disorder.

Mental health researchers will find this an interesting study.

610. DEAN, Alfred, and Walter M. Ensel. "Modeling social support, life events, competence, and depression in the context of age and sex." *Journal of Community Psychology* 10 (October 1982): 392-408.

As part of a longitudinal study, life events, social support, and personal competence are examined in terms of their ability to explain depressive symptomatology in three empirically discerned age groups of males and females.

Research

The major findings point to the centrality of social support in the epidemiology of depression in all age-sex groupings.

Of interest to mental health professionals.

611. ———. "The epidemiology of depression in young adults: The centrality of social support." *Journal of Psychiatric Treatment and Evaluation* 5 (1983): 195-207.

Examines the role of life changes, social support, and psychological resources in predicting depression among young men and women, age 17-24.

Research

Social support was found to be the single most important factor accounting for depression in young males and females (the less support, the more depressed).

Of interest to mental health professionals.

612. DEAN, Alfred, Nan Lin, Walter M. Ensel. "The epidemiological significance of social support systems in depression." *Research in Community and Mental Health* 2 (1981): 77-109.

An attempt to resolve some problems regarding theory and methods in studying social support and the competing causal models of the relationships between stressful life events, social support, and illness.

Research

Persons who perceive their extended kin to be more supportive report fewer symptoms of depression. Number of extended kin and perceived support from non-kin are unrelated to depression. A buffering effect of extended kin support on life events is evident only among males. There is no buffering effect of social support on chronic stressors. Extended kin support appears to be least effective in reducing the risk of depression among young women.

Of interest to mental health professionals and social and behavioral scientists.

613. DRESSLER, William W. "Extended family relationships, social support and mental health in a southern black community." *Journal of Health and Social Behavior.* 26 (1985): 39-48.

The influence on depression of a variety of social relationships, including the number of extended kin and the perceived supportiveness of both kin and non-kin, are examined.

Research

Persons who perceive their extended kin to be more supportive report fewer symptoms of depression. Number of extended kin and perceived support from non-kin are unrelated to depression. A buffering effect of extended kin support on life events is evident only among males. There is no buffering effect of social support on chronic stressors. Extended kin support appears to be least effective in reducing the risk of depression among young women.

Of interest to mental health professionals and social and behavioral scientists.

614. DZIEWAS, Hartmut, and U. Dziewas. "Soziale kontrolle und soziale unterstützung unter den bedingungen gemeindenaher psychiatrischer versorgung." (German) *Psychiatrische Praxis* 11 (1984): 81-85.

A discussion of the potential effects of social control and social support on psychiatric care in areas close to a patient's residence.

Review, Research, and Discussion

Addresses the impact of subtle forms of social control and insufficient social support by conventional psychiatric treatment. Gives some data on how this affects rehospitalization of psychiatric patients living in neighborhoods close to the hospital, and discusses the desirability of more integrated social-psychiatric treatment. Special attention is given to treatment of schizophrenics and alcohol abusers.

Should interest psychiatrists, social workers, and other mental health professionals, as well as (mental) health care planners and policymakers.

615. EISEMANN, M. "The availability of confiding persons for depressed patients." *Acta Psychiatrica Scandia* 70 (1984): 166-169.

The availability of confiding persons, both within and outside the household, was investigated in a series of 110 depressed patients and of 98 nonpsychiatric controls.

Research

Depressives reported lack of confidants to a significantly higher degree. The only difference among the diagnostic subgroups emerged for the bipolar patients who had about the same availability of a confiding relationship outside the household as the controls.

Of interest to mental health professionals.

616. ELMORE, Shawn K. "The moderating effect of social support upon depression." *Western Journal of Nursing Research* 6, no. 3 (Summer 1984): 17-22.

Examines the relationship between life events, social support, and depression.

Research

A panel study of 72 prescreened clinic patients participating in a stress reduction program failed to find an association between depressed and nondepressed subjects in terms of size of social network. Depressed subjects did appear to experience less satisfaction with social support. A significant relationship was found between stress, life events, and depression.

For a general audience.

617. ERNST, Philip, Barbara Beran, Frances Safford, Moris Kleinhauz. "Isolation and the symptoms of chronic brain syndrome." *The Gerontologist* 18 (1978): 468-474.

Studies the correlation between the isolation of elderly patients and the symptoms of chronic brain syndrome.

Literature Review

A study of the mental and emotional status of the elderly shows social and emotional isolation to be the key intervening variables that disclose the functional symptoms of mental disorders. Treatment modalities counteracting isolation may reverse the symptomatic disorders, whether or not due to pathologies of aging.

Of interest to gerontologists and mental health professionals.

618. ESSEX, Marilyn J., Marjorie H. Klein, Mary Jane Lohr, Lorna
      Smith Benjamin. "Intimacy and depression in older women."
      Psychiatry 48 (1985): 159-178.

Examines the effects of the qualities of intimate relationships on
depression in older women.

Research

A group of women over 50 were randomly selected from five census
tracts in Madison, Wisconsin and given questionnaires about depression
and the quality of their intimate relationships in the summer of 1978
and again in the summer of 1979. Results showed that some of the
dimensions of the relationships with their significant others that
were described by the women predicted depression. The more depressed
women reported that they felt that the relationship was less friendly,
their friendly feelings were not reciprocated by the significant
other, their relationship was less consistent and predictable, and
there was less time spend with the significant other in the best
state. The findings are discussed in relationship to the theories of
Seligman, Beck and others.

Should interest social science researchers concerned with social
support and depression.

619. FISHER, Gene A., and Richard C. Tessler. "Family bonding of
      the mentally ill: An analysis of family visits with residents of
      board and care homes." *Journal of Health and Social Behav-
      ior* 27 (1986): 236-249.

The present study examines visitation outside of the hospital for
persons living in the community. Hypotheses are developed to explain
variation among living in the community. Hypotheses are developed to
explain variation among families in level of involvement with mentally
ill relatives.

Research

Family involvement decreases with distance, physical disability, and
impairment, but increases with need for services. Sharp differences
in visiting patterns were found between residents who had at least one
psychiatric hospitalization and residents who had never been hospitalized for mental illness. These differences suggest that the bonding
of families to the chronically mentally ill is quite different from
the bonding of families to patients with organic brain syndromes.

Of interest to mental health professionals and social and behavioral
scientists.

620. FLAHERTY, Joseph A., F. Moises Gaviria, Elizabeth M. Black,
      Edward Altman, Timothy Mitchell. "The role of social support
      in the functioning of patients with unipolar depression."
      American Journal of Psychiatry 140 (1983): 473-476.

Investigates the relationship between social support systems, life events, social adjustment, and depressive symptoms.

Research

Social support had a high correlation with all outcome variables, with the strongest association existing between social adjustment and depressive symptoms.

May be helpful to mental health professionals.

621. FOORMAN, Sydney, and Camille Lloyd. "The relationships between social support and psychiatric symptomatology in medical students." *Journal of Nervous and Mental Diseases* 174 (1986): 229-239.

Investigates the relationship between social support and psychiatric symptomatology among 82 first year medical students at the University of Texas Medical School in Houston.

Research

Data supported the hypothesis that social support and psychopathology were negatively correlated at the beginning of the school year. By midyear, however, social support and symptomatology were positively correlated with each other. Social ties may present competing demands on an individual's time and energy, which have potentially detrimental, as well as beneficial effects on mental health.

Of interest to psychiatrists and medical educators.

622. FRYDMAN, M.I. "Social support, life events and psychiatric symptoms: A study of direct, conditional and interactive effects." *Social Psychiatry* 16 (1981): 69-78.

Examines the relationship of life stress, social support, and coping style to psychiatric symptoms in the parents of chronically ill children.

Research

The data suggest that the impact of life event stress is reduced by the availability of social support. This implies that early intervention to assist these parents might be expected to reduce their psychiatric morbidity.

Of interest to mental health professionals.

623. GOERING, P., D. Wasylenki, W. Lancee, S.J.J. Freeman. "Social support and post hospital outcome for depressed women." *Canadian Journal of Psychiatry* 28 (1983): 612-618.

Describes characteristics of a group of discharged mental patients and their posthospital outcomes with regard to readmissions, social adjustment, and symptoms.

Research

In a larger follow-up study of discharged patients, a subgroup of 87 women with nonpsychotic disorders had an unexpectedly poor outcome at 6 months with regard to readmissions, symptoms, and social adjustment. The only factor that distinguished those who had been readmitted was lack of social support. Lack of social support was also related to poor symptoms and social adjustment outcomes.

Should interest mental health professionals.

624. GOLDBERG, Evelyn L., Pearl Van Natta, George W. Comstock. "Depressive symptoms, social networks and social support of elderly women." *American Journal of Epidemiology* 121 (1985): 448-456.

This cross-sectional analysis of data from 1,144 white women, age 65-75, investigated the relationship of demographic, social network, and social support characteristics to the level of depressive symptoms.

Research

The size and homogeneity of social networks was found to be related to symptoms of depression, with smaller networks more common among the more severely depressed. Women in the lower socioeconomic strata were more likely to be depressed.

Social epidemiologists and other researchers of mental health will benefit from this study.

625. GOLDSTEIN, Jill M., and Carol L.M. Caton. "The effects of the community environment on chronic psychiatric patients." *Psychological Medicine* 13 (1983): 193-199.

Describes a study of the rehospitalization and clinical functioning of psychiatric patients and the factors affecting their adjustment.

Research

There were no significant differences in the rehospitalization rates or clinical functioning of 119 schizophrenics in New York City discharged to various family and community living arrangements. Social support and interpersonal stress were stronger predictors of successful recovery and adjustment than the availability of out-patient treatment programs.

Community psychologists, social workers, and psychiatrists will find this an interesting, although perplexing study.

626. GRUSKY, Oscar, Kathleen Tierney, Ronald W. Manderscheid, David B. Grusky. "Social bonding and community adjustment to chronically mentally ill adults." *Journal of Health and Social Behavior* 26 (1985): 49-63.

Specifies, estimates, and discusses two models of social adjustment and service use among a national sample of 971 chronically mentally ill adults.

Research

Community and work bonding showed strong positive relationships with personal and community adjustment, but the corresponding effects of family bonding are nonsignificant. In addition, the three types of social bonding affected service use differently.

Of interest to mental health professionals and social and behavioral scientists.

627. HALL, Lynne A., Carolyn A. Williams, Raymond S. Greenberg. "Supports, stressors, and depressive symptoms in low-income mothers of young children." *American Journal of Public Health* 75 (1985): 518-522.

Describes a study that investigated the association of social supports and stresses with depressive symptoms in a sample of 111 predominantly low-income mothers of young children.

Research

The prevalence of depressive symptoms was measured by the Center for Epidemiologic Studies--Depression Scale (CES-D). Comparing the relative importance of two different types of support--the quality of primary intimate relationships, and the social network--only the quality of the husband/intimate relationship was associated with CES-D scores among married women. The social network demonstrated a moderate, inverse association with CES-D scores among unemployed women.

Of interest to social and behavioral scientists.

628. HENDERSON, Scott. "Do support systems prevent psychiatric disorders?" *Medical Journal of Australia* 1 (April 30, 1977): 662-664.

This article questions the general agreement in the literature regarding the role of social support in preventing psychiatric disorders, especially neuroses.

Review--Theoretical

This paper reviews the literature on social support in psychiatric disorders and provides a good summary of three components of social support, attachment, cohesion, and affectional functions of social networks. Several areas needing research are described and presented in a refreshing way.

Useful to researchers of social support.

629. ——————. "Personal networks and the schizophrenias."
     Australian and New Zealand Journal of Psychiatry 14 (1980):
     255-259.

Discusses the relationship between schizophrenia and the abnormalities
of personal networks.

Discussion

The construct known as 'social support' has recently been involved as
one such element which, when deficient, may be a causal factor in the
onset of schizophrenia. The evidence for this is unsatisfactory and
likely to remain so. For clinical purposes, it would be more useful
to look at the effect of social relationships in secondary and tertia-
ry prevention.

Of interest to mental health professionals and social and behavioral
scientists.

630. KEANE, Terence M., W. Owen Scott, Gary A. Chavoya, Danuta
     M. Lamparski, John A. Fairbank. "Social support in Vietnam
     veterans with posttraumatic stress syndrome--a comparative
     analysis." *Journal of Consulting and Clinical Psychology*
     53 (1985): 95-102.

A cross-sectional study of the social support systems of Vietnam
veterans.

Research

This study compared the perceived support of three groups of Vietnam
veterans--those diagnosed with posttraumatic stress disorder (PTSD);
those who were well adjusted; and those who saw no combat, but were
receiving hospital services at the time of the study. Assessments of
recall of social support 3 months prior to service, three months after
discharge, and at the time of the study were made. The PTSD group's
social support declined over time and was at lower levels than that of
the comparison groups.

Psychologists, social workers, and others working with veterans will
find this article useful.

631. LAMB, H. Richard, and Roger Peele. "The need for continuing
     asylum and sanctuary." *Hospital and Community Psychiatry*
     35 (1984): 793-797.

Addresses the issues of why asylum should be provided, for what
patients, the relationship between asylum and rehabilitation, and the
implications for mental health professionals.

Essay

The chronically mentally ill are in need of social support, protection, and relief from the pressures of life. Whatever degree of rehabilitation is possible for each patient cannot take place unless support and protection--whether from family, treatment program, board and care home, or public hospital--are provided at the same time.

Should interest mental health professionals and families of the mentally ill.

632. LIEM, Ramsay, and Joan Liem. "Social class and mental illness reconsidered: The role of economic stress and social support." *Journal of Health and Social Behavior* 19 (1978) 139-156.

Reexamines the relationship of psychiatric dysfunction to large-scale social structures and processes in light of recent studies of the psychological consequences of economic stress and social support.

Literature Review

Examines, individually, the relationship of social class, stress, employment related stress, life events, support, and interpersonal relationships to mental illness. Addresses the need to examine the etiology of dysfunction and levels of social organization holistically, rather than separately.

Of interest to mental health professionals and social and behavioral scientists.

633. LIN, Nan, and Alfred Dean. "Social support and depression. A panel study." *Social Psychiatry* 19 (1984): 83-91.

This description of the research program on social support and health at Albany, New York focuses on issues concerning the conceptualization of social support, its measurements, and the modeling of its role in the stressors-illness process.

Essay

Work, so far, has demonstrated the significance of social support as a factor in the etiology of mental illness.

Of interest to mental health professionals and researchers of social support.

634. LIN, Nan, and Walter M. Ensel. "Depression-mobility and its social etiology--the role of life events and social support." *Journal of Health and Social Behavior* 25 (1984): 176-188.

Proposes a research strategy in which the persistence and change in depression can be examined, and explores ways in which persistence and change are influenced by social factors.

Research

Implications from the results are: 1) vulnerable groups and individuals could be alerted to factors that may have detrimental effects on them and explore possible avenues for avoiding certain types of life events or amassing stronger support systems; and 2) given certain information regarding which groups and individuals are most likely to need medical or psychiatric intervention, resources can be more intelligently distributed to meet anticipated needs.

Of interest to counselors, therapists, and social and behavioral researchers of social support.

635. MARSELLA, Anthony J., and Karen K. Snyder. "Stress, social supports, and schizophrenic disorders: Toward an interactional model. *Schizophrenia Bulletin* 7, no. 1 (1981): 152-163.

Proposes a three factor model for research and clinical intervention in schizophrenia, focusing on stressors, social networks and supports, and adaptational patterns to stress states.

Literature Review

Formative, precipitative, expressive, and maintaining factors in schizophrenic-type disorders are described in this interventive model.

Mental health professionals will find this a good general review and model of the dynamic nature of schizophrenia.

636. MONROE, Scott M., Evelyn J. Bromet, Melanie M. Connell, Stephen C. Steiner. "Social support, life events, and depressive symptoms: A 1-year prospective study." *Journal of Consulting and Clinical Psychology* 54 (1986): 424-431.

Provides strong evidence of the association of life events and social support in the etiology of depression.

Research

Four hundred and seventy three women with good marital situations and asymptomatic of depression were assessed one year later. Those with poorer social support resources and disruptive life events were found to have more symptoms of depression.

Researchers will find this a very important methodological paper.

637. MONROE, Scott M., and Stephen C. Steiner. "Social support and psychopathology: Interrelations with preexisting disorder, stress, and personality. *Journal of Abnormal Psychology* 95 (1986): 29-39.

An overview of the different mechanisms for understanding the relation between social support and psychopathology.

Review and Analysis

Recommendations are given to correct measurement redundancies, method limitations, and conceptual ambiguities.

Of interest to social and behavioral scientists.

638. MOSHER, Loren R., and Samuel J. Keith. "Psychosocial treatment: Individual, group, family, and community support approaches." *Schizophrenia Bulletin* 6 (1980): 10-41.

A review of psychosocial treatment of schizophrenia.

Literature Review

The following approaches to the treatment of schizophrenia were compared: individual psychotherapy, group psychotherapy, family therapy, and community support systems. Available evidence indicated that treatments emphasizing the individual patient's social environment reported the most consistent positive findings. The most effective psychosocial treatment of schizophrenia would have to enhance comprehensive, corrective, and sustaining sources of social support.

Of special interest to psychiatrists, psychotherapists, and other mental health professionals, particularly those involved with the treatment of schizophrenics.

639. MUELLER, Daniel P. "The current status of urban-rural differences in psychiatric disorder. An emerging trend for depression." *Journal of Nervous and Mental Disoases* 169 (January 1981): 18-26.

Examines differences in the prevalence of psychiatric disorder by size of community.

Review and Research

It was concluded that psychiatric disorders, particularly nonpsychotic or reactive depression, were more prevalent in urban centers than in smaller communities. Availability of supportive neighborhood ties was offered as a possible explanation.

Of interest to epidemiologists, social scientists, and mental health professionals.

640. MURPHY, Elaine. "The impact of depression in old age on close social relationships." *American Journal of Psychiatry* 142 (March 1985): 323-327.

Changes in the ratings of the intimacy of personal relationships in depressed elderly patients were studied over a one year period.

Research

A significant number of patients who had recovered by the end of the year were more likely to report an improvement in the quality of their close relationships than were patients who had a poor clinical outcome.

Of interest to mental health professionals.

641. NEWMANN, Joy P.   "Gender, life strains, and depression." *Journal of Health and Social Behavior*   27 (1986): 161-178.

Comparative male-female vulnerability to several stressful life circumstances that have been implicated in the development of depression are reported.

Research

Women are more likely than men to suffer hardships associated with the absence of a spouse, social isolation, financial difficulties, and chronic health problems.   However, none of these hardships has a significantly greater impact on depressive syndrome levels for women than for men.

Of interest to mental health professionals.

642. O'CONNELL, R.A., J.A. Mayo, L.K. Eng, J.S. Jones, R.H. Gabel.   "Social support and long-term lithium outcome." *British Journal of Psychiatry*   147 (1985): 272-275.

Psychosocial factors affecting treatment outcome were studied in 60 diagnosed bipolar patients treated with lithium for one year.

Research

Social support was the factor most strongly correlated with good outcome.

Of interest to mental health professionals.

643. O'NEIL, Mary Kay, William J. Lancee, Stanley J.J. Freeman. "Psychosocial factors and depressive symptoms." *Journal of Nervous and Mental Diseases*   174 (1986): 15-23.

Evidence is provided that depression in a college aged population is related to family history of psychiatric illness, stressful life events, and lack of a confidant.

Research

College students suffering depressive symptoms and being treated at a university clinic were compared to a nondepressed group randomly selected from the university general population.   No interaction effect was demonstrated among the psychosocial factors.

Psychologists and others interested in mental health work will benefit from this paper.

644. PAI, Shaila, S.M. Channabasavanna, Nagarajaiah, R. Raghuram. "Home care for chronic mental illness in Bangalore: An experiment in the prevention of repeated hospitalization." *British Journal of Psychiatry* 147 (1985): 175-179.

Examines the use of home care as an alternative to hospitalization for Indian psychiatric patients, and provides an interesting model for other forums of evaluative research on mental health interventions, including social support.

Research

A matched group comparison study of 25 chronic psychiatric patients managed in home care and hospital care situations indicated the importance of family support in the success of home care. Long-term community adjustment was found to be related to the quality of social support experienced by patients.

Of interest to mental health professionals.

645. REISS, Steven, and Betsey A. Benson. "Psychosocial correlates of depression in mentally retarded adults. 1. Minimal social support and stigmatization." *American Journal of Mental Deficiency* 89 (1985): 331-337.

A case-control study of social support and stigmatization and depres-sion among mildly mentally retarded adults.

Research

A powerful association was found between low levels of social support and depression, but none between perceived stigmatization and depression.

Psychologists and others working with mentally retarded people will find this helpful in developing interventions and other programs to promote greater social support for the mentally retarded.

646. ROBERTS, Catherine Ramsay, Robert Edmund Roberts, John M. Stevenson. "Women, work, social support, and psychiatric morbidity." *Social Psychiatry* 17 (1982): 167-173.

Describes a study of psychiatric morbidity in women as a function of work and social support.

Research

A community survey of 1,710 women examined several sociodemographic variables and the prevalence of psychiatric morbidity. Employed women had fewer psychiatric problems, and only social contacts were found to be a significant predictor of psychiatric morbidity.

Community psychologists and others interested in psychiatric epidemiology will find this a valuable study.

647. ROEHL, Janet E., and Morris A. Okun. "Depression symptoms among women reentering college--the role of negative life events and family social support." *Journal of College Student Personnel* 25 (1984): 251-254.

A random sample of 322 female students returning to a large southwestern university was studied to examine the interrelationships between negative life events, family support, and depression.

Research

Family social support, negative life events, and their interaction account for a substantial proportion of the variance in the scores of reentering women students on symptoms of depression. Orientation and counseling programs for reentering women should include discussions of life events and social support.

Of interest to mental health professionals and college counselors.

648. SCHWARTZ, Lee S. "Normalization of dexamethasone test associated with social support system improvement." *Psychiatric Journal of the University of Ottawa* 9 (1984): 45-46.

Outlines the treatment of a patient with a major depressive episode of melancholia, showing the dramatic effect of improved social support.

Case Report

The patient failed to show normalization of the dexamethasone suppression test (DST) after treatment for melancholia with antidepressants despite a clinical remission. However, the DST reverted to normal after a significant improvement in his social support network.

Should interest psychiatrists and other mental health professionals.

649. SOLOMON, Zahava, and Evelyn Bromet. "The role of social factors in affective disorder: An assessment of the vulnerability model of Brown and his colleagues." *Psychological Medicine* 12 (1982): 123-130.

Evidence is presented linking the social environment to affective disorders, especially depression.

Research

The researchers seek to determine if a conceptual model is associated with affective disorders among a sample of residents living near the

Three Mile Island nuclear plant. Findings were not consistent with the vulnerability hypothesis and are attributed to methodological problems in the study.

Researchers interested in factors affecting the etiology of affective disorders should benefit from this study.

650. SURTEES, P.G. "Social support, residual adversity and depressive outcome." *Social Psychiatry* 15 (1980): 71-80.

Investigates the relationship between social support and the severity of symptoms seven months after the onset of a depressive illness.

Research

Results suggest that the presence of social support provides partial immunity against symptoms recurring. Confiding relationships that are reciprocal provide the highest protective qualities.

Of interest to mental health professionals.

651. SURTEES, Paul. "Kith, kin, and psychiatric health: A Scottish survey." *Social Psychiatry* 19 (1984): 63-67.

Four factors (demographic, living group, loss experiences, and social support) and their relationship to the presence of psychiatric disorder were studied.

Research

The social network results suggested that while diffuse support measures distinguished cases from non-cases, a measure of confidant intimacy did not.

Of interest to mental health professionals.

652. TEST, Mary Ann, William H. Knoedler, Deborah J. Allness. "The long-term treatment of young schizophrenics in a community support program." *New Directions in Mental Health Services* 26 (June 1985): 17-27.

A description of a 10 year treatment and follow-up of young adults with schizophrenic disorders to test the effect of the community support model over time.

Descriptive

Training in community living produced two major findings: hospitalization of chronically mentally ill patients could be dramatically reduced through a comprehensive community and support program; and patients in such a system showed less symptomatology, more satisfaction with life, and better work and social functioning than patients treated under the traditional model. However, follow-up on patients discharged from the TCL program after 14 months revealed that many of the positive gains had been lost.

Of interest to mental health professionals.

653. WEISS, Robert J., and Bernard J. Bergen. "Social support and the reduction of psychiatric disability." *Psychiatry* 31 (1968): 107-115.

Hypotheses are formulated about the elements that constitute support-ive relationships, which can serve as a meaningful foundation for future research on social support.

Theoretical

Proposes that the successful efforts of persons with serious emotional impairments to adapt in the community are contingent upon their receipt of gratification for dependency needs without a drastic loss of self-esteem; social supports for the needs of emotionally impaired individuals are possible only if such needs are defined as attributes of socially legitimate roles.

Of interest to psychiatrists and other mental health professionals as well as researchers of social support.

654. WILLIAMS, Christene Blanton. "Dissonance following aggressive behavior with and without social support and choice." *Psychological Reports* 23 (1968): 1343-1350.

This study is one of the first to explore the role of social support and free choice in aggressive behavior.

Research

Sixty females opposed to or neutral to using electroshock in research were placed in situations where they administered shock to another person. In the situation above (no social support), shocks were minimized. Perceived choice not to administer shock and social support were unrelated to changing attitudes about using electroshock in research, devaluation of the shocked individual, or a feeling of obligation to participate.

Psychologists and others interested in aggression will find this interesting.

655. WINEFIELD, H.R. "Social support and the social environment of depressed and normal women. *Australian and New Zealand Journal of Psychiatry* 13 (1979): 335-339.

A brief self-report measure of social support was administered ini-tially to a student population, and then to a sample of hospitalized depressed women.

Research

Comparison of the responses of the 32 patients with 35 student women of similar age showed no differences between the groups in number of cohabitants or of casual friends, or in faith in the value of talking over one's problems. Patients were more likely than controls to report having no or few confidants, nobody confiding in them, and little confidence in being liked by others.

Of interest to mental health professionals.

656. ZIMMERMAN, Mark, William Coryell, Bruce Pfohl, Dalene Stangl. "The validity of four definitions of endogenous depression. II. Clinical, demographic, familial, and psychosocial correlates." *Archives of General Psychiatry* 43 (1986): 234-244.

A survey of the literature and studies examining the correlates of a clinical diagnosis of endogenous or nonendogenous depression. Four definitions of endogenous depression were used.

Research

Some support for the validity of each of the four definitions was found. The validity of the Newcastle scale was the most frequently supported, with the endogenous depressives having a lower rate of personality disorder, marital separations and divorces, familial alcoholism, life events, and nonserious suicide attempts. Contrary to expectation, the DSM-III and Research Diagnostic Criteria endogenous patients were more likely to lack a confidant to whom they spoke at least once per week.

Of interest to mental health professionals.

c. Chapter

657. COOPER, Brian, and Ute Sosna. "The family settings of psychiatrically disturbed aged." *In* Lee N. Robbins, Paula J. Clayton, John K. Wing (Eds.). *The Social Consequences of Psychiatric Illness.* New York: Brunner/Masel, 1980.

Examines the extent to which mental disorders in the elderly are associated with reduced social contacts, and the resultant inadequate level of social support.

Literature Review

Presents a description of alienation and anomie as processes which interrupt social support among the aged. Data from panel studies in Germany are presented in support of the concept that mental illness and social support are related among the elderly.

Students of sociology, social work, and other social sciences will benefit from this chapter.

d. Dissertations

658. FRAZIER, Cynthia L. "Depression, self-esteem, and physical
      health as a function of social support in the elderly." Ph.D.
      dissertation, New School for Social Research, 1982.

Investigates types of social support and several health outcomes in a
geriatric population.

Research

The data suggested that perception of social support plays an important mediating role between actual support and psychological health,
as expressed by depression or self-esteem. Physical health seemed not
to be affected by social support.

Helpful for gerontologists and other health care providers of the
elderly.

659. GOLDING, Jacqueline M. "An integrated role restriction and
      stress approach to gender differences in depression." Ph.D.
      dissertation, University of California, Los Angeles, 1985.

Examines the role restriction hypothesis and the stress model for the
explanation of gender differences in depressive symptomatology.

Research

Results provided some evidence for both the role restriction and the
stress models. Being married and being employed decreased depression,
and employment strain increased depression. Marital support and
employment support were found to be protective against depressive
symptomatology.

Of interest to social scientists, in particular, researchers of
gender differences in health outcomes.

660. LOUIE, Douglas. "Sex difference in the life experience-
      depression relationship among the elderly." Ph.D. disserta-
      tion, Syracuse University, 1984.

A study of the gender differences in life events and social support
among a national sample of community elderly and their correlation
with depression.

Research

Previous psychiatric symptomatology was the strongest predictor of
depression, and social support had a positive effect on depression,
but life events were not significantly associated with depression. No
evidence for a buffer effect of social support was found.

Useful for gerontologists, social scientists, and mental health
practitioners.

661. MOORMAN, Deborah A. "The impact of the perceptions of disease severity, treatment environment, and social support systems on the appointment keeping patterns of patients with psychiatric illness." Ph.D. dissertation, University of Maryland, 1983.

A study of the effect of social support, among other factors, on the appointment keeping patterns of psychiatric patients.

Research

The social support system and perception of treatment environment proved to be the best predictors of appointment keeping patterns.

Should interest mental health professionals and researchers of the utilization of health services.

662. SOLOMON, Zahava H. "Stress, vulnerability and social support: A study of depression and anxiety in mothers of preschool children." Ph.D. dissertation, University of Pittsburgh, 1980.

Examines the stress-illness hypothesis among mothers with preschool children after the Three Mile Island accident.

Research

Results supported the suspected impact of stressful events on symptomatology, but only partially supported the social vulnerability model. Three Mile Island mothers had high rates of disorder, and social support was associated with health outcomes, but independently of stress. The role of social support was not confirmed.

Of interest to social and behavioral scientists, in particular, stress researchers, and family physicians of young mothers.

663. TURNER, Sarah L. "Prevailing disability among schizophrenics in community care: Services utilized, social supports reported. Johnston County, North Carolina." Ph.D. dissertation, University of North Carolina at Chapel Hill, 1977.

Assessed the impact of service utilization and social supports on the presence of disability among noninstitutionalized schizophrenics.

Research

Disability was found to be related to lack of social supports. For example, more of the nondisabled were satisfied with the scope and range of their interpersonal relationships, whereas fewer disabled patients reported the presence of a confidant or other person whom they could depend upon for help. Not much of an effect was found for previously utilized services on present disability status.

Of interest to mental health professionals, especially those concerned with community care.

664. VOORHEES, Deborah J. "The Shetland Islands: Social change
      and psychiatric symptoms." Ph.D. dissertation, California
      School of Professional Psychology, Berkeley, 1985.

A longitudinal study of the effect of economic development and the
related social changes on mental health in two communities.

Research

No statistically significant changes in psychiatric symptoms occurred
as the result of a dramatic economic development in the target community, except among older women. Other variables associated with
increased symptoms were negative attitudes toward the economic development, increased life stress, financial problems, and lack of stable
social support.

Of particular interest to community health researchers and community
development planners.

4. ADDICTIVE BEHAVIOR

a. Articles

665. CAPLAN, Robert D., Sidney Cobb, John R.P. French, Jr.
      "Relationships of cessation of smoking with job stress, per-
      sonality, and social support." *Journal of Applied Psychology*
      60 (1975): 211-219.

A study of the effects of job stress, social support and personality
factors on smoking cessation.

Research

Successful cessation was associated with low levels of social support,
since subjects receiving little social support were thought to be less
influenced by group norms regarding smoking habits. The effects of
decreased job stress on cessation rates were a function of the level of
social support: only low support persons in such conditions were able
to successfully quit the smoking habit.

Helpful to health behavior researchers and professionals involved in
smoking cessation programs.

666. COPPOTELLI, H. Catherina, and C. Tracy Orleans. "Partner
      support and other determinants of smoking cessation mainte-
      nance among women." *Journal of Consulting and Clinical
      Psychology* 53 (1985): 455-460.

A study of how partners may affect maintenance of smoking cessation
among married women.

Research

Maintenance of smoking cessation can largely be attributed to support by a partner. This support is provided by encouraging and rewarding the desired behavior, by avoiding such stressful conditions as interpersonal conflicts, and by offering problem-solving assistance and empathy. Partner support may be decisive in the early maintenance of abstinence from smoking.

Of particular interest to smoking cessation specialists, and researchers interested in changing health behavior.

667. FONDACARO, Mark R., and Kenneth Heller. "Social support factors and drinking among college student males." *Journal of Youth and Adolescence* 12 (1983): 285-299.

This study focused on social support and social competence among male college freshmen and the relation of these variables to alcohol use and psychological adjustment.

Research

Results indicated that alcohol use was positively related to social network characteristics that reflect high levels of social interaction and measures of social competence. Drinking was not significantly related to measures of perceived social support. Psychological symptomatology was negatively related to measures of perceived support, social competence, and network density.

Of interest to social and behavioral scientsts.

668. GARDNER, Russell, Jr., Sharon C. Wilsnack, Henry B. Slotnick. "Communication, social support and alcohol use in first-year medical students." *Journal of Studies of Alcohol* 44 (1983): 188-193.

This study of 22 first-year medical students examined the amount of strain that occurred in response to curricular stress as well as mediating variables that influenced drinking behavior.

Research

Communication with others and perceived interpersonal supports only had a significant inverse correlation with alcohol use during the first 12 weeks of the school year. However, faculty support correlated with progressively reduced student drinking throughout the year.

Student services providers, abuse counselors, and others working with students in high stress situations may benefit from this study.

669. GLASGOW, Russell E., Robert C. Klesges, H. Katherine O'Neill. "Programming social support for smoking modification: An extension and replication." *Addictive Behaviors* 11 (1986): 453-458.

A study was carried out to replicate and extend an earlier investigation of social support in worksite smoking programs.

Research

Twenty-nine employees were assigned to either a basic smoking control program or a basic treatment plus significant other support condition. Both treatment conditions were equally successful in producing abstinence or reduction in smoking behavior at posttest and six-month follow-up assessments. In contrast to previous research, there was considerable relapse in both conditions by follow-up. Consistent with previous findings, supportive social interactions were not related to treatment outcome, but the level of non-supportive social interactions was inversely correlated with treatment success. Implications of the findings and directions for future research are discussed.

Of interest to social and behavioral scientists and health professionals concerned with behavior modification.

670.   GREY, Carolyn, Elizabeth Osborne, Marvin Reznikoff. "Psychosocial factors in outcome in two opiate addiction treatments." *Journal of Clinical Psychology* 42 (1986): 185-189.

The present study investigated the relationship of somatization, stress, and perceived social support to short-term outcome in naltrexone versus methadone treatment.

Research

In the methadone group, drug abuse was correlated significantly with somatization, stress, and family support. In the naltrexone group, retention was correlated significantly with somatization and stress.

Of interest to drug counselors and researchers.

671.   JOHN, Ulrich. "Soziale unterstützende personen in der rehabilitation alkoholabhängiger." (German) *Zeitschrift für Klinische Psychologie und Psychotherapie* 30 (1982): 40-51.

The effects of supportive families and self-help groups on the social rehabilitation of alcoholics were examined.

Research

It was concluded that successful rehabilitation, as measured by abstinence, development of social networks, and supportive relationships or job situations, was approximately the same for those who primarily relied on family members for support and those who sought support in self-help groups.

Of particular interest to rehabilitation specialists working with alcoholics.

672.   MERMELSTEIN, Robin, Sheldon Cohen, Edward Lichtenstein,
       John S. Baer, Tom Kamark. "Social support and smoking
       cessation and maintenance. *Journal of Consulting and Clinical
       Psychology* 54 (1986): 447-453.

Evidence is provided that social support is important in smoking
cessation and maintenance, although in different ways and at different
times in the process.

Research

Support from a partner and general perceptions of support were important in the initial decision and short term maintenance of cessation.
Smokers in the social network were found to hinder maintenance and
significantly affect relapse and long-term abstainers.

Very important to those attempting to quit smoking and those attempting to help them.

673.   MERMELSTEIN, Robin, Edward Lichtenstein, Karen McIntyre.
       "Partner support and relapse in smoking-cessation programs."
       Journal of Consulting and Clinical Psychology 51 (1983):
       465-466.

Examines a partner's helpfulness in smoking cessation.

Research

Successful cessation was significantly related to the amount of
helpfulness experienced from a partner. Partners of successful
participants were more reinforcing and less punishing than the partners of subjects who did not succeed in quitting smoking.

Useful to researchers and conductors of smoking cessation programs.
May also be helpful for smokers who are trying to quit and their
partners.

674.   PAGE, Ronald D., and Sharman Badgett. "Alcoholism treatment
       with environmental support contracting." *American Journal of
       Drug and Alcohol Abuse* 10 (1984): 589-605.

Evidence suggests that contracting with alcoholics to enhance their
environmental (social) supports is beneficial in treating their
alcoholism.

Research--Evaluation

Eighty-eight male alcoholics were divided into an experimental and
control group. Each group received routine care for alcoholism, but
the experimental group additionally completed training to improve
environmental support. Both groups showed improvement in support with
the experimental group showing the most improvement on the outcome
variables of the environmental deprivation scale, maladaptive behavior
rating, and employment.

Alcohol counselors and others affected by this disease will benefit from this work.

675. RHOADS, Deborah L. "A longitudinal study of life stress and social support among drug abusers." *International Journal of the Addictions* 18 (1983): 195-222.

Forty-nine clients, recently discharged from heroin detoxification programs, were interviewed at monthly intervals for three months, and information was gathered on drug use, stressful life events, the availability of social support, and the presence of psychiatric symptomatology.

Research

Clients who reentered treatment reported increasing social support over the three month period, decreased their use of heroin and other drugs, and evidenced decreased depression and anxiety. The remainder of the sample evidenced no significant changes. The results of separate cross correlation analysis of the data for males and females suggested that women addicts are especially sensitive to the effects of life stressors and tend to lack the support systems which are available to the men. The female addicts, in the absence of social support, appear to try to cope by "self-medicating" with illegal drugs.

Should interest mental health professionals.

676. ROSENBERG, H. "Relapsed versus non-relapsed alcohol abusers--coping skills, life events, and social support." *Addictive Behaviors* 8 (1983): 183-186.

Examines coping skills, life events, and social support as differentiating factors in relapsed and nonrelapsed alcohol abusers.

Research

Results indicate that nonrelapsers experienced fewer negative and more positive life events, and were less compliant in their coping style in problem situations than relapsed alcohol abusers. The social support findings were inconclusive.

Substance abuse researchers may find this article helpful.

677. SCHILIT, Rebecca. "Childhood social support deficits of alcoholic women." *Social Casework* 67 (1986): 579-586.

Examines the childhood social support deficits of a sample of alcoholic women.

Research

Three hundred and one alcoholic women were compared with 137 nonalcoholic women. The alcoholic women reported feeling less comfortable with and experiencing less support from both the family and peer group during their childhood than did the control group. The limitations of the study are discussed, and suggestions made for future research.

Should interest social and behavioral scientists and mental health professionals.

678.   SORENSON, James L., David Gibson, Guillermo Bernai, David Deitch.   "Methadone applicant dropouts: Impact of requiring involvement of friends or family in treatment." *International Journal of the Addictions*   20 (1985): 1273-1280.

Examines attrition among applicants to a methadone maintenance program before and after it began to require that applicants have a relative or close friend willing to act as a treatment sponsor.

Research

Few applicants were unable to locate sponsors.   The dropout rate was greater for blacks than for Hispanics and whites, both before and after the sponsor requirement was introduced.   Young addicts with recent drug histories and singles were somewhat less likely to enter treatment after the requirement was introduced.

Of interest to drug counselors and mental health professionals.

679.   STAHL, Claus D., and Werner Panzer.   "Soziales umfeld und familiensituation bei drogengefährdeten jugendlichen." (German)   *Praxis der Kinderpsychologie und Kinderpsychiatrie* 22 (1973): 230-235.

A study of drug addiction endangered adolescents and their family environment.

Research

The results show that both a disrupted, insupportive family and individual problems, particularly identity crises, contribute to increased vulnerability to drug addiction.   The role of authoritarian and extremely permissive parents is discussed.

Helpful to mental health professionals and policymakers concerned with the prevention of adolescent drug abuse.

680.   STEPHENS, Cheryl J.   "Perception of pregnancy and social support as predictors of alcohol consumption during pregnancy." *Alcoholism: Clinical and experimental research*   9 (1985): 344-348.

This study sought to determine the association of perceptions of pregnancy and social support to alcohol consumption during pregnancy.

Research

Using standard multiple regressions, two components of social support (general support and pregnancy support) were found to be working in opposite directions prior to pregnancy, with general support showing a positive association with alcohol consumption. Findings suggest that social support may be an important predictor of alcohol consumption, both prior to and during pregnancy, and merits further investigation.

Of interest to researchers of stress, social support, and alcoholism.

681. WERMUTH, Laurie, and Susan Scheidt. "Enlisting family support in drug treatment." *Family Process* 25 (1986): 25-33.

Describes general principles and specific techniques for recruiting family members in drug abuse programs and in other treatment settings.

Descriptive

Eight principles are discussed, including: focusing on family members who live with the client, tailoring recruitment to the needs of individual families, emphasizing how the family member will benefit, helping families to build a support network, and informing family members of what is expected of them.

Of interest to drug and alcohol counselors.

b. Dissertations

682. BENSON, Carole S. "Coping and support among daughters of alcoholics." Ph.D. dissertation, Indiana University, 1980.

Examines whether the offspring of alcoholics are, themselves, at high risk of developing psychiatric symptoms or becoming alcoholics.

Research

Daughters of alcoholic fathers and psychiatrically disturbed fathers showed more adjustment problems in terms of neurotic symptoms, acting-out pathology, or depressive symptoms than did daughters of normal fathers. Furthermore, family climate and social support proved to be better predictors of a daughter's adjustment status than the father's history of alcoholism or psychiatric illness.

Useful to social scientists interested in mental health or alcoholism, and psychiatrists.

683. STEPHENS, Cheryl J. "Alcohol consumption, perception of pregnancy and social support: A study of pregnant women in a southern city." Dr. P.H. dissertation, University of California, Berkeley, 1984.

A study of drinking patterns prior to and during pregnancy among

Southern women and the effects on perception of pregnancy and social support.

Research

There was no evidence for a higher proportion of heavy drinkers among Southern women than among non-Southern women. Southern women decreased alcohol consumption significantly more during pregnancy. Only weak effects were found for the relationship between alcohol consumption and the perception of pregnancy and social support.

For nurses, social scientists, and public health officials.

684. WRIGHT, Barbara S. "A comparative study of the psychosocial network of the acute and recovered alcoholic." Ph.D. dissertation, United States International University, 1976.

Examined the differences in the psychosocial networks of acute and recovered male alcoholics.

Research

The results indicated that recovered alcoholics had close to normal size networks, whereas acute alcoholics had significantly smaller networks. Acute alcoholics had less contact with the members of their networks, and the contacts were generally limited to family members and, sometimes, a few friends. Other network characteristics demonstrated similar trends. The acute alcoholic had a poorly developed psychosocial network.

Of special interest to alcohol rehabilitation specialists.

5. SOCIAL ISOLATION AND LONELINESS

a. Books

685. BERNIKOW, Louise. *Alone in America.* New York: Harper & Row, 1986.

A collection of essays dealing with loneliness and its expression in American life.

Book of Readings

Provides fresh insights into loneliness, which has been the subject of much social science research. This book is extremely readable, and provides a thorough review of the literature on loneliness in teens, men, women, the family, the widowed, and in work or community settings.

Should be required reading for students of social support, especially those who wish to investigate its mechanisms.

686.   WEISS, Robert S.   *Loneliness: The Experience of Emotional and Social Isolation.*   Cambridge, MA: MIT Press, 1973.

A collection of papers to capture the phenomena of loneliness and to provide some explanation for those phenomena.

Book of Readings

Organized into seven sections, this book considers possible explanations for the neglect of loneliness in professional journals; suggests mechanisms underlying one form of loneliness; presents discussions of situations in which loneliness seems commonly found, the loneliness of emotional isolation, and the loneliness of social isolation, focusing on geographical uprooting; considers the resources available to the lonely; and outlines important issues to be dealt with and suggestions for managing loneliness.

This book is primarily addressed to social and behavioral scientists and mental health professionals.

b. Articles

687.   ANDERSSON, Lars.   "Intervention against loneliness in a group of elderly women: An impact evaluation."   *Social Science and Medicine*   20 (1985): 355-364.

An intervention program, based on an interpretation of everyday loneliness as consisting of two parts—emotional and social estrangement—is discussed.

Research

Subjects had fewer feelings of loneliness, and of meaninglessness, more social contacts, higher self-esteem, greater ability to trust, and lower blood pressure after the intervention. Women with several years of adult employment on the same job experienced the greatest decrease in feelings of loneliness. Women who had had much contact with their grandparents, and women who had experienced a serious or protracted illness in the family during childhood had the greatest decline in blood pressure.

Of interest to social and behavioral scientists.

688.   ————.   "Loneliness, birth order and social loss among a group of elderly women."   *Journal of Psychosomatic Research*   29 (1985): 33-42.

A study of birth order as a childhood experience, social loss, and loneliness among older adults.

Research

Social loss did not change health status in this population. Loneliness was associated with depressive disorder, but not with physical complaints. One interaction effect, found only for firstborns, indicated that firstborns who are less lonely despite a social loss and those who experience loneliness without a social loss are likely to report physical symptoms.

Of interest to psychiatrists and developmental psychologists.

689. BUHLER, Charlotte. "Loneliness in maturity." *The Journal of Humanistic Psychology* 9 (Fall 1969): 167-181.

A discussion of the normal aspects of loneliness.

Theoretical

A discussion of the development of identity and loneliness, the image of man and loneliness, meaning, contemporary values and loneliness, and the completion of the life cycle and loneliness.

Of interest to developmentalists, gerontologists, and social and behavioral scientists.

690. CZERNIK, Adelheid, and Eckhard Steinmeyer. "Zur frage des einsamkeitserlebens gesunder und neurotiker." (German) *Archiv fuer Psychiatrie und Nervenkrankheiten* 218 (1974): 141-159.

A study of loneliness in normal and neurotic persons.

Theoretical and Research

Discusses loneliness, being alone, and isolation as philosophical and sociological concepts. An empirical investigation showed that neurotic subjects suffer significantly more from loneliness than do normal subjects, and that they are less communicative and less willing to attempt new contacts.

Of particular interest to sociologists and anthropologists.

691. DASBERG, H. "Belonging and loneliness in relation to mental breakdown in battle. (With some remarks on treatment.)" *Israel Annals of Psychiatry and Related Disciplines* 14 (1986): 307-321.

A study of psychosocial factors, intensive loneliness, and mental breakdown in battle.

Research

Mental breakdown resulting from from extreme loneliness occurs predominantly among soldiers who are unable to develop a sense of belonging in the army. The perception of having a special bond with the military family was one of the most effective means to prevent battle breakdown.

Particularly of interest to psychiatrists working in the military.

692. HOOVER, Stephanie, Andrus Skuja, Joseph Cosper. "Correlates of college students' loneliness." *Psychological Reports* 44 (1979): 1116.

The present study sought to identify the relationships demographic, social, and interpersonal adjustment variables have with subjective ratings of loneliness and time spent alone among college students.

Research

Results suggest that while there was some overlap between ratings of loneliness and time spent alone, the measures of time alone had a more consistent association with social and emotional isolation variables than did the subjective ratings of loneliness. The number of casual friends, social club membership, attendance at religious activities imply the presence of a social network, but were not significantly related to loneliness or to time spent alone.

Of interest to social and behavioral scientists.

693. KOHN, Melvin L., and John A. Clausen. "Social isolation and schizophrenia." *American Sociological Review* 20 (1955): 265-273.

Reports on the findings of a study designed to ascertain the extent and significance of social isolation in adolescence in a sample group of schizophrenic patients and a matched group of normal controls.

Research

Approximately one-third of the schizophrenic and manic depressive patients gave evidence of having been socially isolated at age 13-14, whereas appreciably none of the normal controls gave evidence of having been isolated at that age. There was no evidence that isolated patients were prevented from interacting with their peers because of a lack of available playmates, excessive residential mobility, severe illness, or parental restrictions, nor was there evidence of a correlation between social isolation and familial relationships.

Of interest to mental health professionals and social and behavioral scientists.

694. LOWENTHAL, Marjorie Fiske. "Social isolation and mental illness in old age." *American Sociological Review* 29 (1964): 54-70.

The relation between isolation and mental disorders in old age is analyzed to assess the prevalent assumption that age-linked isolation is an important correlate of mental illness in old age and to contribute to further understanding of social isolation in general.

Research

Lifelong extreme isolation (or alienation) is not necessarily conducive to the development of mental disorders that bring persons to the psychiatric ward in their old age; life-long marginal social adjustment may be conducive to the development of such disorders. Late-developing isolation is apparently linked with mental disorders, but is of no greater significance among those with psychogenic disorders than among those with organic disorders, and may be more of a consequence than a cause of mental illness in the elderly.

Of interest to mental health professionals, gerontologists, and social and behavioral scientists.

695. NIEMI, Timo. "Effect of loneliness on mortality after retirement." *Scandinavian Journal of Social Medicine* 7 (1979): 63-65.

Examines the effect of interests and relationships on post-retirement mortality.

Research

Men who had retired on old-age pensions in 1964, were divided into three groups--792 married, 119 widowed or divorced, and 77 single--to investigate the hypothesis that people who have fewer available sources of interest and support are at greater risk of death after retirement. No statistically significant differences in mortality on the basis of marital status could be found between the groups, although the results tended to favor the hypothesis. The number of suicides and accidents among the men who died within two years of retirement exceeded the expected values, but the increase was distributed fairly evenly between the groups.

Should interest social and behavioral scientists.

696. QUALLS, Phyllis E., Blair Justice, Richard H. Allen. "Isolation and psychosocial functioning." *Psychological Reports* 46 (1980): 279-285.

Examines the relationship between social isolation from family and from friends and social functioning, personality characteristics, and symptomatology.

Research

A strong association was found between isolation and impairment in social functioning.

Of interest to mental health professionals.

697. REVENSON, Tracey A., and Jeffrey L. Johnson. "Social and
      demographic correlates of loneliness in late life. *American
      Journal of Community Psychology* 12 (1984): 71-85.

This study analyzed survey data from newspaper questionnaires circu-
lated in three North American cities in order to examine the
prevalence of loneliness across the life-span and some of its
correlates in late life.

Research

Loneliness decreased across the adult life-span, with respondents age
65 and older the least lonely; elders were also more satisfied with
their social relationships. Neither gender nor living alone was
related to loneliness for older people. The data also suggest that
desolation or the loss of an intimate attachment, rather than isolation per se, is a major correlate of loneliness in late life.

Of interest to gerontologists.

698. SCHMIDT, Donald E., Michael K. Conn, Lawrence D. Greene,
      Kay E. Mesirow. "Social alienation and social support."
      Personality and Social Psychology Bulletin 8 (1982): 515-521.

This study was based on an alteration of the common notion that
alienation is consistently related to interpersonal withdrawal. Forty
males and 63 females were surveyed and the concepts of alienation and
social support were measured.

Research

Results suggest that men and women employ different strategies in
response to alienation. Although women, in general, seem no more
likely than men to become alienated, they may have different interpersonal orientations to help them cope. While men may be more likely to
withdraw, women may be more likely to seek better coordination with
the group.

Of interest to researchers of social support.

699. STOKES, Joseph P. "The relation of social network and
      individual difference variables to loneliness." *Journal of
      Personality and Social Psychology* 48 (1985): 981-990.

Focuses on the relationship of loneliness to social network variables
and to three individual difference measures: extraversion,
neuroticism, and willingness to self-disclose.

Research

Both social network variables and individual difference measures were
predictive of loneliness in a college student sample. The social
network variable showing the strongest and most consistent relation to

loneliness was network density; denser networks were associated with less loneliness. Both extroversion and neuroticism were correlated with loneliness. The relation of extroversion and loneliness was mediated by social network variables, but that of neuroticism and loneliness was not. Implications of these results are discussed, and cautions about the limitations of this study are offered.

Of particular interest to mental health professionals and social and behavioral scientists.

700. WILKINSON, Gregg S. "Isolation and psychological disorder." *Psychological Reports* 36 (1975): 631-634.

Data are presented on the relationship between interpersonal isolation immediately prior to contact with a hospital and psychological disturbance as reported by psychiatric diagnosis.

Research

A significant association was found between the presence of isolation, psychosis, and high disturbance, indicating that isolation, in an interpersonal sense, may be detrimental to psychological well-being.

Of interest to social and behavioral scientists.

c. Chapter

701. ROOK, Karen S. "Research on social support, loneliness, and social interaction: Toward an integration." *In* Philip Shaver (Ed.). *Review of Personality and Social Psychology*, Vol. 5, Beverly Hills: Sage, 1985.

Contrasts the conceptual frameworks that guide research in the areas of social support, loneliness, and social isolation.

Literature Review

Begins with an overview of the conceptual frameworks for research on social support, loneliness, and social isolation, considering how each of these areas has been defined, what fundamental provisions are believed to be supplied by social relationships, and what consequences are predicted when these provisions are lacking. Systematically compares the major features of these frameworks, and suggests directions for future research.

Of particular interest to researchers of social support, loneliness, and social isolation.

d. Dissertation

702. AUSTIN, Adriana G. "The relationship of social support and creative potential to loneliness in older women." Ph.D. dissertation, New York University, 1984.

Examines the influence of social support and creative potential on loneliness in older women, using an interactional theoretical framework.

Research

Both social support and creative potential had direct inverse effects on loneliness, but the data did not suggest an interaction effect between support and creative potential.

Of interest to social scientists and gerontologists.

6. SUICIDE

a. Books

703. DURKHEIM, Emile. *Suicide: A Study in Sociology*. New York: The Free Press, 1951.

An analysis of the interconnectedness of suicide with social and natural phenomena.

Research

Provides a classification of suicide (egoistic, altruistic, and anomie) based on societal conditions or rules and individual behavior patterns. Durkheim proposed that the basic problem must be to interrelate the life histories of individual suicides and attempted suicides with sociological variables on the hypothesis that certain social environments may: a) induce, b) perpetuate, or c) aggravate the suicide-potential.

A classic, first published in 1897, which is of interest to social and behavioral scientists and mental health professionals.

704. HALBWACHS, Maurice, translated by Harold Goldblatt. *The Causes of Suicide*. New York: Free Press, 1978.

A follow-up study to Durkheim's classic *Suicide: A Study in Sociology*, published in 1897.

Research

Argues that we are justified in using official statistics as an index of the phenomenon of suicide, but considers possible sources of unreliability in them. Proposes a sociological definition of suicide and states that every reason for suicide has the common element of isolation of the victim from his social milieu.

Should interest social and behavioral scientists.

b. Articles

705. BARUK, Henri. "La solitude daus le monde d'aujourd'hui et le développement du suicide." (French) *Bulletin de l'Académie Nationale de Médecine* 168 (1984): 726-732.

Discusses modern day loneliness and the rise of suicide.

Essay

Describes several contexts of loneliness in contemporary times: loneliness among the elderly, among the sick in hospitals, in modern families, and in the face of death. Individuals in such situations may be more likely to attempt suicide.

Of general interest to psychiatrists, psychologists, social workers, and social scientists working in the field of mental health.

706. BOCK, E. Wilbur. "Aging and suicide: The significance of marital, kinship, and alternative relations." *The Family Coordinator* 21 (1972): 71-79.

A random sample of the aged population in a retirement community in Florida provided a normative group with which elderly suicides were compared.

Review and Analysis

A study of suicide in a retirement community demonstrated that elderly married individuals need to be involved in such relationships as kin networks, friendships, and community organizations. These social ties can provide alternatives to each other, counteract the isolation of the elderly widowed, and significantly reduce their potentially suicidal behavior.

Of interest to mental health professionals, social workers, and gerontologists.

707. BURCH, Jane. "The bereavement in relation to suicide." *Journal of Psychosomatic Research* 16 (1972): 361-366.

Recently bereaved people who committed suicide were compared with a recently bereaved group in the general population who did not.

Research

The bereaved who committed suicide seemed to have received less support from their relatives; their bereavement caused them more social disruption and was more likely to leave them living alone.

Of interest to mental health professionals.

708. SLATER, Judith, and Richard A. Depue. "The contribution of environmental events and social support to serious suicide attempts in primary depressive disorder." *Journal of Abnormal Psychology* 90 (1981): 275-285.

An analysis of serious suicide attempts in the context of preceding environmental events.

Research

Serious suicide attempts were strongly related to an increase in events that were beyond the control of the patient, in the year preceding the attempts. Events that involved the loss of an important social support were particularly significant as predictors of suicide attempts. The results also suggested a buffering role of social support on suicidal risk in the presence of an increase in stressful events.

Useful to stress researchers as well as researchers and clinicians interested in suicide.

709. TROUT, Deborah L. "The role of social isolation in suicide." *Suicide and Life Threatening Behavior* 10 (1980): 10-23.

Investigates the extent to which social isolation may be a direct causal factor in suicidal behavior.

Literature Review

Reviews theories on suicide and social isolation, measures of social isolation, and empirical studies which concern the relationship of social isolation to suicide. Concludes that social isolation has a primary and direct role in suicide, and discusses implications for helping contacts, family and group therapy, and supportive and educational public programs.

Should interest mental health professionals, planners, and policymakers.

CHAPTER 5

SOCIAL SUPPORT AND LIFE CYCLE ISSUES

a. Article

710. LOWENTHAL, Marjorie Fisk, and Clayton Haven. "Interaction and adaptation: Intimacy as a critical variable." *American Sociological Review* 33 (1968): 20-30.

Analyzes the relationship between adult socialization patterns and adaptation.

Research

The presence of an intimate relationship serves as a buffer to gradual social role losses and to traumatic losses accompanying widowhood and retirement. Age and sex differences may also have implications in the relationship between socialization patterns and adaptation at earlier stages of the life span.

Of special interest to psychologists.

b. Chapters

711. KAHN, Robert L. "Aging and social support." *In* Matilda White Riley (Ed.). *Aging from Birth to Death.* Boulder, CO: Westview Press, 1979.

Proposes a conceptual approach for studying the process of aging and other life-course changes.

Theoretical and Conceptual

Implies that each individual moves through life surrounded by a set of significant other people who give or receive social support, and that the adequacy of the support determines individual well-being, social performance, and success in managing life changes and transitions.

Should interest social and behavioral scientists.

712. ———, and Toni C. Antonucci. "Convoys over the life course: Attachment, roles, and social support." *In* Paul B. Baltes and O.G. Brim (Eds.). *Life Span Development and Behavior (Vol. III)*. New York: Academic Press, 1980.

Concerned with social support as an important determinant of well-being, both for its direct contribution and its ability to moderate stress.

Review

Reviews the research on social support in terms that integrate theories of attachment and theories of role. Describes the function of social support and well-being throughout the life cycle.

Should interest social and behavioral scientists, social workers, and mental health professionals.

713. ———. "Convoys of social support: A life-course approach." *In* Sara B. Kiesler, James N. Morgan, Valerie Kincaid Oppenheimer (Eds.). *Aging: Social Change.* New York: Academic Press, 1981.

Explores social support across the life course and discusses how demands for and expectations might change at various times in an individual's life.

Literature Review

Discusses social support from a social role point of view, and introduces some new mechanisms for thinking about social support. The concept of conveying social support, as it relates to process and methodological issues of studying social support through the life cycle, is discussed.

Essential reading for researchers interested in social support, especially sociologists and social psychologists.

1. BONDING

a. Books

714. BOLTON, Frank G., Jr. *When Bonding Fails: Clinical Assessment of High Risk Families.* Beverly Hills, CA: Sage, 1983.

A synthesis of sociology, attachment theory, and existing child

maltreatment knowledge. A clinical/academic approach to the problem
of violent families.

Theoretical

The twelve chapters are grouped into four parts: introduction, behavioral observation of attachment capacity, the premature child, failure
to thrive child, premature parent, and resource scarcity. Addresses
the mystery of why some families engage in violence when confronted
with certain stresses and others do not.

Of interest to mental health professionals, social workers, and child
development specialists.

715. PARKES, Colin Murray, and Joan Stevenson-Hinde (Eds.). *The
      Place of Attachment in Human Behavior.* New York: Basic
      Books, 1982.

A consideration of infant-mother attachment, problems in parenting,
bonding in adult life, and disorders in adult life related to
attachment.

Book of Readings

The book is divided into four parts: the nature of child-mother
attachments, the various forms they may take, and how they develop
under normal conditions; how attachments develop under abnormal
conditions and the problems that result; the implications of childhood
attachments for the occurrence and development of attachments in adult
life; and the influence of early or current attachments on incidence
and cause of psychiatric disorders in adulthood.

Of interest to mental health professionals and child development
specialists.

b. Articles

716. ANISFELD, Elizabeth, and Evelyn Lipper. "Early contact,
      social support, and mother-infant bonding." *Pediatrics* 72
      (1983): 79-83.

A study of 59 new mothers, investigating the effects of extra contact
immediately following birth and of the interaction between variables
in the labor and delivery situation and the extent of social support
available to the mother.

Research

Those mothers who had been allowed extra contact with their newborn
infants immediately postpartum, when compared to those who were
subject to routine hospital procedures, exhibited significantly more
affectionate behavior. More affectionate behavior was observed in
mothers with less, rather than more social support; there was no

observable difference between multiparous and primiparous mothers; and mothers of female infants exhibited more affectionate behavior toward their infants, regardless of which procedure they experienced.

Should interest physicians and other health care workers in the obstetric and pediatric specialties.

717.   BOWLBY, John.   "The making and breaking of affectional bonds: Aetiology and psychopathology in the light of attachment theory."   *British Journal of Psychiatry*   130 (1977): 201-210.

An account of attachment theory as a way of conceptualizing the propensity of human beings to make strong affectional bonds to particular others is given, explaining the many forms of emotional distress and personality disturbance to which unwilling separation and loss give rise.

Theoretical

Describes certain common patterns of personality development, both healthy and pathological, with respect to attachment theory, as well as some of the common patterns of parenting contributing to them.

Of special interest to individuals concerned with human development and early childhood development.

718.   COLLETTA, Nancy Donohue.   "Social support and the risk of maternal rejection by adolescent mothers."   *Journal of Psychology*   109 (1981): 191-197.

Adolescent mothers were used to test the hypothesis that variations in amounts, sources, and kinds of support would be related to maternal rejection.

Research

The results indicate that both emotional support and the total amount of support received have an inverse relationship with maternal rejection. Relatives and a partner or spouse were found to be the most important sources of support. It was concluded that when young mothers are isolated from a supportive social environment, their children run a greater risk of maternal rejection.

Of interest to social and behavioral scientists and mental health professionals.

719.   CRANLEY, Mecca S.   "Social support as a factor in the development of parents' attachment to their unborn."   *Birth Defects*   20, no. 5 (1984): 99-124.

Two studies are discussed, which have investigated the association between aspects of social support and parents' attachment to their unborn children.

Research

Overall social support was positively associated with the woman's attachment to her fetus; support from health care professionals was more highly correlated with attachment than was support from family and friends. The second study found a positive association between marital relationship and attachment to the fetus for both men and women.

Of interest to obstetricians, pediatricians, nurses, and child development experts.

720. CROCKENBERG, Susan B. "Infant irritability, mother responsiveness and social support influences on the security of infant-mother attachment." *Child Development* 52 (1981): 857-865.

Investigates the influence of infant irritability, maternal responsiveness, and social support on the development of secure and anxious infant-mother attachments at one year.

Research

Results indicate that social support is the best predictor of secure attachment, and that it is most important for mothers with irritable babies. Some evidence suggests that social support may mitigate the effects of unresponsive mothering by providing the infant with a responsive substitute.

Of interest to child development specialists, especially child psychologists and pediatricians.

2. CHILD DEVELOPMENT

b. Articles

721. BRYANT, Brenda K. "The neighborhood walk: Sources of support in middle childhood." *Monographs of the Society for Research in Child Development* 50, no. 3 (1985): 1-122.

A study of children's perceptions of their social network involvement and how that relates to their social-emotional functioning.

Special Issue

Perception of social support was associated with social-emotional functioning of children in relatively secure and low-stress conditions. Broad-based and informal sources of support were better predictors of social-emotional functioning than limited network and formal sources of support. The results showed the importance of active development in social contacts during middle childhood.

Of special interest to all researchers of child development and health care professionals/educators with children in this age group.

722. DUNST, Carl J., Carol M. Trivette, Arthur H. Cross. "Mediating influences of social support: Personal, family, and child outcomes." *American Journal of Mental Deficiencies* 90 (1986): 403-417.

The mediating influences of social support were examined in a study of 137 parents of mentally retarded, physically impaired, and developmentally at-risk children.

Research

More supportive social networks were associated with better personal well-being, more positive attitudes, and more positive influences on parent-child play opportunities and child behavior and development.

Of interest to child psychologists, social workers, and professionals working with the mentally retarded.

723. FLAHERTY, Joseph A., and Judith A. Richman. "Effects of childhood relationships on the adult's capacity to form social supports." *American Journal of Psychiatry* 143 (1986): 851-855.

Psychoanalytic perspectives suggest that the quality of adult relationships is derived from earlier childhood attachment experiences. The authors tested this thesis by correlating medical students' perceptions of their earlier relationships with the perceived quality of their current social support networks.

Research

The data suggest the need for a more complex and psychodynamically relevant conceptualization of social supports, which has implications for therapeutic interventions to ameliorate support deficits.

Of interest to psychiatrists and other mental health professionals.

724. JOHNSON, David W., and Roger T. Johnson. "Social interdependence and perceived academic and personal support in the classroom." *Journal of Social Psychology* 120 (1983): 77-82.

Responses made to a classroom climate instrument by 859 students in grades five through nine in three urban and suburban school districts were analyzed to determine correlations between attitudes toward social interdependence and attitudes toward relationships with peers and teachers.

Research

Cooperativeness and frequent participation in cooperative learning stituations were positively related to perceptions of support, help, and friendship from teachers and peers.

Of interest to social psychologists.

725. PASCOE, John M., and Jo Anne Earp. "The effect of mothers' social support and life changes on the stimulation of their children in the home." *American Journal of Public Health* 74 (1984): 358-360.

The relationship of maternal life change, social support, and pre-school home environment was examined.

Research

Mothers reporting more social support provided a more stimulating home environment for their children, despite the number of life changes they had experienced.

Child development specialists and others interested in maternal-child interactions will find this an interesting study.

726. PASCOE, John M., Frank A. Loda, Valerie Jeffries, Jo Anne Earp. "The association between mothers' social support and provision of stimulation to their children." *Developmental and Behavioral Pediatrics* 2 (1981): 15-19.

Specific forms of maternal social support were analyzed for their relationship to a validated measure of home stimulation.

Research

The data suggest that augmentation of specific aspects of mothers' social support networks may increase their children's informal learning opportunities.

Of interest to pediatricians, child psychologists, and social workers.

727. PELLIGRINI, David, Shelley Kosisky, Debra Nackman, Leon Cytryn, Donald H. McKnew, Elliot Gershon, Joel Hamovit, Karen Cammuso. "Personal and social resources in children of patients with bipolar affective disorder and children of normal control subjects." *American Journal of Psychiatry* 143 (1986): 856-861.

The authors examined the personal resources and social resources of 23 children of patients with bipolar affective disorder and 33 children of normal control parents.

Research

Positive resource profiles were related to psychiatric well-being in the offspring. Nondisordered probands, in particular, demonstrated a

strikingly positive profile of personal resources, as well as a wide
range of peer, sibling, and other kin supporters.

Of interest to psychiatrists and other mental health professionals.

728. QUINTON, David, Michael Rutter, Christine Liddle. "Institu-
      tional rearing, parenting difficulties and marital support."
      Psychological Medicine 14 (1984): 107-124.

This study focused on the possible role of marital support as a factor
that might ameliorate or mitigate the influence of adversities in
childhood.

Research

Institution-reared women showed a markedly increased rate of poor
psychosocial functioning and of severe parenting difficulties in adult
life. However, the support of a non-deviant spouse and of good living
conditions in adult life provided a powerful predictive effect.

Of interest to child development and mental health professionals.

729. SÉGUIN, Louise, Marie-Patricia Gagné, Huguette Crête.
      "L'importance de la préparation au rôle de parents et de son
      support." (French) *Union Médicale du Canada* 113 (1984):
      755-761.

Describes the importance of the parent-child relationship in the
development of the child.

Theoretical

Parents can be prepared for educating children, and their psychosocial
environment can be a source of support in bringing up children. This
may lead to healthier child development, and may help prevent major
childhood and adolescent health problems. The role of health professionals in this context is discussed.

May interest family sociologists, child psychologists, and parents of
young children.

3. THE ELDERLY

a. Books

730. ATCHLEY, Robert C. *Social Forces and Aging: An Intro-
      duction to Social Gerontology*. Fourth Edition. Belmont, CA:
      Wadsworth, 1985.

Provides a brief, comprehensive introduction to social gerontology.

Text

This major reorganization and expansion of *Social Forces in Later Life* is divided into an introductory section on the scope of social gerontology, the demography of aging, and the history of aging in America plus sections on individual aging, aging and the social situation, personal adaptation to aging, aging and society, and aging and the future. Several of the chapters touch upon issues related to social support, and Chapter 7 specifically deals with "Family, friends, and social support."

Useful to students and teachers of social gerontology, gerontologists, and social scientists.

731. PETERSON, Warren A., and Jill Quadagno. *Social Bonds in Later Life: Aging and Interdependence*. Beverly Hills: Sage, 1985.

The theme of this book is aging and interdependence.

Text

Organized into areas of interdependence: intimate relationships, social support systems, and community supports, especially those dealing with health and social integration issues. The conceptual framework of interdependence grows naturally out of exchange theory and the focus on support systems.

Of interest to gerontologists and social and behavioral scientists.

732. TIMSIT, Karl-Georg, Ulrich Lange, Norbert Erlemeier, Ingrid Timser-Puschner. *Psychosoziale Aspecte der Situation Älterer Menschen*. (German). Stuttgart: W. Kohlhammer, 1975.

A report on a large survey of West German elderly regarding a number of psychosocial and demographic variables.

Research

Data were collected on social networks and social interaction, and on needs and goals of this elderly population. Demographic variables included age, sex, self-rated health, education, and household situation. The extent of social contacts was positively associated with general well-being, and it was concluded that more efforts should be undertaken to keep the elderly in the community as long as possible.

Of interest to gerontologists and policymakers/planners.

b. Articles

733. BALTES, Margret M., Th. Kindermann, R. Reisenzein. "Die
      beobachtung von unselbstständigem und selbstständigem
      verhalten in einem Deutschen altersheim: Die soziale umwelt
      als einflutzgrötze." (German) *Zeitschrift für Gerontologie*
      19 (1986): 14-24.

A study of the nature of the interactions between residents in a
nursing home and their social partners.

Research

Supportive behavior by either fellow residents or nursing personnel
was dependent upon the kinds of behavior exhibited by a resident.
Dependent behaviors were answered by dependence-supportive behaviors;
independent self-care behaviors or passive and destructively engaged
behaviors usually received no response, while constructively engaged
behaviors sometimes met engagement-supportive behaviors. Results were
compared with those of a similar study in the United States.

Especially interesting to nursing home health professionals and
gerontologists.

734. CHAPPELL, Neena L. "Social support and the receipt of home
      care services." *Gerontologist* 25 (1985): 47-54.

Examines the differences between the elderly in Manitoba who use
formal home care services and those who do not.

Research

Analysis showed users as less healthy and less active than nonusers.
Users interacted as much as did nonusers with the informal networks
available to them, suggesting that formal and informal services
complement rather than substitute for each other.

Of interest to social science researchers and gerontologists.

735. COE, Rodney M., Fredric D. Wolinsky, Douglas K. Miller, John
      M. Preadergast. "Elderly persons without family support
      networks and use of health services. A follow-up report on
      social network relationships." *Research on Aging* 7 (1985):
      617-622.

Compares the use of health services by a random sample of 394 noninstitutionalized elderly.

Research

Although elderly persons without family used hospital emergency rooms
7 to 30 times more often than those with family in the area, differences in physicians' visits or hospital utilization were not
statistically significant. Since elderly without family in the area

had similar health status to those with family, the increased use of emergency room services, especially for nonurgent care, is thought to be due to the lack of family access to a lay referral system.

Should interest social scientists.

736. DOOLIN, Joseph. "Planning for the special needs of the home-less elderly." *Gerontologist* 26 (1986): 229-231.

The special needs of the homeless elderly are discussed, followed by the presentation of a program to augment the work of public shelters.

Descriptive

It is possible to develop a program within the infrastructure of the aging service network, and funded largely by existing resources, that meets some of the basic needs of homeless older adults.

Of interest to gerontologists and public health professionals.

737. GOLDBERG, Gertrude S., Ruth Kantrow, Eleanor Kremen, Leah Lauter. "Spouseless, childless elderly women and their social supports." *Social Work* 31 (1986): 104-112.

A study of spouseless, childless elderly women living in a metropoli-tan area to determine the sources of social support they use to provide companionship and socialization, and cope with illness, social-psychological problems, and financial need, and to discover whether there are differences in the support provided by kin and friends.

Research

Most of the sample of 52 single, childless elderly women (65 and older) had developed substitute supports for the close kin they lacked. Most respondents were younger elderly (65 to 74) and consid-ered themselves in good health; however, informal support was also being provided to nearly all the women in the sample who were over 80. The women relied more on primary-group than on formal supports, yet the very poor women in the sample were receiving very little primary-group support. It is suggested that social policy be guided by research that focuses on the more vulnerable groups of spouseless, childless elderly women--the very old, the ill, the poor, and the divorced or separated--and that patterns of support among elderly lesbians be investigated.

Of interest to social scientists, gerontologists, and public policymakers.

738. HAUTZINGER, Martin, A. Boenigk-Berghöfer, G. Thoms. "Soziale kontakte und depressivität im alter." (German) *Aktuelle Gerontologie* 12 (1982): 67-71.

Investigates the association between social relationships and depression-proneness among residents in homes for the aged.

Research

The results indicated that there was a strong inverse relationship between amount of social contacts and depressive symptoms. This relationship was particularly strong for those who had social contacts with family and friends outside their homes.

Should be interesting to gerontologists.

739. HENDERSON, A.S., D.A. Grayson, R. Scott, J. Wilson, D. Rickwood, D.W.K. Kay. "Social support, dementia and depression among the elderly living in the Hobart community." *Psychological Medicine* 16 (1986): 379-390.

A systematic description of the social environment of the elderly, both in mental health and in states of depression or impaired cognition.

Research

Cases of dementia and depression were ascertained in a community sample of 274 elderly people living in Hobart, Tasmania by the Canberra Geriatric Mental State and the Mini Mental State Examinations, and social relationships and support were measured with the Interview Schedule for Social Interaction. The elderly were found to have fewer social relationships than younger adults, but to be more satisfied with what they had. The presence of offspring in the same town increased the number of close ties and social relationships, but was more important for men than for women. Elderly women had more affectional ties than elderly men. Persons with cognitive impairment or dementia reported having less social interaction than they would like, and depressed subjects reported having markedly less social interaction than the mentally healthy elderly, but did not complain that it was too little.

Should interest gerontologists and social scientists.

740. HENDERSON, A.S., Ruth Scott, D.W.K. Kay. "The elderly who live alone: Their mental health and social relationships." *Australian and New Zealand Journal of Psychiatry* 20 (1986): 202-209.

Surveys of the mental health status of elderly persons who lived alone were compared to those who lived with others.

Research

Elders living alone were found to have social networks and social interactions similar to those of other elderly persons even though they reported fewer close relationships and much more loneliness. There was no difference in the prevalence of depressive disorders or dementia on DSM-III criteria, although elders living alone had a higher frequency of neurotic depression.

Of interest to gerontologists and mental health professionals.

741. LEFOY, R.B. "The elderly person and family life." *Australian Journal of Social Issues* 12 (1977): 33-42.

A discussion of how the process of growing old is affected by being in the family group and is reinforced by the association with younger members of the family.

Review

Evidence from industrialized societies shows that the elderly can gain considerable support during the process of aging by being included in the modified extended family. While institutions for the elderly are necessary, more elderly people could remain integrated in the normal community providing family life survives and is supplemented by an active policy of home help.

Of interest to gerontologists and social and behavioral scientists.

742. LEVITT, Mary J., Toni C. Antonucci, M. Cherie Clark, James Rotton, Gordon E. Finley. "Social support and well-being: Preliminary indicators based on two samples of the elderly." *International Journal of Aging and Human Development* 21 (1985-1986): 61-77.

The structure of social support and its relation to health, affect, and life satisfaction are compared for two samples of the elderly.

Research

Older men in poor health and without supportive relationships are targeted as a particularly high risk group. The discussion includes a focus on personal, situational, and life span differences related to variations in support and well-being.

Of interest to gerontologists.

743. LOHR, M.J., M.J. Essex, M.H. Klein. "Life satisfaction and subjective health among older women--the importance of social support and coping." *Gerontologist* 25, Supplement 1 (1985): 265-266.

Studies the mediating effects of social support and coping among older populations.

Research

Studies show that quantity of social support is directly related to life satisfaction, while quality of support is mediated by health status. Among coping techniques, health maintenance behavior is the most effective. Findings emphasize the joint effects of health status, social support, and coping on life satisfaction.

Of interest to gerontologists.

744. McGHEE, Jerrie L. "The effects of siblings on the life satisfaction of the rural elderly." *Journal of Marriage and the Family* 47 (1985): 85-91.

The hypothesis that geographic proximity of same-sex siblings exerts a positive influence on life satisfaction is tested, employing data from a sample of 231 rural elderly.

Research

Regression analysis revealed that the importance of a sister's availability was second only to physical mobility in predicting higher life satisfaction among older rural women. Among men, the availability of a brother was positively associated with life satisfaction, but the effect was negligible. Cross-sex siblings and sibling interaction had relatively minor effects on the life satisfaction of older men and women. Results indicated a need for further study, particularly of the bonds between sisters.

Of interest to social scientists.

745. MORABIA, Alfredo, Francois Loew, Hilke Takla. "Medical care and social support for the elderly in Switzerland: Imbalance and mix." *Social Science and Medicine* 23 (1986): 1327-1332.

Discusses the social and physical needs of Switzerland's elderly citizens, current policy for meeting those needs, and a proposed alternative policy for the future.

Review and Theoretical

The current practice of providing medical solutions to broad social problems facing the old will bring about serious economic and sociocultural dilemmas in future decades due to the aging trends in Switzerland. Social support to the elderly by a well-balanced system of health and social welfare, emphasizing their autonomy and dignity, would provide a desirable alternative to medicalization. The goals of such a system should include reducing inequalities, lowering financial burdens, rationalizing medico-social support, and creating conditions indispensable to an active independent life for the aged.

Should interest gerontologists and public policymakers.

746. MORGAN, Thomas J., Robert O. Hansson, Monica J. Indart, Donald M. Austin, Marcia M. Crutcher, Peter W. Hampton, Karen M. Oppegard, Victor E. O'Daffer. "Old age and environmental docility: The roles of health, support and personality." *Journal of Gerontology* 39 (1984): 240-242.

Examines the environmental docility hypothesis concerning the adaptability in terms of physical, social, and psychological factors to increasing environmental demands of elderly persons.

Research

The results generally supported the hypothesis, only less competent individuals, as expressed by a poorer state of health, a lack of supportive networks, and a lack of personality resources, demonstrated more adjustment problems when faced with increases in environmental demands.

Helpful to stress researchers, gerontologists, and sociologists.

747. OPPEGARD, K., Robert O. Hansson, Thomas Morgan, Monica Indart, Marcia Crutcher, Peter Hampton. "Sensory loss, family support, and adjustment among the elderly." *Journal of Social Psychology* 123 (1984): 291-292.

A study of the effect of social caregiving support on psychological consequences of hearing and vision loss among the elderly.

Research

Results indicated that sensory loss was associated with depression and anxiety among older adults, but that social and caregiving support of a family network seemed to moderate these relationships.

Helpful to stress and social support researchers.

748. POULIN, John E. "Age segregation and the interpersonal involvement and morale of the aged." *Gerontologist* 24 (1984): 266-269.

Examines the relationships between residential age segregation and the interpersonal involvement and morale of the elderly, focusing on the effect of age segregation upon interpersonal involvement with close friends and relatives and overall life satisfaction.

Research

The interpersonal involvement and morale of 232 elderly persons living in the community were contrasted with that of 78 persons in senior citizens' housing. Residents of senior citizens' housing were found to have slightly larger, more supportive interpersonal networks, but less contact with their closest friends than community residents. There was no difference between the two groups in life satisfaction.

Of interest to gerontologists, social workers, community planners, and social scientists.

749. REMPEL, Judith. "Childless elderly: What are they missing?" *Journal of Marriage and the Family* 47 (1985): 343-348.

The subjective and objective experiences of noninstitutionalized childless and parent elderly are compared, using the 1979 Social Change in Canada data base, in an attempt to determine the value of the mutual support relationship provided by children.

Research

The results show few statistically significant differences between the two categories of elderly. The childless are more financially secure and in better health, but parents tend to be surrounded by greater numbers of friends and have more general satisfaction with life.

Should interest social scientists.

750. REVICKI, Dennis A. "Social support factor structure in the elderly." *Research on Aging* 8 (1986): 232-248.

This research examines the factor structure of social support measures using the responses of a sample of 210 elderly.

Research

Results suggest that social support is a multidimensional construct. There are clear direct relationships between the different support factors and physical health, mental health, life satisfaction, and self-esteem in the elderly.

Of interest to social and behavioral scientists.

751. ———, and J.P. Mitchell. "Social support factors in the rural elderly." *Gerontologist* 25, Supplement 1 (1985): 97.

Examines the factor structure of social support measures in a sample of 210 elderly people.

Research Abstract

Significant correlations were found between social support and mental health, physical health, life satisfaction, and self-esteem. A moderate positive relationship was found between participation in church and other groups and perceptions of social support.

Of interest to gerontologists and social support theorists.

752. RUBINSTEIN, Robert L. "The elderly who live alone and their social supports." *Annual Review of Gerontology and Geriatrics* 5 (1985): 165-193.

This chapter discusses the antecedents, correlates, and outcomes of living alone in old age.

Theoretical and Analytical

Living alone may itself not induce loneliness and low life satisfaction, but it may eventuate in a degree of social estrangement which, in turn, has been found to be associated with reduced life satisfaction. The potential negative effects of living alone are mitigated by regular phone or face-to-face contact with family or neighbors.

Of interest to gerontologists and social and behavioral scientists.

753. SHEEHAN, Nancy W.   "Informal support among the elderly in
      public senior housing." *Gerontologist*   26 (1986): 171-175.

Informal support among tenants in public senior housing was assessed
through self-administered questionnaires by key informants and through
in-depth interviews with tenants.

Research

Although informal assistance was reported, more impaired tenants
received little assistance.   The interviews also revealed minimal
social involvement of frail tenants. Frail tenants reported a variety
of reasons for avoiding relationships with other tenants.

Of interest to gerontologists and social and behavioral scientists.

754. SOSNA, Ute, and H.W. Wahl.   "Soziale belastung, psychische
      erkrankung und körperliche beeinträchtigung im alter:
      Ergebnisse einer felduntersuchung."   (German)   *Zeitschrift
      für Gerontologie* 16 (1983): 107-114.

An epidemiological study of social conditions, psychiatric illness,
and physical impairment among the elderly.

Research

Psychiatric illness and physical impairment were significantly related
to unfavorable housing conditions and declining social class membership, although the significant association with physical health status
was eliminated for the latter variable after controlling for mental
health symptoms.   Only subjective reports of social isolation were
significantly associated with both health outcomes; for objective
indices of isolation, no such relationships were found.

Particularly useful to epidemiologists and social scientists.

755. STOLLER, Eleanor P.   "Self-assessments of health by the
      elderly: The impact of informal assistance." *Journal of Health
      and Social Behavior* 25 (1984): 260-270.

Explores the impact of informal networks on the relationship between
health status indicators and self-assessments of health.

Research

Self-ratings of health by older people are influenced by age and sex,
independent of objective health indicators. Informal assistance has
an indirect negative effect on self-rated health, through its depress-
ing effects on psychological morale.   The recipient of informal
assistance is placed in the role of a dependent individual.

Particularly useful to researchers of health and social support in old
age.

756. THOMAS, Paula D., and Elizabeth M. Hooper. "Healthy elder-
      ly: Social bonds and locus of control." *Research in Nursing
      and Health* 6 (1983): 11-16.

An investigation into social relationships and their connection with
health was integrated into a five year study of nutrition in 300
healthy elderly persons.

Research

The elderly subjects in this study were characterized by adequate,
satisfying social bonds and by an internal locus of control orientation, both in general and specific to health. They maintained active
social interaction patterns in the face of advancing age, and they
believed that they exercised some control over their lives and health.

Of interest to health professionals and to gerontologists in
particular.

757. VEYLON, Roger. "Les interactions entre la société et les
      personnes agees." (French) *La Nouvelle Presse Médicinale*
      6 (1977): 1777-1779.

A discussion of the social status of the elderly in modern society.

Comment

The author argues that the elderly become more and more segregated
from modern society and describes ways through which their social
environment, in particular, family members, tries to isolate them.

Of interest to gerontologists.

758. WARD, Russell A. "Informal networks and well-being in later
      life: A research agenda." *Gerontologist* 25 (1985): 55-61.

Identifies several problems of definition common to research on social
support networks and their impact on the elderly.

Literature Review

Informal social support networks are prevalent among the elderly, but
their contribution to well-being is not clear. A conceptual model is
suggested as a foundation for operationalizing and measuring aspects
of social support.

For a general research audience.

759. ZUCKERMAN, Diana M., Stanislav V. Kasl, Adrian M. Ostfeld. "Psychosocial predictors of mortality among the elderly poor: The role of religion, well-being, and social contacts. *American Journal of Epidemiology* 119 (1984): 410-423.

Explores selected psychosocial variables as possible predictors of mortality among the elderly.

Research

This study isolated three psychosocial variables that are significant predictors of mortality: religiousness, presence of living offspring, and happiness. The first and third reduced the risk of mortality primarily among the elderly who were in poor health. The presence of living offspring had a broader effect independent of health status.

Of interest to gerontologists and social and behavioral scientists.

c. Chapters

760. CHIRIBOGA, David A. "Social supports." *In* George Maddox (Ed.). *The Encyclopedia of Aging.* New York: Springer, 1986.

Reviews recent and past literature on social supports and the elderly.

Review

In addition to empirical findings, contributions of three theoretical formulations are emphasized: social exchange, equity, and stress. Family members, including both spouse and adult children, are presented as a critical source of support in later life.

Intended for general audiences, undergraduate, and graduate students of geriatrics and gerontology.

761. DUNKEL-SCHETTER, Christine, and Camille B. Wortman. "Dilemmas of social support: Parallels between victimization and aging." *In* Sara B. Kiesler, James M. Morgan, Valerie Kincaid Oppenheimer (Eds.). *Aging: Social Change.* New York: Academic Press, 1981.

Explores the parallels of research on social support and victimization and social support in old age.

Literature Review

Describes the adaptiveness of social support, the needs for specific types of social support, and the factors which interfere with the provision and adequacy of social support. The implications of these parallels are discussed in light of new research initiatives.

Essential reading for social psychologists and sociologists interested
in social support, victimization, and aging.

762. MECHANIC D. "Social factors affecting the mental health of the
     elderly." *In* H. Häfner, G. Moshel, N. Sartorius (Eds.).
     Mental Health in the Elderly. Berlin: Springer-Verlag, 1986.

Reviews the social factors that affect the health and welfare of a
rapidly increasing elderly population and its psychological vulnerability and makes suggestions for social policy.

Review

Utilizing the skills, experience, and wisdom of the elderly in voluntary activities would contribute in many ways to their health and
vitality. Better quality assessment and screening devices for access
to long-term care services should be developed, and incentives designed to encourage isolated elderly to live together, thereby increasing their financial resources, social supports, and control over
their lives.

Of interest to gerontologists, mental health professionals, human
service workers, and public policymakers.

763. SPENCE, Donald L., and John J. Cunningham. "Social factors
     and family supports." *In* Evan Calkins, Paul J. Davis,
     Amasa B. Ford (Eds.). *The Practice of Geriatrics.* Philadel-
     phia: W.B. Saunders, 1986.

Concerned with the involvement of community and family in the support
of geriatric patients.

Essay

Professional and lay people need to understand that many assumptions
related to the inevitable decline of old age are untrue--chronic
health and age-related mental health problems can be managed. The
disabilities of aging are predominantly the result of an impairment in
interaction with the environment. Both functional and social assessments should be used to identify disabilities, and health and social
services should be combined in a new approach to long-term care of the
elderly that is both beneficial to quality of life and economically
feasible.

Of interest to geriatricians and public policymakers.

764. TAYLOR, R.C. "Environmental and behavioral factors in
     psychiatric disorders in the elderly. An approach through
     risk groups." *In* H. Häfner, G. Moshel, N. Sartorius
     (Eds.). *Mental Health in the Elderly.* Berlin:
     Springer-Verlag, 1986.

Examines factors associated with losing independent functioning and needing various forms of home or institutional care in ten groups of elderly inhabitants of Aberdeen, Scotland living in their own homes.

Research

The three groups which are minimally disadvantaged—the isolated, never married, and childless—have little social support available to them compared to the rest of the sample, but there is no evidence that their health or psychological functioning is worse than that of the sample as a whole. The recently widowed, those living alone, and those from among the manual, nonskilled social class are close to the sample mean and have both strengths and weaknesses. The groups characterized by poor health and/or psychological functioning include the recently moved, recently discharged from hospitals, and the very old.

Of interest to social and behavioral scientists, gerontologists, social service workers, and mental health professionals.

765. VEIEL, H.O.F. "Social support and mental disorder in old age: Overview and appraisal." *In* H. Häfner, G. Moshel, N. Sartorius (Eds.). *Mental Health in the Elderly*. Berlin: Springer-Verlag, 1986.

Discusses the lack of evidence documenting the beneficial influence of supportive social structures and transactions on the mental health of the elderly, and suggests directions for future research.

Review

The opportunity for preventive and therapeutic intervention offered by the social support concept underscores the need for more precise empirical data concerning the effects of social support on the mental health of the elderly. Meaningful research will have to take into account the particular conditions of elderly populations and be able to demonstrate causal effects.

Of interest to gerontologists, mental health professionals, and social and behavioral scientists.

d. Dissertations

766. CASTELMAN, Karen O. "The effect of kin and friend support systems on the subjective well-being of elderly widows." Ph.D. dissertation, University of South Florida, 1984.

Examines the nature of social support provided by kin and friends and the effects upon the well-being of elderly widows.

Research

No difference was found between the importance of support from kin or friends to the well-being of elderly widows. Quality of a confidant relationship was highly related to well-being. Confidential interactions usually took place with kin, and sociable and recreational interactions with friends.

Of interest to gerontologists.

767. RICE, Susan. "Single, older, childless women: A study of social support and life satisfaction." D.S.W. dissertation, University of California, Los Angeles, 1982.

A study of social support and life satisfaction in the single, elderly, childless population.

Research

A couple of social support variables, as well as several background variables, including age, self-reported health, education, and socioeconomic status, were related to life satisfaction. The never married generally fared better in terms of life satisfaction than did divorced or widowed women. This was explained, using the concepts of role creation and role substitution.

Helpful for counselors of lonely elderly people and gerontologists.

768. TOLEDO, Sarah T. "Housing satisfaction, supportive services and social networks as related to life satisfaction of the elderly." Ph.D. dissertation, Oklahoma State University, 1982.

A study of the life satisfaction of elderly people living in two different housing projects.

Research

Results indicated that housing satisfaction and use of social networks were the most important factors in exploring life satisfaction. Better housing conditions may mediate the negative effects of fewer neighborhood services on life satisfaction.

Of interest to gerontologists, health care planners, and policymakers.

A. CAREGIVERS

a. Books

769. CHAFFIN, Bethany. *Caring for Those You Love.* Bountiful, UT: Horizon, 1985.

A very thorough and compassionate guide to caregiving for cognitively impaired elders.

Guide--Literature Review

Describes several categories of senile dementia and cognitive impairment, and reviews the state-of-the-art and science in treating these conditions. Also provides very helpful approaches to the caregiver's need to cope with the burden of caregiving. Appendices are important in that they reflect other sources for help, including reading lists and other items.

Caregivers--family and professional--will benefit from this useful book.

770. GILLIES, John. *A Guide to Compassionate Care of the Aging.* New York: Thomas Nelson, 1985.

This book, based on Maslow's needs hierarchy, deals with caring for an elder.

Text-Handbook

Book's units are devoted to fulfilling needs--physiologic, security, emotional, esteem, and growth. Provides useful information on everything from compassionate responses, to dependency, to federal funding for adult day care programs.

Excellent overview and practical guide to providing or mobilizing social support for all readers.

771. HORNE, Jo. *Care-giving: Helping an Aging Loved One.* Glenview, IL: American Association of Retired Persons and Scott, Foresman, 1985.

A guide written for family and/or friends considering taking care of an aging loved one.

Handbook

Deals with the things which should be considered in caring for an elder, such as living arrangements, financial and legal problems, physical and emotional disability, and community support services. The book is written with the caregiver(s) in mind and has excellent sections dealing with coping and social support mechanisms.

Intended for general audiences, but a very good source for health professions students caring for elders.

b. Articles

772. BLASS, John P. "Caring for demented patients and their families." *Archives of the Foundation of Thanatology* 12, no. 1 (1986): 25.

Discusses techniques which can help demented patients and their families.

Review Abstract

Dementing illnesses lead to progressively increasing disabilities in
the patients and strains on the family or other support systems.
Techniques which can help include optimal medical care including
pharmacology, rehabilitation techniques, and counseling and social
supports. Social supports are critical, both for the patient and
caretakers, replacing the self-care necessary for survival of the
patient and allowing the caretakers to cope with the intense strain of
caring for the patient.

Of interest to geriatricians, social workers, and mental health
professionals.

773. BRAUN, Hans. "Verwandtschaftliche hilfe für ältere menschen.
      Eine explorative untersuchung des handlungfeldes weiblicher
      helfer." (German) *Zeitschrift für Gerontologie* 16 (1983):
      210-215.

A study of women who care for an elderly relative, the types of care
they offer, the context in which the care takes place, and the relationships between the care-provider and care-recipient.

Research

Five types of care were described: basic care and nursing,
psychosocial care, obligatory attendance, housekeeping, and supportive
contacts with the social environment. Care-providers usually received
material and/or emotional gratification for their efforts. Several
negative experiences for the care-provider, e.g. awareness of the
decrepitude of a relative and fear of the future, were described.

Of interest to gerontologists, health care planners and providers for
the elderly, and lay people taking care of themselves or an elderly
relative.

774. COHEN, Shirley. "Supporting families through respite care."
      Rehabilitation Literature 43 (1982): 7-11.

Evidence is provided emphasizing the value to caregivers of respite
care.

Literature Review

Respite care is defined and a brief review of its effectiveness is
provided. Suggestions for who should consider respite care services
and how to find them are provided.

Respite care providers, caregivers in need, and researchers will
benefit from this article.

775. GENDRON, C.E., L.R. Poitras, M.L. Engels, D.P. Dastoor,
     S.E. Sirota, S.L. Barza, J.C. Davis, N.B. Levine. "Skills
     training with supporters of the demented." *Journal of the
     American Geriatrics Society* 34 (1986): 875-880.

This study examined the effects of Supporter Endurance Training (SET)
on family caregivers of elderly demented patients.

Research

Eight supporters were provided eight weekly training sessions in
meditative relaxation and assertiveness, while four caregivers received no special training. A videotape dramatizing typical problem
situations encountered with a demented family member was used to
elicit information about the supporters' coping styles. Post-training
and six-month followup evaluation indicated improvements among the
trained individuals on measures related to assertiveness, problem
solving, and stress reduction as well as increases in the length of
time supporters estimated they would be able to cope with the problems
involved with caregiving. Few such improvements occurred among the
untrained subjects, suggesting that brief, structured skills training
programs help caregivers to improve their coping skills.

Of interest to mental health practitioners, geriatricians,
gerontologists, and public policymakers.

776. GILLEARD, C.J. "Problems posed for supporting relatives of
     geriatric and psychogeriatric day patients." *Acta
     Psychiatrica Scandia* 70 (1984): 198-208.

Examines the types of problems faced by caring relatives and the
strain imposed by their dependents, and, more specifically, compares
and contrasts the problems and strains associated with geriatric
versus psychogeriatric day care patients.

Research

While differences emerged in the type of problems these two groups of
supporters experienced with their dependents, the overall prevalence
of emotional disturbance was high in both groups.

Of interest to gerontologists and nursing home administrators.

777. JARRETT, William H. "Caregiving within kinship systems: Is
     affection really necessary?" *Gerontologist* 25 (1985): 5-10.

Suggests that filial affection for aged descendents is not always
sufficient to enable caregivers to cope with the strain of caregiving.

Literature Review

A reorientation of social values pertaining to caregiving. Kinship is
suggested as an important aspect of the social rationale for supporting the caregiver and thus aiding in the coping process and adjustment
to burden.

For general audiences, but of particular interest to human service providers.

778. JONES, Dee A., and Norman J. Vetter. "A survey of those who care for the elderly at home: Their problems and their needs." *Social Science and Medicine* 19 (1984): 511-514.

An examination of the network of informal and formal care, the problems and morbidity of informal carers who assist and support the dependent elderly in the community, and the implications of these problems for health and social services.

Research

Evidence supports the view that the family is the main source of assistance to the dependent elderly, usually the woman in the family. Very little assistance, either informal or formal, is received by the caregivers.

Of interest to gerontologists, social workers, mental health professionals, and health care planners and policymakers.

c. Chapter

779. MEDERER, Helen Jeanne. "The transition to a parent-caring role by adult children." *In* Vernon L. Allen, and Evert van de Vliet (Eds.). *Role Transitions.* New York: Plenum, 1983.

Reports on research-testing propositions that describe change within parent-child helping patterns over time.

Research

Findings indicate that, contrary to expectation, the possession of greater resources by the child does not make the transition to a parent-caring role easier--the opposite emerged. The higher the level of commitment to the role of parent caring, the easier the transition. Most adult children possess a high level of filial obligation and are willing to help parents.

Should interest social workers and social and behavioral scientists.

4. DEATH AND DYING

A. PALLIATIVE CARE

a. Books

780. CAUGHILL, Rita E. (Ed.). *The Dying Patient: A Supportive Approach.* Boston: Little, Brown, 1976.

An attempt to help nursing personnel develop the necessary knowledge and skills to give supportive care to dying patients.

Book of Readings

Readings focus on improving the quality of living for the dying and providing needed support for their relatives.

Intended for nurses and student nurses, but should also be useful to medical students, physicians, and allied health personnel.

781. GARFIELD, Charles A. (Ed.). *Psychosocial Care of the Dying Patient.* New York: McGraw-Hill, 1978.

Guidelines to help health professionals provide effective emotional support to terminal patients and their families.

Book of Readings

Chapters written by terminal patients, family members, caregivers, and social and behavioral scientists support the themes of "an apprecia-tion of the emotional realities of dying" and "the undeniable human need for caring." Guidelines for terminal care; patients and families facing death; the emotional impact of doctor-patient relationships; recognition and confrontation of psychological needs; counseling the family; specific issues regarding terminal care; and recent develop-ments in caring for the dying patient, including a community model of psychosocial support for patients and families facing life-threatening illness, are included within this volume.

Intended for physicians, nurses, and allied health professionals, especially those who work with the terminally ill.

782. LAMERTON, Richard. *Care of the Dying.* London: Priory Press, 1973.

Guidelines and practical advice for all concerned with helping dying patients.

Resource Book

Stresses the importance of attention, friendship, relief, and comfort; the need for teaching nurses and medical students how to meet both the medical and the emotional needs of the patient; and the need for the kind of services provided by the hospice. Contains an extensive list of references and bibliography.

Should be helpful to medical and nursing students, nurses, physicians, and other caregivers.

b. Articles

783. FOUNTAIN, Marsha Jean. "Psychosocial support for the person experiencing cancer." *Orthopedic Nursing* 4, no. 5 (September-October 1985): 33-35.

Delineates the psychosocial support necessary to care for a person with cancer, which will best meet the needs of the patient and family, while also supporting the nurse.

Descriptive

Discusses loss of control, patient/family support, maladaptive patient behavior, and the dying patient. Two major points are made: 1) one of a cancer patient's greatest fears is that of abandonment; and 2) allowing staff to grieve is important and should be encouraged.

Of interest to oncologists, nurses, and other health professionals providing care to cancer patients.

B. BEREAVEMENT COUNSELING

a. Books

784. KALISH, Richard A. *Death, Grief, and Caring Relationships.* Second Edition. Monterey, CA: Brooks/Cole, 1985.

Deals with understanding death, the process of aging, and grief.

Text

Divided into five sections: the meaning of death, the process of dying, grief and bereavement, a life-span perspective, and caring relationships. The section on caring relationships contains chapters on roles and relationships, health and educational programs, and providing for emotional well-being.

Intended for professionals and volunteers who work with the dying and bereaved, students in classes on death and grief, and lay persons who wish to learn and understand more about death and grief.

785. OSTERWEIS, Marian, Fredric Solomon, Morris Green (Eds.). *Bereavement: Reactions,   Consequences,   and   Care.* Washington, DC: National Academy Press, 1984.

A synthesis of the nature and consequences of bereavement, its underlying biologic and psychologic mechanisms, and the factors that protect some individuals, but leave others at risk for poor outcomes.

Report

Useful background papers and critical reviews from a variety of professionals on the reactions and consequences of bereavement, perspectives on bereavement, and assisting the bereaved.

Of interest to all health professionals.

786. SCHOENBERG, Bernard, Irwin Gerber, Alfred Weiner, Austin
     H. Kutscher, David Peretz, Arthur C. Carr. (Eds.).
     Bereavement: Its Psychosocial Aspects. New York: Columbia
     University Press, 1975.

A multidisciplinary approach to the examination of the psychosocial
aspects of bereavement.

Book of Readings

Divided into sections on fundamental concepts, the bereavement process, the bereaved family, the health professional, and therapeutic
intervention. Addresses such significant topics as the value of
interdisciplinary health support systems, the usefulness of self-help
groups, the prospects of methods of crisis intervention and the
development of human support services for the bereaved that are
integrated into health service planning, community organization, and
the roles and training of health workers.

Should interest social scientists, members of the caring professions,
public policymakers, and laypersons interested in the issues of death
and dying.

b. Articles

787. BANKOFF, Elizabeth A. "Social support and adaptation to
     widowhood." *Journal of Marriage and the Family* 45 (1983):
     827-839.

This study examined the effects of social support on the psychological
well-being of 245 women who had been widowed for less than three
years.

Research

Whether social support is helpful, harmful, or inconsequential to
widows' psychological well-being seems to depend on such factors as
where the widows are in the adjustment process, the type of support
given, and its source.

Of interest to counselors and mental health professionals.

788. BERARDO, Felix M. "Survivorship and social isolation: The
     case of the aged widower." *The Family Coordinator* 19
     (1970): 11-25.

Examines the environmental conditions surrounding the aged male
survivor and assesses his accommodation to widowhood status.

Review and Analysis

Evidence indicates the the aged male survivor experiences a different
impact from spousal loss than does his female counterpart and that he

encounters severe difficulties in adapting to the single status. Adjustment problems are especially compounded by the loss of his occupational role, which abruptly removes him from meaningful contact with friends and co-workers. Social isolation among aged widowers leads to a precarious condition that is reflected in unusually high rates of mental disorders, suicide, and mortality risk.

Of interest to gerontologists and social and behavioral scientists.

789. BRYAN, Elizabeth M. "The death of a newborn twin: How can support for parents be improved?" *Acta Geneticae Medicae et Gemellologiae* 35 (1985): 115-118.

Explores the experiences and needs of mothers who lose a newborn twin.

Research

Semistructured questionnaires were sent to 14 bereaved mothers. All mothers continued to think of the surviving child as a twin, and six had feelings of resentment to the survivor. All felt their loss had been underestimated. Support could be improved by acknowledging the mother's grief and encouraging her to talk about the dead baby. Reminders, such as photographs, could be provided. Parents should be offered counseling and the opportunity to meet similarly bereaved parents.

Of interest to bereavement counselors, social workers, and other mental health professionals.

790. FERRARO, Kenneth F., Elizabeth Mutran, Charles M. Barresi. "Widowhood, health, and friendship support in later life." *Journal of Health and Social Behavior* 25 (1984): 245-259.

Examines the effect of widowhood on future health and friendship support, using a national sample of the low-income aged.

Research

Not many differences were noted in the health-friendship support relationships between older married and widowed persons. An important finding was that recency of widowhood seemed to be a significant predictor of acquiring friendship supports: recently widowed persons may go through a period of adjustment to that life event by augmenting certain types of social support.

Particularly interesting to gerontologists and social scientists.

791. HELMRATH, Thomas A., and Elaine M. Steinitz. "Death of an infant: Parental grieving and the failure of social support." *Journal of Family Practice* 6 (1978): 785-790.

Explores the events and personal interactions that help or hinder parents following their infants' deaths.

Research

The seven bereaved couples in this study encountered significant problems with their resolution of guilt following the loss of their infants. The failure of society to support them during this critical period forced these parents to experience the mourning process in relative isolation.

Helpful to mental health professionals.

792. HOHENBRUCK, B.G., M.Y.M. de Kleine, L.A.A. Kollée, L.M.H. Robbroechk. "Rouwverwerking en begeleiding bÿ het overlÿden van pasgeborenen." (Dutch) *Nederlands Tÿdschrift voor Geneeskunde* 129 (1985): 1582-1585.

A study of coping with mourning and care and support after neonatal death.

Research

In general, it was found that parents experiencing the death of a newborn infant did not receive satisfactory emotional support and guidance from medical specialists (pediatrician, obstetrician). Follow-up care by primary care medical workers (the general practitioner and district nurse) was also often lacking, although many parents expressed a need for such care.

Of special interest to obstetricians, pediatricians, general practitioners, and other medical or para-medical professionals involved in neonatal care.

793. LEHMANN, Darrin R., John H. Ellard, Camille B. Wortman. "Social support for the bereaved: Recipients' and providers' perspectives on what is helpful." *Journal of Consulting and Clinical Psychology* 54 (1986): 438-445.

This study describes helpful and unhelpful attempts at support for people who had recently lost a spouse or a child.

Research

Those support providers who had backgrounds similar to those of the bereaved and allowed the expression of feelings were most helpful. Those support providers who gave advice and encouraged recovery were less helpful. The relationship and ability to provide support were unrelated to the provider's experience with bereavement.

Thanotologists, hospice workers, and others dealing with bereavement will find this an interesting article.

794. ROSS-ALAOMOLKI, Kathleen. "Supportive care for families of dying children." *Nursing Clinics of North America* 20, no. 2 (1985): 457-466.

A review of the disruptive effects to families of dying children, which discusses the importance of supportive care.

Review

Discusses parental anticipatory grief, the development of the concept of illness and death in children, last phases of the life process, and the importance of communication. Except for the general notion that strong supportive relationships with family, friends, etc. should be incorporated in supportive care programs, little social support information is provided.

Nurses and others providing care to families with dying children may find this article useful.

795. VAN DE VEN, Luc, and Ria Hectors.   "Reflecties over de begeleiding van familieleden van dementerende bejaarden." (Dutch). *Tÿdschrift voor Gerontologie en Geriatrie* 14, no. 4 (1983): 149-156.

Discusses the emotional problems of the relatives of patients suffering from senile dementia.

Theoretical

Some reactions of the relatives of demented old people are interpreted as manifestations of a mourning process. The typical grief reactions may not only be the result of real loss, but also of anticipated loss, the imminent death of a relative. Psychotherapeutic help may be appropriate, and relatives of demented old people may support each other in group meetings.

Of interest to gerontologists, psychotherapists dealing with mourning processes, and lay people who care for a relative suffering from senile dementia.

c. Dissertations

796. FEINSON, Marjorie Chary.   "Distress and social support: A needs assessment of bereaved older adults." Ph.D. dissertation, Rutgers University, The State University of New Jersey, New Brunswick, 1982.

Investigates the prevalence of psychological distress and the impact of health status and social support on distress in bereaved older adults.

Research

The sample was significantly more distressed than a nonbereaved control sample. Health and social support variables were important predictors of distress among widows. For widowers, however, social support, religious preference, and employment status contributed most to the alleviation of psychological distress.

Particularly useful to gerontologists and other professionals concerned with the mental health of the aged, but also of interest to
stress researchers.

797. KEITH, Judy, G.B. "The relationships between the adjustment
of the widowed and social support, self-esteem, grief experience, and selected demographic variables." Ed.D. dissertation, University of Tennessee, 1982.

A study of the relationship between the adjustment of the widowed and
a number of social and psychological variables.

Research

No particular effects of social support or demographic variables on
long term adjustment to widowhood were found. Females appeared to
have more interpersonal support, and personal self-esteem was found to
be more important for adjustment than general or social self-esteem.

Useful for bereavement counselors.

1. EFFECT OF LOSS ON MORBIDITY AND MORTALITY

a. Articles

798. JACOBS, Selby, and Adrian Ostfeld. "An epidemiological
review of the mortality of bereavement." *Psychosomatic
Medicine* 39 (1977): 344-357.

Epidemiological literature revealing excess mortality in the newly
widowed is reviewed.

Literature Review

Factors and mediating processes that need to be considered in clarifying the effect of bereavement on the mortality of the survivor are
those that characterize the survivor's environment or other sources of
social stress and those that characterize the survivor's susceptibility and life expectancy, such as the nature of the attachment to the
deceased, depression, and health practices.

Of interest to social and behavioral scientists.

799. MADDISON, David and Agnes Viola. "The health of widows in
the year following bereavement." *Journal of Psychosomatic
Research* 12 (1968): 297-306.

Explores the physical and psychological consequences of conjugal
bereavement.

Research

Widows experienced significantly more physical and psychological symptoms and illnesses during the 13-month period following their spouses' deaths than did their matched controls. These findings are discussed in view of the bereavement process and normal grief reactions.

Of interest to general practitioners, bereavement counselors, and medical sociologists.

800. NIEMI, Timo. "The mortality of male old-age pensioners following spouses' death." *Scandinavian Journal of Social Medicine* 7 (1979): 115-117.

The effect of the death of a spouse on the mortality of retired men was investigated using a sample of 939 married, retired men, 174 of whom had lost their spouse after retirement.

Research

A larger than anticipated number of retired men died during the first six months following bereavement, but no increase in mortality could be shown over a longer term. Circulatory diseases and tumors were over-represented as causes of death among those who died following the loss of their wives. Loss of an important relationship may lead to sudden cardiac death or accelerate the development of a disease.

Should interest epidemiologists, medical researchers, and social scientists.

801. PARKES, C. Murray, B. Benjamin, R.G. Fitzgerald. "A broken heart: A statistical study of increased mortality among widows." *British Medical Journal* 1 (1969): 740-743.

Investigates the correlation between the death rate of widowers, 55 years of age and older, and the death rate of married men of the same age.

Research

The greatest increase in the mortality rate of widowers occurs during the first six months following the death of a spouse. A larger than chance number of the causes of death of these widowers fall within the same diagnostic groups as those of their deceased wives. There is no evidence of increase after the initial six month period.

Of interest to social and behavioral scientists, nursing home administrators, and health professionals caring for the elderly.

802. PENNEBAKER, James W., and Robin C. O'Heeron. "Confiding in others and illness rate among spouses of suicide and accidental death victims." *Journal of Abnormal Psychology* 93 (1984): 473-476.

The present survey examined the degree to which confiding in others was associated with health problems in the year following the death of a spouse.

Research

Results indicated that the more that subjects discussed their spouse's death with friends and the less they ruminated about the death, the fewer were the increases in health problems reported.

Of interest to mental health professionals.

803. REES, W. Dewi, and Sylvia G. Lutkins. "Mortality of bereavement." *British Medical Journal* 4 (October 7, 1967): 13-16.

A survey was carried out to assess the effect of bereavement on the mortality of close relatives in a small semirural community.

Research

A sevenfold increase in risk among the bereaved over that of the control group was found, indicating that bereavement carries a considerably increased risk of mortality. This risk was found to be greater for male than for female relatives. The increased risk was greatest for the widowed and least for female children.

Of interest to health professionals in general.

b. Chapter

804. STROEBE, Wolfgang, Margaret S. Stroebe, Kenneth J. Gergen, Mary Gergen. "The effects of bereavement on mortality: A social psychological analysis." *In* Alan Monat, and Richard S. Lazarus (Eds.). *Stress and Coping. An Anthology.* Second Edition. New York: Columbia University Press, 1986.

A discussion of the cognitive and social psychological processes which account for the "loss effect" among spouses.

Theoretical/Analytical

The consequences of losing a marital partner should be the more severe, the closer the relationship between the partners, the greater the role differentiation within the marital group, and the fewer alternative persons available who could serve part of the functions formerly fulfilled by the partner. While the absence of strong positive affective bonds between the partners may imply that they will no longer serve each other as sources of social and emotional support, it should leave their willingness and ability to fulfill task-related and social protective functions for each other unimpaired.

Of general interest to all health professionals.

2. BEREAVEMENT COUNSELING

a. Book

805. SCHOENBERG, B. Mark (Ed.). *Bereavement Counseling: A Multidisciplinary Handbook*. Westport, CT: Greenwood Press, 1980.

A multidisciplinary attempt to offer guidelines to persons engaged in providing support to the dying and the bereaved.

Book of Readings

Presents a broad perspective, which includes thanatology, counseling models, the role of the nurse and of the clergy in working with the dying and their families, preparing a child for facing death, bereavement in the elderly, and supporting a friend who is in mourning.

Should be helpful to members of the various caring professions as well as laypersons interested in the issues of death and dying.

b. Articles

806. BEHNKE, Marylou, Emmalee Setzer, Pauline Mehta. "Death counseling and psychosocial support by physicians concerning dying children." *Journal of Medical Education* 59 (1984): 906-908.

Reports on the content of death education in residency training.

Research

A small group of residents were surveyed regarding their previous training in death counseling, to assess the need for residents to provide such counseling, and to define the self-perceived confidence of residents in their ability to provide counseling. The study found little previous training in death education and little confidence in the ability to provide counseling, although the need was perceived.

Medical educators, thanatologists, and others working with the hospice movement would find this report interesting.

807. HERMANN, Joan F. "Psychosocial support: Interventions for the physician." *Seminars in Oncology* 12 (1985): 466-471.

Addresses the psychosocial tasks of patients and families anticipating a death and the specific strategies a physician may employ to facilitate that process.

Review

Reviews the components of successful palliative care, and focuses on the role of the physician and health care team in providing the patient and family with information and counseling, helping them with decision-making, and preparing them for the postdeath bereavement process.

Of interest to physicians, other health care professionals, social workers, and clinical psychologists.

808. PARKES, Colin Murray. "Bereavement counseling: Does it work? *British Medical Journal* 281 (1980): 3-10.

A study of the effectiveness of various forms of counseling that focus on the increased risk of psychiatric and psychosomatic disorders associated with the death of a loved one.

Research

The evidence shows that professional services and self-help services are capable of reducing the risk of psychiatric and psychosomatic disorders resulting from bereavement. Services are most beneficial among those who perceive their families as unsupportive.

Of interest to mental health professionals.

c. Chapter

809. PARKES, Colin Murray. "Evaluation of a bereavement service." *In* A. De Vries, and A. Carmi (Eds.). *The Dying Human.* Ramat Gan, Israel: Turtledove, 1979.

A bereavement service was studied to determine the impact of supportive intervention on the health of the bereaved.

Research

Results indicated that the introduction of the service for bereaved people at St. Christopher's Hospice in London produced a real improvement in health outcome. The need for drugs, alcohol, and tobacco among the bereaved was reduced along with the number of symptoms attributable to anxiety and tension.

Of particular interest to mental health professionals.

CHAPTER 6

SOCIAL AND CULTURAL FACTORS AND SOCIAL SUPPORT

1. ETHNIC AND CROSS-CULTURAL ISSUES

a. Books

810. LOMNITZ, Larissa A. *Networks and Marginality: Life in a Mexican Shantytown.* New York: Academic Press, 1977.

A broad and thorough coverage of the unique features of institutionalized social support in the Mexican culture, which provides important insights for bicultural studies of social support among Mexican-Americans.

Resource Book

Takes a classic approach in its descriptions of institutionalized support, describing the influence of the setting, migration, family network interactions, and mechanisms which effect social reciprocity.

Anyone who is involved in bicultural research or provides human services to Mexican clients will benefit from this book.

811. STACK, Carol. *All Our Kin.* New York: Harper and Row, 1974.

An anthropological study of the social networks in a section of a poor black community in the Midwest.

Research

Black familes in The Flats have evolved patterns of co-residence, kinship-based exchange networks linking multiple domestic units, elastic household boundaries, life-long bonds to three-generation households, social controls against the formation of marriages that could endanger the network of kin, the domestic authority of women, and limitations on the role of the husband or male friend within a woman's kin network. These highly adaptive features of urban black families comprise a resilient response to the conditions of poverty and unemployment.

Of interest to social and behavioral scientists.

b. Articles

812. ANTONUCCI, T.C. "Cross-cultural issues in the concept of social support." *Gerontologist* 25, Supplement 1 (1985): 264-265.

Reviews studies of social support in different cultural settings.

Literature Review/Abstract

Informal comparisons of the data show that there are distinct issues among cultures and subcultures regarding perception, expectation, and assessment of social support. Conceptions of social support, the role of family and friends, and intra-family issues involving social support need to be investigated.

Of interest to researchers of social support.

813. BARANOWSKI, Thomas, David E. Bee, David K. Rassin, C. Joan Richardson, Judy P. Brown, Nancy Guenther, Philip R. Nader. "Social support, social influence, ethnicity, and the breastfeeding decision." *Social Science and Medicine* 17 (1983): 1599-1611.

Describes a survey of mothers to determine factors related to their decision to breastfeed.

Research

Results found the most supportive person in the decision of Black-American mothers was a close friend; among Mexican-American mothers it was the mother's mother, and among Anglo-Americans, the male partner.

Pediatricians and others interested in factors affecting breastfeeding decisions may benefit from the results of this survey.

814. CHATTERS, Linda M., Robert Joseph Taylor, James S. Jackson. "Aged blacks' choices for an informal helper network." *Journal of Gerontology* 41 (1986): 94-100.

An exploration of the relationship of sociodemographic, health, and family factors to informal helper choice among a nationally representative sample of 581 older (55 and over) blacks.

Research

Logistic regression analysis revealed that marital status is important in determining the selection of sister, friend, or neighbor. The presence of children decreased the likelihood that siblings and friends would be chosen. Perceived family closeness facilitated the selection of siblings, but inhibited the choice of friends. Regional differences suggested a greater likelihood that the category of sister, friend, or neighbor would be selected by Southern residents.

Of interest to gerontologists and social and behavioral scientists.

815. ———. "Size and composition of the informal helper networks of elderly blacks." *Journal of Gerontology* 40 (1985): 605-614.

Examines the relationship of health, family composition, and availability factors related to the size and composition of the informal support networks of older blacks.

Research

A national representative survey of 581 older blacks found associations between the size and composition of social networks and marriage, sex, and regional variations. Health factors were found not to be related to either size or composition of the informal social support networks.

Those interested in minority health factors, support patterns, and family interactions will find this an important paper.

816. CROUCH, Ben M. "Age and institutional support: Perceptions of older Mexican-Americans." *Journal of Gerontology* 27, no. 4 (1972): 524-529.

Reports findings on how older Mexican-Americans view old age and perceive three primary institutions from which informal and formal programs of aid arise—the family, the church, and the government.

Research

This sample had a decidedly negative evaluation of the status of old age. Data on the perception of support institutions suggest that older Mexican-Americans generally recognize a de-emphasis of the extended family, feel that the church has a social action as well as a sacred function, and believe that the Anglo government could be a potent agency for support.

Useful to gerontologists, cultural anthropologists, and social and behavioral scientists.

817. CRUZ-LOPEZ, Miguel, and Richard E. Pearson. "The support
      needs and resources of Puerto Rican elders." *Gerontologist*
      25 (1985): 483-487.

Describes a study of the natural support systems available to elderly
Puerto Ricans and their relationship to physical and emotional
well-being.

Research

Examines the support needs, resources, and natural systems that
trained helpers can affect in improving the social support available
to Hispanic and other elderly.

Of interest to social workers and other health professionals working
with the elderly.

818. DAVIS, Robert. "Black suicide and social support systems--an
      overview and some implications for mental health practi-
      tioners." *Phylon* 43 (1982): 307-314.

A review of the rates of suicide among blacks, etiological factors,
and preventive models. The external restraint theory, which holds
that suicides vary inversely with restraining factors such as low
social status and the insulation that strong communal and family ties
provide, is examined.

Review and Analysis

There is no organized interest group or research structure that can
disseminate current information on the nature and pattern of suicide
among blacks and its implications for mental health practitioners.
Similarly, there is no evidence that black professional organizations
have assigned this problem a high priority. Hence, there has been no
apparent surge of public opinion designating suicide as a problem
within the black community.

Of interest to mental health professionals and social and behavioral
scientists.

819. DELGADO, Melvin. "Ethnic and cultural variations in the care
      of the aged Hispanic elderly and natural support systems: A
      special focus on Puerto Ricans." *Journal of Geriatric Psy-
      chiatry* 15 (1982): 239-255.

Presents an overview of Puerto Rican/Hispanic demographic trends in
the United States, an outline of key factors in addressing the needs
of this population, a framework from which to examine natural support
systems, and a series of recommendations on how best to utilize
Hispanic elders as a human service resource.

Descriptive

Hispanic elders perform important natural support functions within the

Hispanic community. However, the functions of natural support systems traditionally held by Hispanic elders may be in danger of disappearing.

Of interest to social and behavioral scientists.

820. ———. "Hispanic natural support systems: Implications for mental health services." *Journal of Psychosocial Nursing and Mental Health Services* 21, no. 4 (April 1983): 19-24.

Defines natural support systems and outlines the services they provide, examines the cultural value underpinnings that make them the first alternative for assistance, and presents a typology for assessing the causes of natural support systems' inability to provide aid.

Descriptive

Hispanic natural support systems and mental health settings must work together in attempting to meet the mental health needs of this group. The mental health settings must work together in attempting to utilize the strengths of clients. Natural support systems are probably the greatest resource within Hispanic communities.

Of interest to social and behavioral scientists.

821. DRESSLER, William W. "The social and cultural context of coping: Action gender and symptoms in a southern black community." *Social Science and Medicine* 21 (1985): 499-506.

Evidence suggests that differences exist in the coping styles employed by males and females in black communities and their effectiveness.

Research

Generally, males can rely on extended family to help them cope with economic and social stressors, but active coping usually provides deleterious effects. Females are better able to use active coping, relying on their own abilities. This paper underscores the need to interpret coping in light of the broader, cultural background.

Sociologists, anthropologists, and others interested in the cultural factors that affect coping styles may find this helpful.

822. ———, Jose Ernesto Dos Santos, Fernando E. Viteri. "Blood pressure, ethnicity, and psychosocial resources." *Psychosomatic Medicine* 48 (1986): 509-519.

Examines the extent to which the effect of "race" or "ethnicity" on blood pressure may be modified by the presence or absence of psychosocial resources.

Research

Results support the hypothesis that the risk of high blood pressure associated with mixed black ethnic status is modified or buffered by the availability of psychosocial resources. Psychosocial resources provide protective functions against high blood pressure that are enhanced for persons of mixed black ethnic status.

Of interest to researchers in psychosomatic and behavioral medicine.

823. DURRETT, Mary Ellen, Phyllis Richards, Midori Otaki, James W. Pennebaker, Linda Nyquist. "Mother's involvement with infant and her perception of spousal support, Japan and America." *Journal of Marriage and the Family* 48 (1986): 187-194.

Investigates the differences between Japanese and American mothers' perceptions of support from their husbands, and the relationship between those perceptions and the mothers' involvement with their infants.

Research

Significant differences were found between the two cultures for the mothers' perceptions of support from the husband and the infants' early home environments. Findings indicate that the more a mother perceives support from her husband, the more apt she is to become involved with the infant when they are together and the less she feels that she needs to be in the presence of the infant at all times.

Of interest to pediatricians and child development specialists.

824. FARRELL, Janice, and Kyriakos S. Markides. "Marriage and health: A three-generation study of Mexican-Americans." *Journal of Marriage and the Family* 47 (1985): 1029-1036.

An investigation of the relationships between health, marital status, and marital satisfaction, using data from a three-generation study of Mexican-Americans.

Research

There were few consistent differences found in physical health symptoms and self-rated health by marital status once the effects of sex, age, income, and education were held constant. The significant differences were generally found in the midlife and younger generations. Women of all generations reported poorer health than men. Marital satisfaction was related to the health of the middle and younger generation, but not the older generation. Marriage and good marriage appear to have more protective influences on younger Mexican-Americans, but generational differences may reflect selection effects.

May interest sociologists and anthropologists.

825. FEAGIN, Joe R. "Social sources of support for violence and nonviolence in a Negro ghetto." *Social Problems* 15 (1968): 432-441.

A classic study of the factors associated with violence orientation among American blacks after the 1964 New York's Bedford-Stuyvesant Riots.

Research

Confirms the relationship of numerous social/demographic factors associated with violence orientation. Those respondents with high indices of communal participation (social support) were less likely to be violence oriented.

Sociologists, social planners, police, and others working in socioeconomically deprived areas should read this paper.

826. ———. "A note on the friendship ties of black urbanites." *Social Forces* 49 (1970): 303-308.

A research note dealing with the friendship ties of black urbanites that emphasizes the need for more systematic and comparative work on the social networks of urban blacks.

Research

This paper documents the importance of friendship as an integral factor in linking an individual to a specific community. The findings are not dissimilar from those of previous studies, but they do document the tendency of blacks to have small, encapsulated social support networks.

Social workers, sociologists, and others interested in urban studies and research on minority groups will benefit from this study.

827. FLEISHMAN, R., and A. Shmueli. "Patterns of informal social support of the elderly: An international comparison." *Gerontologist* 24 (1984): 303-312.

Compares the patterns of affective and instrumental mutual support of the elderly and their primary helpers in Baka, Jerusalem, and examines the role of ethnicity, sex, and age in explaining manifest differences is Israeli and foreign patterns of informal social support.

Review

An Israeli study has found that the elderly of Baka, a Jerusalem neighborhood, like those in other Israeli studies, receive strong, family-oriented informal support with little participation by non-kin. Similar family-oriented patterns of support, reported in foreign studies, are coupled with substantial assistance from non-kin. The authors suggest ways in which such strong, family-oriented support systems might be used as a complement to formal services and an alternative to institutionalization.

Of interest to health planners and policymakers and social service professionals.

828. GAUDIN, James M., Jr., and Katheryn B. Davis. "Social networks of black and white rural families: A research report." *Journal of Marriage and the Family* 47 (1985): 1015-1020.

Examines the structural characteristics and supportiveness of the social networks of 175 black and white rural, lower SES mothers.

Research

Black mothers reported their networks to be significantly less supportive than did white mothers. Networks of black families were significantly smaller than those of whites and more kin dominated. Black mothers' networks were less heterogeneous than those of whites, but were more durable. Rural, lower SES black families reported less help available and fewer persons to call upon for help in times of need than did whites. Professional helpers were absent from the social networks of both blacks and whites.

Should interest social scientists.

829. GRAVES, Theodore D., and Nancy B. Graves. "Stress and health among Polynesian migrants to New Zealand." *Journal of Behavioral Medicine* 8 (1985): 1-19.

A group of 228 Samoans, 212 Cook Islanders, and 224 native-born New Zealanders of European background, all living in the same working class neighborhoods in Auckland, were interviewed to determine the effect of cultural differences on adaptation to life in a major industrial city.

Research

There were strong positive associations between reported symptoms of poor health and both the frequency of external situational stressors and the strength of Type A psychological attributes, which together account for 25% of the variance in health status in all the ethnic and sex groups. Social support systems, however, did not provide the anticipated stress-buffering effects. In fact, evidence seems to suggest that traditional practices of obligation and reciprocity by members of the Polynesians' ethnic communities, particularly in the case of the Samoans, are costly and stressful, thereby offsetting their social support systems' stress-buffering role.

Of interest to anthropologists and sociologists.

830. GRIFFITH, James. "Emotional support providers and psychological distress among Anglo and Mexican-Americans." *Community Mental Health Journal* 20 (Fall 1984): 182-201.

Compares emotional support network characteristics of Anglo-Americans to those of Mexican-Americans, and examines the relationship between the reliance on specific support providers and psychopathological symptoms for both groups.

Research

Both Anglos and English-speaking Mexican-Americans reported significantly larger networks and more cumulative contact and reciprocity with network members than did Spanish-speaking Mexican-Americans, and named significantly more friends and neighbors as emotional support providers. Spanish-speaking Mexican-Americans, on the other hand, more often depended on extended kin and spouses than did the other two sub-groups.

Of interest to social and behavioral scientists.

831. HENDRICKS, Leo E. "Unwed adolescent fathers: Problems they face and their sources of social support." *Adolescence* 15 (Winter 1980): 861-869.

A pilot study to identify and describe, quantitatively, problems encountered by a selected sample of black, unwed adolescent fathers and possible sources of social support in resolving those problems.

Research

Ninety-five percent of the young fathers expressed a high degree of readiness to attend a teenage parenting agency if it offered services for unwed adolescent fathers. Agencies and institutions serving family planning needs should provide services for unwed adolescent fathers as well as unwed adolescent mothers.

Of use to mental health professionals and health professionals providing direct services to adolescents, as well as those in preventive medicine and public health.

832. JAMES, Alice, William L. James, Howard L. Smith. "Reciprocity as a coping strategy of the elderly: A rural Irish perspective." *Gerontologist* 24 (1984): 483-489.

A longitudinal study of the aging process in western Ireland, which addresses the questions of how the elderly use informal support networks to cope with the problems of aging; what personal mechanisms people use to adapt to the aging process, and which of these mechanisms are most effective; and whether intergenerational social exchange is a constructive process that reinforces the independence of the elderly.

Research

Reciprocity, fostered through the stem family, sibling relations, pets, neighbors, parental caretakers, financial resources, and variations in family configurations, was found to be one of the major forces that reinforce independence in the aged in Ireland. The policy implications of reciprocity as a coping strategy are discussed.

Of interest to social and behavioral scientists.

833. KEEFE, Susan E., Amado M. Padilla, Manuel L. Carlos. "The Mexican-American extended family as an emotional support system." *Human Organization* 38 (1979): 144-152.

Compares and contrasts the Mexican American and Anglo American family structure and reliance on kin for emotional support, and examines the utilization of other sources of support for emotional problems compared with the tendency to rely on relatives.

Research

Data on family and mental health, gathered over three years from both Mexican Americans and Anglo Americans in Santa Barbara, Santa Paula, and Oxnard, California demonstrated that although the kinship structure of the two ethnic groups is fundamentally different, both groups rely on family for help. However, Anglos are more likely to seek help from friends, neighbors, coworkers, and groups, while Mexican Americans' main resource is their extended kin network, and relatively little support is derived from other informal sources. Both Anglo and Mexican Americans often seek aid from more formal sources of support. Mental health professionals need to be aware of the probability that the absence or malfunction of the supportive family is far more distressing for Mexican Americans, to whom it is the primary source of informal support, than for Anglo Americans in similar circumstances, and the implications this has for treatment.

Of interest to social and behavioral scientists and mental health professionals.

834. KEEFE, Susan Emley. "Southern Appalachia: Analytical models, social services, and native support systems." *American Journal of Community Psychology* 14 (1986): 479-498.

A theoretical model of ethnicity, covering structural, cultural, and symbolic aspects, is developed for the analysis of social services in southern Appalachia, and results of an exploratory study of ethnic differences between Appalachians and non-Appalachians in a mountainous North Carolina county, lending validity to the model, are presented.

Theoretical/Research

The author argues that the analysis of social services in southern Appalachia benefits more from a model based on ethnicity than from more commonly used models based on lower socioeconomic status or rural residence. Educational and mental health services are discussed in the context of Appalachian ethnicity and the potential for using native support systems in improving these services.

Of interest to anthropologists, sociologists, and health care planners and providers.

835. KENDIG, Hal L., and Don T. Rowland. "Family support of the
      Australian aged: A comparison with the United States."
      Gerontologist 23 (1983): 643-649.

Findings on the involvement of older Australians with members of their
modified extended families, especially adult children, are presented.

Research

The relationships between the aged and their children are shown to
entail close emotional bonds and a regular, two-way flow of instrumental support. Although most of the results are similar to those of
American studies, older Australians more frequently live in joint
households and make greater use of community and institutional
services.

Of interest to gerontologists and family sociologists.

836. LINDBLAD-GOLDBERG, Marion, and Joyce Lynn Dukes. "Social
      support in black low-income, single-parent families."
      American Journal of Orthopsychiatry 55 (1985): 42-58.

Structural and functional features of social networks and demographic
variables were explored in a study of 50 clinic-referred and 76
nonclinic, black, low-income, single-parent families.

Research

Dysfunctional families evidenced asymmetrical reciprocity within
network relationships and had more stressful home environments than
did nonclinical families.

Of interest to social workers, mental health professionals, and
professionals working with low-income, single-parent families.

837. LINDSEY, Ada M., Marylin J. Dodd, Shin-Gon Chen. "Social
      support network of Taiwanese cancer patients." *International
      Journal of Nursing Studies* 23, no. 2 (1985): 149-164.

A study designed to determine the nature and characteristics of the
social support network, as perceived by Taiwanese hospitalized with
cancer.

Research

The findings provide evidence that, in this sample of hospitalized
Taiwanese cancer patients, the spouse, family members, and other
relatives are perceived to be the predominant and almost sole social
support network. The stability of the subjects' perceived network is
characterized by the greater than five year duration of the
relationships.

Of interest to nurses, oncologists, social workers, and others caring
for cancer patients.

838. MARKIDES, Kyriakos, Joanne S. Boldt, Laura Ray. Sources of helping and intergenerational solidarity: A three-generations study of Mexican Americans." *Journal of Gerontology* 41 (1986): 506-511.

Reports on an investigation of sources of help and advice (excluding that of spouses) and degree of intergenerational solidarity in a three-generational sample of Mexican Americans.

Research

Elderly Mexican Americans were found to be involved in strong helping networks with their children, who heavily rely upon them for help and advice. Family is the predominant source of support in all three generations, with women being relied upon for help regarding health matters, and men for help regarding home repairs and upkeep. Help and advice regarding financial and personal problems are generally sought from family members of the same sex. All female dyads were shown by scales measuring intergenerational solidarity to have greater associational solidarity than all-male or cross-sex dyads, but few differences appeared in affectual solidarity, which was uniformly high. There appeared to be minimum association and intergenerational helping between grandparents and grandchildren.

Of interest to social and behavioral scientists.

839. MARKIDES, Kyriakos S., and Janice Farrell. "Marital status and depression among Mexican-Americans." *Social Psychiatry* 20 (1985): 86-91.

An attempt to study the stress buffering role of marriage among Mexican-Americans.

Research

Using data from a cross sectional study of three generations, women, widowed, and divorced/separated persons had significantly higher scores on the CES-D depression scale than did men and married persons. This effect remained after the introduction of controls, and marital status did not matter in older generations.

An important contribution to the literature on social support among minority groups, which may be used with students of the social sciences and health.

840. MATSUMOTO, Y. Scott. "Social stress and coronary heart disease in Japan: A hypothesis." *Milbank Memorial Fund Quarterly* 48 (1970): 9-36.

A theory based on a review of the literature on studies of coronary heart disease, suggesting that cultural mechanisms have protective effects against heart disease, is proposed.

Review--Theoretical

Diet, social stress, work group characteristics, group structure and social support are reviewed from the perspective of the protective institutions in Japanese culture such as tea rooms, baths, after work male socializing, etc. A thesis of stress reduction, high cohesion, and strong, constant social support and integration is offered.

Researchers and cultural anthropologists will find this very interesting.

841. MINDEL, Charles H., Roosevelt Wright, Jr., Richard A. Starrett. "Informal and formal social support systems of black and white elderly: A comparative cost approach." *Gerontologist* 26 (1986): 279-285.

Focuses on the types and amount of support provided by the social support subsystems of elderly blacks and whites.

Research

Multiple classification analysis indicated racial differences in types and amount of support provided by the informal and formal social support systems, but not to the degree suggested by previous research.

Of interest to social and behavioral scientists and gerontologists.

842. MURDOCK, Steve H., and Donald F. Schwartz. "Family structure and the use of aging services: An examination of patterns among elderly Native Americans." *Gerontologist* 18 (1978): 475-481.

Examines the social service needs and use rates of elderly Native Americans and their relationship to family structure.

Research

Data from interviews of 160 elderly Native Americans living in a reservation setting were examined. Although levels of objective need were uniformly high, they were especially high for elderly persons living alone. Levels of perceived service needs, awareness of service agencies, and use of agency services, however, were higher for those living in extended family settings. Family structure appears to be an important factor in the provision of services to elderly Native Americans.

Of interest to sociologists, anthropologists, and health professionals working with Native Americans.

843. MUTRAN, Elizabeth. "Intergenerational family support among blacks and whites: Response to culture or to socioeconomic differences." *Journal of Gerontology* 40 (1985): 382-389.

An investigation of the factors that influence family helping behavior within black and white families.

Research

Black families were found to give and receive more help than their
white counterparts when the variables of age and sex were controlled.
These results were interpreted on the basis of black cultural attitudes of respect for each generation.

Those interested in exchange relations, social support, or minority
relations will benefit from this study.

844. NEIGHBORS, Harold W., and James S. Jackson. "The use of
      informal and formal help: Four patterns of illness in the black
      community." *American Journal of Community Psychology* 12
      (1984): 629-644.

Explores factors related to the use of informal and professional help,
both separately and in combination, by members of the black community,
and investigates ways in which friendship- and kin-based networks
influence the use of professional helping services, using data from
the National Survey of Black Americans.

Research

The findings indicated that most blacks use informal help, alone, or a
combination of informal and professional help. Women use professional
services at higher rates than men and are more likely to use formal
and informal help, combined. Older, low-income blacks are likely not
to seek any help at all. People with physical health problems are apt
to use formal and informal help in combination, while those with
emotional problems are unlikely to seek any help at all.

Of interest to health care planners and policymakers and social and
behavioral scientists.

845. NESER, W., H. Tyroler, J. Cassel. "Social disorganization and
      stroke mortality in the black population of North Carolina."
      American Journal of Epidemiology 93 (1971): 166-175.

An analysis of the relationship of mortality rates to indicators of
social and familial disorganization.

Research

The relationship between the stroke mortality of young blacks and
levels of social disorganization was studied. Mortality rose in
steady increments as family disorganization increased. The findings
may reflect a physiological response to the constraints imposed on
subordinated members of society.

Of interest to epidemiologists and health professionals.

846. ORPEN, Christopher. "The effect of social support on reactions to role ambiguity and conflict: A study of white and black clerks in South Africa." *Journal of Cross Cultural Psychology* 13 (1982): 375-384.

Examines the negative effects of role conflict and role ambiguity on satisfaction and performance.

Research

Social support significantly reduced the negative effect of job stress among the black clerks, but failed to do so among the white clerks. The data does not provide reasons for the differences found in perceived role ambiguity and conflict and in perceived peer and leader support between the white and black clerks.

Of interest to social and behavioral scientists.

847. PHILIPS, Billy U., and John G. Bruhn. "Smoking habits and reported illness in two communities with different systems of social support." *Social Science and Medicine* 15A (1981): 625-631.

A retrospective comparison of smoking habits and reported illness in Roseto, Pennsylvania and Tecumseh, Michigan, undertaken to determine the role of different systems of social support in abating the consequences of risk behaviors, such as smoking, or chronic disease.

Research

Results lend support to the hypothesis that social support is a protective factor against coronary heart disease.

Of interest to researchers of chronic disease, stress, and social support.

848. REED, Dwayne, Daniel McGee, Katsuhiko Yano. "Psychosocial processes and general susceptibility to chronic disease." *American Journal of Epidemiology* 119 (1984): 356-370.

The concept of general susceptibility to disease has developed as a unifying explanation for the findings that a variety of diseases are associated with certain social and cultural situations. This hypothesis was tested in a prospective study of 4,251 men of Japanese ancestry in Hawaii who answered a psychosocial questionnaire in 1971.

Research

There was no support for the hypothesis that social networks are especially protective among persons having the highest levels of mobility and inconsistency. The inclusion of known health hazards did not alter these findings.

Useful to epidemiologists and social and behavioral scientists studying coronary heart disease.

849.　ROSENTHAL, Carolyn J.　"Family supports in later life: Does ethnicity make a difference?" *Gerontologist* 26 (1986): 19-24.

The implications of ethnicity and social support in later life are discussed, particularly with respect to their conceptualization.

Review and Analysis

The author argues that the dimensions of culture, structure, and behavior must be kept conceptually and analytically distinct, and the analysis of the relationship between any two must control for the effects of the third.

Of interest to gerontologists and to social and behavioral scientists.

850.　ROWLES, G.D.　"The church as a focus of support for the rural elderly." *Gerontologist* 25, Supplement 1 (1985): 97.

Examines the current and future roles of the rural church as a source of support for the elderly in settings of few institutional alternatives.

Research Abstract

Four options for enhancing the role of the rural church are proposed--increasing accessibility, complementing existing programs, enhancing support systems, and providing gerontology education and training.

Of interest to rural medical community.

851.　SMITH-RUIZ, Dorothy.　"Relationship between depression, social support, and physical illness among elderly blacks: Research notes." *Journal of National Medical Association* 77 (1985): 1017-1019.

A study of depression in relation to social support and physical illness among elderly blacks.

Research

Social support had a strong beneficial effect on psychological well-being. However, depressive symptoms did not seem to be related to the presence of physical illness in this population. It was suggested that social supports, as important determinants of overall social and psychological well-being, should receive more attention from health care professionals.

Of interest to physicians, gerontologists, and health care planners, particularly those concerned with the black elderly.

852. STARRETT, Richard A., Charles H. Mindel, Roosevelt Wright, Jr. "Influence of support systems on the use of social services by the Hispanic elderly." *Social Work Research and Abstracts* 19, no. 4 (1983): 35-40.

Examines the relationship between informal and formal social support systems and the use of social services by the Hispanic elderly.

Research

Informal support systems do not directly affect the use of formal social services; rather, through their influence on other factors, they exert significant indirect effects.

Of special interest to social service workers.

853. STRAYHORN, Gregory. "Social supports, perceived stress, and health: The black experience in medical school: A preliminary study." *Journal of the National Medical Association* 72 (1980): 869-881.

A preliminary attempt to determine possible relationships among stressors, social supports, and health outcome.

Research

While black students had higher perceived stressor scores, their perceptions of social supports did not differ significantly from those of white medical students. There were no significant differences in systolic and diastolic blood pressure among the high and low stress groups. The interaction of stressors and social supports did not predict blood pressure.

Of interest to medical educators.

854. TAYLOR, Robert Joseph. "The extended family as a source of support to elderly blacks." *Gerontologist* 25 (1985): 488-495.

Describes the results of the National Survey of Black Americans regarding family, demographic, and social support factors and health.

Research

Social support was found to correlate with income, education, region, degree of family interaction, and proximity of relatives. The study clarifies the role of social support and health among black Americans.

Of interest to medical sociologists, cultural anthropologists, and others working in the area of health, social networks, and ethnicity.

855. ———. "Receipt of support from family among black Americans: Demographic and familial differences." *Journal of Marriage and the Family* 48 (1986): 67-77.

The impact of familial and demographic factors on the receipt of support from family members was examined among a sample of blacks.

Research

The findings indicated that income, age, family contact, subjective family closeness, and proximity of relatives were determinants of receiving support. In addition, an interaction was revealed between age and the presence of a child in determining support from family members.

Of interest to social and behavioral scientists.

856. ———, and Linda M. Chatters. "Patterns of informal support to elderly black adults: Family, friends, and church members." *Social Work* 31 (1986): 432-438.

Examines patterns of concomitant support to elderly blacks from family, friends, and church members using the National Survey of Black Americans.

Research

Eight out of ten respondents reported receiving assistance from friends, six out of ten from church members, and over half from family. Few respondents were "socially isolated." The formal support system does not substitute for informal support. Formal programs and services should be examined and instituted to aid and complement the informal support system, relieving the stresses and strains of caregiving and encouraging network members to assist in the care of the elderly.

Of interest to social workers, health professionals, and public policymakers.

857. van HAM APT, Nana. "Quellen von unterstüzung und formen des wohlbefindens bei alten menschen in Ghana (Sources of support and forms of satisfaction of the elderly in Ghana)." (German) *Zeitschrift für Gerontologie* 19, no. 2 (March-April 1986): 90-95.

Examines the living conditions and sources of support for the elderly in Ghana.

Research/Descriptive

Surveys the status of old people in traditional tribal structures and describes their present situation with recourse to economic problems and social changes. Based on data from seven studies carried out between 1962 and 1985, the position of the elderly is described within the roles of parent, kinsman, spouse, member of the household, worker, friend, and citizen. The sources of support and possibilities of the elderly fulfilling what they regard as the most important requirements made of them is discussed for each role. Attention is drawn to the limits of the family support system and the necessity for further research, particularly from the perspective of welfare workers.

Of interest to anthropologists, sociologists and social welfare workers.

858. VEGA, William A., Bohdon Kolody, Juan Ramon Valle. "The relationship of marital status, confidant support, and depression among Mexican immigrant women." *Journal of Marriage and the Family* 48 (1986): 597-605.

A survey of 1,915 Mexican women living in San Diego County was undertaken in order to examine the role of confidant support in moderating depressive symptoms among low-income immigrant women of discrete marital status.

Research

Multiple regression analyses of the data revealed that the presence of a confidant relationship has the single strongest reducing effect upon depression scores. Income and education both have a predictable inverse effect, while disrupted marital statuses increase depression scores. Women in disrupted marital status have higher levels of depressive symptoms than married women, and the never married have lower levels of depression. The scores of widows are similar to those of married women.

Of interest to social and behavioral scientists.

859. VERNON, Sally W., and Robert E. Roberts. "A comparison of Anglos and Mexican-Americans on selected measures of social support." *Hispanic Journal of Behavioral Sciences* 7 (1985): 381-399.

Differences between Anglos and Mexican-Americans were examined for three measures of social support.

Research

Most initial ethnic differences disappeared when the effects of age, gender, education, income, and marital status were controlled. There were some differences in the pattern and magnitude of association between measures of social support and demographic variables when analyses were stratified by ethnicity.

Of interest to social and behavioral scientists.

860. WALSH, Anna C., and Jeanne Simonelli. "Migrant women in the oil field: The function of social networks." *Human Organization* 45 (1986): 43-52.

Describes informal social networks of women associated with migrant oil workers and tests the efficacy of ethnographic methods in predicting the social planning needs of specific communities.

Research

Participation in informal support networks is an important factor in the social and economic survival of both men and women in the boom/ bust cycle of oil and gas exploration. An active support network can eliminate certain of the more detrimental aspects of boomtown living. When a woman is excluded from various support activities, the stability of the migrant household may be threatened.

Of interest to social and behavioral scientists.

861. WOLF, Jacquelyn H., Naomi Breslau, Amasa B. Ford, Henry D. Ziegler, Anna Ward. "Distance and contacts: Interactions of black urban elderly with family and friends." *Journal of Gerontology* 38 (1983): 465-471.

Evidence suggests that black, working class elderly have fewer contacts as income increases than do their white counterparts.

Research

The frequency of social interaction with family and friends for elderly whites is related to the geographical distance from them. To determine the factors affecting social interaction of elderly blacks, a survey of 655 black urban residents over 60 was taken. The neighborhood was found to be an important factor affecting social interaction of blacks.

Sociologists, community psychologists, and others interested in minority/cultural factors in social support will benefit from this study.

c. Chapter

862. BRYER, Kathleen B. "The Amish way of death: A study of family support systems." *In* Rudolf H. Moos (Ed.). *Coping with Life Crises: An Integrated Approach.* New York: Plenum Press, 1986.

A study of the way of life and death within the traditional society of the Amish.

Descriptive

In Amish society, most individuals can face death confidently with the assurance that they will be able to live out their days at home, surrounded by loved ones who will help them to plan and organize their own deaths. Their strong religious belief system provides a framework for calm acceptance of the impending death. In keeping with their concept of death as a natural part of the rhythm of life, the Amish people have a deep sense of continuity across generations; they know that their families will receive massive community support when they die.

Of interest to medical anthropologists, medical historians, and social and behavioral scientists.

d. Dissertations

863. CHAPARRO, Linda L. "Predicting health preventive and health protective behaviors among Mexicano/Chicanos." Ph.D. dissertation, University of Michigan, 1985.

Examines determinants of medical and self-care health behaviors in a Mexicano/Chicano population.

Research

Social support and health satisfaction had a positive influence on protective (self-care) behaviors, whereas concern about health was negatively associated with protective behaviors. Concern about health was positively associated with preventive (medical/dental) behaviors.

Of interested to social and behavioral scientists, public health officials, and social workers.

864. CUNNINGHAM, Rhonda C. "Racial dimensions of life stress and social support in the prediction of health changes." Ph.D. dissertation, University of Houston, 1980.

The effect of life events and social support on subsequent health change among a black and an Anglo sample were compared.

Research

Both the Holmes and Rahe Social Readjustment Rating Scale and a revised life event scale, tested in a pilot-study among blacks and Anglos, were significant predictors of health changes, although the revised scale proved to be more sensitive when useful primary prevention considerations were attended to. There was no evidence of any effect of social support.

Of interest to social scientists and stress researchers.

865. WISE, Frederick. "Mental health and support systems among urban Native Americans." Ph.D. dissertation, Michigan State University, 1981.

This study stemmed from the assumption that Native Americans have a high incidence of mental health problems and their subculture provides strong familial and informal support networks.

Dissertation

Results indicated weaker than expected traditional, familial, and informal support systems, accompanied by minimal reliance on formal supports. Considering the relatively high degree of pathology observed and its lack of correlation with help-sources, there appears to be a marked discrepancy between the help Native Americans need and the help they obtain.

Of interest to social and behavioral scientists and to mental health professionals, especially those working with ethnic groups.

866. WOO, Deborah A. "Social support and the imputation of mental illness: Chinese Americans and European Americans." Ph.D. dissertation, University of California, Berkeley, 1983.

A study of perceptions of intimacy, support, and mental health problems in the context of the Chinese American and the European American cultural orientation.

Research

Individual and social self did not have the same importance in the two cultural orientations. In the European American orientation, individual identity and independence were emphasized, whereas in the Chinese American orientation, more emphasis was put on the social self, as articulated in social roles. As a result, intimacy and social support were differently related to mental health problems.

Of particular interest to anthropologists, medical sociologists, and mental health professionals.

2. LIFE EVENTS, CHANGE, AND STRESS

a. Books

866. DOHRENWEND, Barbara Snell, and Bruce P. Dohrenwend (Eds.). *Stressful Life Events and Their Contexts. Monographs in Psychosocial Epidemiology 2.* New York: Neale Watson Academic Publications, 1981.

The second in a series of monographs on themes of particular interest to investigators in the field of psychosocial epidemiology. Discusses the interrelationships between life events and changes in health.

Book of Readings

The 15 articles in this monograph discuss a variety of issues related to measuring life events, social support, and their interrelationships.

Especially useful to social and behavioral scientists and others interested in stress and its measurement.

867. ELLIOTT, Glen R., and Carl Eisdorfer (Eds.). *Stress and Human Health. Analysis and Implications of Research.* New York: Springer, 1982.

A National Academy of Sciences' Institute of Medicine study of

Research on Stress in Health and Disease. Defines research issues, delineates desirable and adverse aspects of stress in its various forms, and examines biomedical, behavioral, and sociological approaches to the description and alleviation of excessive stresses.

Report

Chapter seven, devoted to the panel report on psychosocial assets and modifiers of stress, reviews what is known about psychosocial assets and modifiers, discusses the methodological problems involved in studying their relationships to stress, and pinpoints research strategies that will further our understanding in this area.

Of use to researchers of stress and social support.

868. HOBFOLL, Stevan E. (Ed.). *Stress, Social Support and Women*. New York: Hemisphere, 1986.

This book is concerned with the stressors women undergo from adolescence to old age and the resources women use to cope with these stressors.

Book or Readings

A central goal of this volume is to draw implications from research on social support for clinical and other interventions as they concern women. A second goal is to encourage new research in the areas of social support, and to suggest methodological and theoretical directions this research might take. Each of the 15 chapters in this volume follows an ecological life-span approach, addressing the problems women normally confront in each life stage.

Of interest to researchers of stress and social support.

869. LAZARUS, Richard S., and Susan Folkman. *Stress, Appraisal, and Coping*. New York: Springer, 1984.

A theory of stress, focusing on cognitive appraisal and coping, is described. Major movements within the field, including issues of behavioral medicine, are examined.

Theoretical and Analytical

An integrative theoretical analysis, which pulls together two decades of research and thought on issues in behavioral medicine, emotion, stress management, treatment, and life span development. The work is multidisciplinary with an emphasis on the psychological aspects of stress. Chapter 8 contains a valuable discussion on social resources and supports.

Of interest to social and behavioral scientists, physicians, nurses, social workers, and researchers in these fields.

b. Articles

870.   ALBRECHT, Terrance L., and Mara B. Adelman.   "Social
       support and life stress--new directions for communication
       research."   *Human Communication Research*   11 (1984): 3-32.

A critical review of the broad research literature on social support.
Includes hypotheses for future research and a review of some central
dilemmas of supportive relationships.

Review

An attempt to bring the area to the attention of communication
researchers. Further inquiry is needed by those equipped to study the
nature of the communication process with the requisite theoretical and
methodological tools.   Several key directions for research were
delineated, including theoretical foundations and dilemmas of the
support process.

Of interest to social and behavioral scientists and researchers of
social support.

871.   BURK, Ross W., and Ross D. Parke.   "Behavioral and physio-
       logical response to the presence of a friendly or neutral
       person in two types of stressful situations."   *Journal of
       Personality and Social Psychology*   24 (1972): 143-153.

Simultaneous measures of physiological arousal and affiliative behavior were taken, while subjects waited for a threatening event.   One
hundred and twenty males were randomly distributed over a 2x2x3
design.

Research

The major findings were: a) embarrassment subjects were less
affiliative with and more aroused by the other person than were fear
subjects, b) firstborns engaged in more affiliative behavior, particularly with the supportive person, but were not more calmed by the
other person than later-borns, c) subjects with the supportive other
were more affiliative and more aroused than subjects with the neutral
other.

Of particular interest to social psychologists.

872.   BURKS, Nancy, and Barclay Martin.   "Everyday problems and
       life change events: Ongoing versus acute sources of stress."
       Journal of Human Stress   11 (Spring 1985): 27-35.

Examines a relatively neglected source of stress: everyday problems,
defined as ongoing, often chronic situations, which are stressful for
a substantial period of time.

Research

Everyday problems were more effective than life events in predicting psychological symptoms. A significant interaction between everyday problems and life events was found. An interaction was found between everyday problems and nonfamily social support, as predicted by the buffering hypothesis.

Of interest to researchers of stress and social support.

873. COYNE, James C., and Anita De Longis. "Going beyond social support: The role of social relationships in adaptation." *Journal of Consulting and Clinical Psychology* 54 (1986): 454-460.

Explores the relationship of stress, support, and adaptational outcomes.

Theoretical

Marriage is used as an example of the stress providing and support productivity relationship. Therapeutic intensity of family therapy is described, which highlights paradoxes of these types in social relations.

Marital therapists will find this an interesting paper.

874. GAD, Marsha Treadwell, and James H. Johnson. "Correlates of adolescent life stress as related to race, SES and levels of perceived social support." *Journal of Clinical Child Psychology* 9 (1980): 13-16.

Assesses the relationship between life changes, socioeconomic status, and social support to life stress for black and white adolescents.

Research

Findings suggest that adolescents from lower socioeconomic groups, regardless of race, experience higher levels of negative life change related to perceived health status. The absence of any correlation to social support is believed to stem from inadequate measurement of social support.

Of interest to counselors, physicians, and social workers working with adolescents.

875. GRACE, Glenn D., and Thomas Schill. "Expectancy of personal control and seeking social support in coping style." *Psychological Reports* 58 (1986): 757-758.

A number of potential locus of control differences in coping styles were examined to determine whether subjects with high expectations of personal control report seeking significantly more social support in coping than do subjects with low expectancies of personal control.

Research

Results indicate a significantly greater initiation of contact with others during periods of distress for subjects with high as opposed to those with low personal control.

Of interest to social and behavioral scientists.

876. HOLAHAN, Charles J., and Rudolf H. Moos. "Personality, coping, and family resources in stress resistance: A longitudinal analysis." *Journal of Personality and Social Psychology* 51 (1986): 389-395.

Employing a longitudinal analysis, stress-resistance factors in the areas of personality, coping, and family support were used to predict psychological and physical adjustment.

Research

Findings demonstrated that feelings of self-confidence, an easy-going disposition, a disinclination to use avoidance coping, and the availability of family support operate jointly to protect individuals from negative psychological consequences of life stress. For women, the stress-resistance index also predicted psychosomatic complaints experienced one year after initial testing.

Of interest to researchers of social support and stress.

877. KELLY, Karen E., and B. Kent Houston. "Type A behavior in employed women: Relation to work, marital, and leisure variables, social support, stress, tension, and health." *Journal of Personality and Social Psychology* 48 (1985): 1067-1079.

The Jenkins Activity Survey (JAS) and the Framingham Type A Scale (FTAS) were administered to 91 women who are employed full time, and questionnaires or interviews were used to obtain information concerning varying work and non-work related variables to determine the relationship of various social factors to Type A behavior.

Research

Type A women had higher occupational levels and reported more demanding jobs and higher stress and tension than Type B women. Type A and B women did not differ in their reports of marital adjustment or time spent in leisure activities. Type A behavior was related to both self-reported stress and tension, and--for married women, only--poorer self-reported health. Social support from various sources was not found to be related to Type A or Type B, although Type A was related to more reported stress and tension for women who believed they had many sources of support, but not for women who did not perceive having many sources of support.

Of interest to behavioral and social scientists.

878. KESSLER, Ronald C., Richard H. Price, Camille B. Wortman. "Social factors in psychopathology--stress, social support, and coping processes." *Annual Review of Psychology* 36 (1985): 531-572.

A summary of the state-of-the-science of social factors in psychopathology.

Review

Deals with the vulnerability factors associated with stress, coping processes, and social support.

Psychologists and others interested in a broad view of social factors in psychopathology will benefit from this work.

879. McFARLANE, Allan H., Geoffrey R. Norman, David L. Streiner, Ranjan Roy, Deborah J. Scott. "A longitudinal study on the influence of the psychosocial environment on health status: A preliminary report." *Journal of Health and Social Behavior* 21 (1980): 124-133.

Describes a prospective study that examines various aspects of the psychosocial environment and their relationship to health status.

Research

Preliminary results indicate that desirable (positive) life events do not have a significant statistical correlation with the measure of strain, whereas undesirable (negative) life events do. Furthermore, two dimensions of life events, anticipation and control, add substantial and interactional information about these relationships.

Of interest to researchers of stress and social support.

880. MEDALIE, Jack H. "Stress, social support, coping, and adjustment." *Journal of Family Practice* 20 (1985): 533-535.

To place stress and support into an overall concept, a diagram of an adjustment model is presented to demonstrate how and where support enters the picture.

Editorial

An adjustment model is offered to integrate some of the inconsistencies in research of social support.

Of interest to researchers of stress and social support.

881. PARKES, Katherine R. "Coping in stressful episodes: The role of individual differences, environmental factors, and situational characteristics." *Journal of Personality and Social Psychology* 51 (1986): 1277-1292.

Examines individual differences (extraversion and neuroticism), environmental factors (social support and work demand), and situational characteristics (type of stressful episode and its perceived importance) as predictors of three self-report measures of coping (general coping, direct coping, and suppression) derived from the Ways of Coping Questionnaire.

Research

Individual differences in 135 first-year female student nurses were assessed prior to exposure to the ward environment, and information about stressful episodes was obtained during the initial period of nursing practice. Multiple regression analysis showed that individual differences and environmental and situational factors were significant predictors of the coping scores and that patterns of main and interactive effects were different for each type of coping. For both direct coping and suppression, predicted interactions across person, environmental, and situational variables contributed significantly to the explained variance, and curvilinear interactions between work demand and neuroticism were significant. Interactions of social support and extraversion with perceived importance predicted direct coping, and interactions between neuroticism and extraversion and between work demand and importance predicted suppression.

Of interest to researchers of stress and coping.

882. PORRITT, D. "Social support in crisis: Quantity or quality?:
      Social Science and Medicine 13A (1979): 715-721.

Data from a controlled trial of crisis intervention with males hospitalized for treatment of road injuries were used to test the prediction that the availability of sources of potential help will be unrelated to crisis outcome, but that the quality of support received will be a determinant of outcome.

Research

Results confirm the predictions that source availability is unrelated to outcome, that source quality is related to outcome, and that crisis intervention has a highly significant effect on the reported quality of support received.

Of interest to researchers of stress and social support.

883. SANDLER, Irwin N., and Manuel Barrera, Jr. "Toward a
      multimethod approach to assessing the effects of social
      support." *American Journal of Community Psychology* 12
      (1984): 37-52.

Two studies assessed the direct and stress-buffering effects of social support on psychological symptoms of college students.

Research

Results indicated a significant direct and stress-buffering effect for support satisfaction in reducing psychological symptomatology.

Of interest to researchers of social support.

884. THOITS, Peggy A. "Life stress, social support, and psychological vulnerability: Epidemiological considerations." *Journal of Community Psychology* 10 (October 1982): 341-362.

A test of the hypothesis that disadvantaged sociodemographic groups are reactive to the effects of life events and that the psychological vulnerability of these groups may be due to the joint occurrence of major stress events and few available social support resources.

Research

The greater vulnerability to life difficulties displayed by disadvantaged groups cannot adequately be explained by the higher incidence of events or the lack of social support, either singly or in combination.

Of interest to researchers of stress and social support.

885. ———. "Social support as coping assistance." *Journal of Consulting and Clinical Psychology* 54 (1986): 416-423.

Deals with social support as a form of coping assistance.

Review--Theoretical

Integration of models of support and coping are useful in explaining normal adjustments to life as well as stress buffering aspects of coping useful to distressed persons. Several supportive strategies are suggested for use in helping relationships.

Consulting and clinical psychologists, social workers, and other theorists will find this a useful article.

886. TYERMAN, Andrew, and Michael Humphrey. "Life stress, family support, and adolescent disturbance." *Journal of Adolescence* 6 (1983): 1-12.

A study of the life stresses and family supports of a group of adolescent psychiatric outpatients.

Research

The adolescent patients reported significantly more negative life events in the previous two years and significantly less satisfaction with family support than a matched control group. The authors discuss these findings in the context of the developmental stresses of this age group.

Of particular interest to psychiatrists and other mental health professionals dealing with adolescents.

887. WEINBERGER, Morris, Jeffrey C. Darnell, B.L. Martz, Sharon
      L. Hiner, Peggy C. Neill, William M. Tierney. "The effects
      of positive and negative life changes on the self-reported
      health status of elderly adults." *Journal of Gerontology*
      41 (1986): 114-119.

This paper examined the effects of positive and negative life changes
and social support upon the self-reported health status of 187 elderly
public housing tenants.

Research

Social support had neither a direct or interactive effect (with life
change) upon health. The authors conclude that studies on life
changes should separate positive from negative effects, and that more
research on the measurement of social support for elderly adults is
needed.

Of interest to gerontologists and social and behavioral scientists.

c. Chapters

888. FIGLEY, Charles R. "Traumatic stress--The role of the family
      and social support system." *In* Charles R. Figley (Ed.).
      *Trauma and its Wake. Volume 2. Traumatic Stress Theory,
      Research and Intervention.* New York: Brunner/Mazel, 1986.

Answers questions regarding what qualifies as a catastrophe that may
result in traumatic or post-traumatic stress reactions, and the role
of family support in preventing and abating traumatic and post-
traumatic stress impairments.

Review

The family is a critical support system to human beings before,
during, and after stressful times, and the system and its members are
also affected, sometimes even more than the victim. By adequate
attention to the health and vitality of the family system, victims of
catastrophe may rely on a powerful stress-coping resource. It is
possible, by supplemental consultation to families regarding
functional methods of coping with catastrophic stress, to more effectively care for victims of traumatic events.

Of interest to practitioners and researchers in the human service
professions.

889. LIEBERMAN, Morton A. "The effects of social supports on
      responses to stress." *In* Leo Goldberger, and Shlomo
      Breznitz (Eds.). *Handbook of Stress: Theoretical and
      Clinical Aspects* New York: Free Press, 1982.

Examines social supports using research findings from the author's
ongoing studies of life cycle transitions, crises, role strains, and
self-help organizations.

Research and Review

Social networks, social resources, and specific ways in which individuals use their social networks for help are examined, and the role
of social support in mitigating the effects of social stress or in
facilitating positive change is addressed.

Of interest to mental health professionals and social and behavioral
scientists.

d. Dissertations

890. COPPEL, David B. "The relationship of perceived social support and self-efficacy to major and minor stresses." Ph.D.
dissertation, University of Washington, 1980.

The relationship between major life events, minor stresses (daily
hassles), social support variables, and personality (intra-personal
support) variables, physical health, and psychological adjustment,
were examined.

Dissertation

Social support and intrapersonal support variables (self-esteem,
self-efficacy, and locus of control) each accounted for a significant
increment in the variance of psychological and health adjustment
measures. Subjects' perception of the quality of their social support
was found to be more strongly related to adjustment than was a quantitative measure of social support.

Of interest to researchers of stress and social support.

891. HABIF, Valerie L. "The role of life stress, social support, and
depression as predictors of health care utilization in a health
maintenance organization." Ph.D. dissertation, University of
Georgia, 1983.

A study of the effect of stress on health care utilization.

Research

Life stress was positively, but moderately, associated with physician
utilization, but this relationship was substantially higher for
individuals with low levels of social support, than for individuals
with high levels of social support.

Of interest to social scientists, in particular medical sociologists
concerned with health care utilization.

892.   LINDNER, Karen C.   "Life change, social support, and cognitive problem solving skills."   Ph.D. dissertation, University of Washington, 1982.

A study of the ways problem-solving thinking is affected by life change, actual social support, and experimentally manipulated social support.

Research

The data indicated that both social support available in everyday life and social support interventions had an effect on problem-solving thinking. People with less actual support responded more favorably to experimentally induced social support than people who experienced higher levels of social support outside the experimental setting.

Of most interest to cognitive psychologists.

893.   PEARSON, Judith Elizabeth.   "The relationship between social support and Type A behavior pattern on appraisal accuracy."   Ph.D. dissertation, The Catholic University of America, 1983.

Examined relationships among coping style, emotional supports, social network morphology, stressful events, and their impact on appraisal accuracy.

Research

The degree of social support did not affect appraisal accuracy.   As network size increased, emotional supports increased.   Type A's and B's reported no differences in social support systems.

Of interest to researchers of stress and social support.

894.   THOITS, Peggy A.   "Life events, social integration, and psychological distress."   Ph.D. dissertation, Stanford University, 1978.

A test of the relationship between life events, psychological distress, and possible mediating conditions.

Research

Data were interpreted in terms of two alternative hypotheses, one concerning a sense of social identity, the other concerning self-esteem. For married men, the social identity hypotheses was strongly supported; changes in social integration lead to changes in distress. For married and formerly married women, the self-esteem hypothesis was supported; changes in prestige were inversely related to distress.

Of interest to social and behavioral scientists.

A. THE STRESS/ILLNESS RELATIONSHIP

a. Book

895. BELLE, Deborah (Ed.). *Lives in Stress. Women and Depression.* Beverly Hills, CA: Sage, 1982.

A study of the stresses which lead to high rates of depression among low-income mothers with young children in an attempt to develop knowledge on which to base future mental health services and public policy decisions.

Research

A sense of mastery was the most consistent correlate of the forms of social support, suggesting that women who receive more support from others feel more in control of their own lives. Finding basic security in other people does not appear to sap individual strength. However social ties are a two edged sword. While social support can be productive of better mental health, relief from the pressures of intensive social involvement can also be productive of better mental health.

Of interest to social and behavioral scientists and mental health professionals.

b. Articles

896. ANDREWS, Gavin, Christopher Tennant, Daphne M. Hewson, George E. Vaillant. "Life event stress, social support, coping style, and risk of psychological impairment." *Journal of Nervous and Mental Diseases* 166 (May 1978): 307-316.

The effects of life event stress, coping style, and social support on psychological impairment were examined in a survey of a representative Australian suburban sample.

Research

Life event stress, coping style, and crisis support/were related to impairment. There was no evidence that coping style or social support become associated by moderating the relationship between life event stress and impairment.

Of interest to social and behavioral scientists, mental health professionals, and researchers of stress.

897. COHEN, Lawrence H., Jack McGowan, Stephanie Fooskas, Sandra Rose. "Positive life events and social support and the relationship between life stress and psychological disorder." *American Journal of Community Psychology* 12 (1984): 567-587.

Describes the investigation of the relationship between negative life events and psychological disorders as these are moderated by social support and positive life events.

Research

Negative life events were significantly related to psychological disorders. A cross-sectional analysis provides evidence for the stress-buffering effects of positive life events and perceived social support. There was no evidence supporting the stress-buffering effects of the actual social support received by the subjects.

Appropriate for research oriented clinical and community psychologists.

898. COMPAS, Bruce E., Barry M. Wagner, Lesley A. Slavin, Kathryn Vannatta. "A prospective study of life events, social support, and psychological symptomotology during the transition from high school to college." *American Journal of Community Psychology* 14 (1986): 241-257.

This prospective study of life events, perceived social support, and psychological symptoms suggests a reciprocal relationship among these variables supporting a transactional model of stress and social support.

Research

Suggests that negative life events result in psychological symptoms when perceived social support is low, and that the converse is also true. These relationships were found to vary in as little as six months and to be amenable to intervention with combinations of counseling and other mental health services.

Of interest to general audiences, although counselors and mental health professionals will benefit most.

899. COOPER, C.L., R.F. Davies Cooper, E.B. Faragher. "A prospective study of the relationship between breast cancer and life events, Type A behaviour, social support and coping skills." *Stress Medicine* 2 (1986): 271-278.

Investigates the link between psychosocial factors and breast cancer in a large sample of women attending breast-screening clinics.

Research

completed by 2,163 women prior to a breast examination. The women were subsequently diagnosed as having cancer, a cyst, benign breast disease, or normal breasts. The cancer group was found to have experienced significantly more loss- or illness-related events, perceived life events generally as more stressful, used fewer and poorer coping skills, and were significantly lower on Type A behavior.

Of interest to researchers of the stress/illness/social support relationships.

900. DOHRENWEND, Bruce P. "The social psychological nature of stress: A framework for causal inquiry." *Journal of Abnormal and Social Psychology* 62 (1961): 294-302.

Investigates studies that show relationships between social environmental factors and mental illness.

Literature Review

Suggests that correlations between sociocultural factors and mental illness do not demonstrate causal relationships. In contrast to community studies, are laboratory investigations of stress, which is often concurrent with social and cultural factors.

Of interest to mental health professionals and researchers studying stress.

901. EATON, William W. "Life events, social supports, and psychiatric symptoms: A re-analysis of the New Haven data." *Journal of Health and Social Behavior* 19 (June 1978): 230-234.

Longitudinal data on life events and psychiatric symptoms are reanalyzed using the panel regression technique.

Research

Analysis shows that life events are fairly independent of each other over a two-year time period. The effect of recall distortion on the life events/mental disorder relationship is negligible. The data provide some evidence that life events are more likely to cause mental disorder if the individual has not experienced similar stresses before.

Of interest to researchers of stress and social support.

902. FULLER, Sarah S., and Sandra B. Larson. "Life events, emotional support, and health of older people." *Research in Nursing and Health* 3 (1980): 81-89.

The effects of life events, emotional support, interaction of life events and emotional support, and age on indices of physical and psychological health were examined.

Research

The results indicate that no general statement about the effects of life events and emotional support on the physical and mental health of older people would be appropriate. There was no evidence that emotional support would protect an individual from the negative consequences of stressful life events. The relatively high morale and generally high perceptions of emotional support among the subjects in this study is worthy of note.

Of interest to nurses, gerontologists, and social and behavioral scientists.

903. GREENE, John Gerald. "Bereavement and social support at the climacteric." *Maturitas* 5 (1983): 115-124.

The relationship between life events and symptoms was examined in a general population sample of Scottish climacteric women.

Research

At least some of the increase in symptoms at that time of life was due to the occurrence of stressful life events. A bereavement involving a close family member and the consequent loss of social support, were found to be significant factors in provoking physical symptoms, but only in the presence of other life stress.

Of interest to gynecologists, family physicians, and researchers of stress and social support.

904. HAGGERTY, Robert J. "Life stress, illness and social supports." *Developmental Medicine and Child Neurology* 22 (1980): 391-400.

Reviews stress as a factor in the etiology of disease; shows the role of stress in altering when and where families use health services; and discusses ways we can protect against the harmful effects of stress, emphasizing social supports.

Review

The author suggests that social support systems should play an increasing part in health services.

Useful to teachers and researchers interested in social support and its relationship to stress.

905. HAUTZINGER, Martin. "Kritische lebensereignisse, Soziale unterstützung und depressivitat bei älteren menschen." (Stressful life events, social support and depression in elderly people.) *Zeitschrift fur Klinische Psychologie-Forschung und Praxis* (German) 14 (1985): 27-38.

Examines the effects of social support and stressful life events on depression and psychotic experiences among a community sample of adults, aged 50 and older.

Research

Social support had an independent effect on depression. Having a partner was protective against depressive symptomatology for males, but, for females, having a partner was associated with more depressive symptoms. Life events were positively related to depression. No significant effects were obtained for psychotic experiences.

Of interest to social and behavioral scientists, in particular stress researchers.

906. LIN, Nan, Walter M. Ensel, Ronald S. Simeone, Kuo Wen. "Social support, stressful life events, and illness: A model and an empirical test." *Journal of Health and Social Behavior* 20 (June 1979): 108-119.

The effects of social support and stressful life events on psychiatric symptoms are examined in a model with data from a representative sample of the Chinese-American adults in Washington, D.C.

Research

Analysis showed that stressors are positively related to the incidence of psychiatric symptoms and social support is negatively related to psychiatric symptoms. The contribution of social support to the predicting of symptoms is greater than that of stressful life events.

Of interest to social and behavioral scientists and researchers of stress.

907. McFARLANE, Allan H., Geoffrey R. Norman, David L. Streiner, Ranjan G. Roy. "The process of social stress: Stable, reciprocal, and mediating relationships." *Journal of Health and Social Behavior* 24 (June 1983): 160-173.

Reports on a prospective longitudinal study in which various aspects of the stress process were examined.

Research

The stress-illness relationship was not mediated by either expectations of control or effectiveness of social supports. A reciprocal relationship was found between social supports and stressful events. An individual with helpful social supports was less likely to experience subsequent stressful events.

Of interest to researchers of stress.

908. MILLER, P.McC., J.G. Ingham, S. Davidson. "Life events,
      symptoms and social support." *Journal of Psychosomatic
      Research* 20 (1976): 515-522.

A comparative study of general practice consultant with non-consultant
provided the opportunity to examine the relationships between the
severity of each of nine common symptoms and the long term threat of
any events experienced in the three months prior to interview.

Research

The most striking findings are the highly significant correlations
between threatening events and psychological symptoms in the consultant sample. There is an almost total absence of any evidence that
non-threatening events are in any way related to symptomatology. This
would suggest that there is a stress threshold which must be exceeded
before any event has ill effects.

Of interest to researchers of stress and social support.

909. MITCHELL, Roger E., and Rudolf H. Moos. "Deficiencies in
      social support among depressed patients: Antecedents or
      consequences of stress?" *Journal of Health and Social
      Behavior* 25 (1984): 438-452.

A two-wave, two-variable panel model was used to examine longitudinal
relationships between stress and support in a sample of 233 clinically
depressed patients.

Research

Changes in levels of strain and in positive life events were significantly associated with changes in family support over a one-year
follow-up period. There was less evidence of an effect of social
support on negative life change events, ongoing strains, or positive
life change events. Analyses are described that examined differences
in the pattern of results as a function of the occurrence of exit or
loss events, the timing of events, and the use of nonlinear models.

Of particular interest to researchers of the relationship of stress
and social support.

910. MONROE, Scott M., Donald F. Imhoff, Beverly D. Wise, Joyce
      E. Harris. "Prediction of psychological symptoms under high
      risk psychosocial circumstances--life events, social support,
      and symptom specificity. *Journal of Abnormal Psychology* 92
      (1983): 338-350.

Describes a prospective study of life events, the perceived dimension
of the events, and social support as predictors of psychological
symptoms.

Psychosocial Research

A relationship was found between the perception of the dimensions of life events and social support, as these factors predict psychological symptoms of depression. Chance life events were unaffected by either perception or social support in their influence on psychological distress.

Psychologists and others interested in personality factors and psychopathology will find this article helpful.

911. MYERS, Jerome K., Jacob J. Lindenthal, Max P. Pepper. "Life events, social integration and psychiatric symptomatology." *Journal of Health and Social Behavior* 16 (1975): 421-427.

Data are presented on the relationship between life events, social integration, and psychiatric symptoms in a community.

Research

Findings support previous literature that points to salutary effects gained by people who are integrated within the social system. The socially integrated apparently have lower rates of psychiatric symptomatology as well as suicide and other anomalies.

Of interest to mental health professionals and researchers studying life stress.

912. PARRY, Glenys. "Paid employment, life events, social support and mental health in working-class mothers." *Journal of Health and Social Behavior* 27 (1986): 193-208.

The authors tested for direct effects of employment and examined these effects in interaction with life event stress, social support, and the presence of a preschool child.

Research

No overall effect of paid employment or preschool children was found. Mothers who had suffered a severely stressful life event in the previous year had higher levels of psychiatric symptomatology. Employment reduced this risk when social support was available, but, in the absence of social support, was associated with high symptom levels.

Of interest to mental health professionals and social and behavioral scientists.

913. PRESTON, Deborah Bray, and Phyllis Kernoff Mansfield. "An exploration of stressful life events, illness, and coping among the rural elderly. *Gerontologist* 24 (1984): 490-494.

Explores the relationship among stressful life events, coping mechanisms, and illness in a sample of 200 rural elderly, and examines the hypothesis that coping acts as a moderate in the stress-illness relationship.

Research

Cluster analysis was used to identify four groups of subjects exhibiting different degrees of stress and health and distinct patterns of coping. The group with the least amount of stress appeared to be the healthiest, suggesting a decided relationship between high stress and poor health. The group employing such "take charge" coping styles as keeping active and managing without much help also seemed to have above average health, despite higher levels of stress, indicating that such coping mechanisms may moderate the stress-illness relationship. The third group, which reported some inhibition of activity due to health, employed the largest repertoire of coping mechanisms, had a larger helping network than the first two groups, and had a reasonably good health status. Members of group four, all of whom were women, mostly widowed and living alone, had high stress, poor health, limited activity, and a below average range of coping mechanisms, but had the largest helping networks.

Of interest to social and behavioral scientists.

914. SARASON, Irwin G., Barbara R. Sarason, Earl H. Potter, Michael H. Antoni. "Life events, social support, and illness." *Psychosomatic Medicine* 47 (March-April 1985): 156-163.

Positive and negative life events and social support were correlated with illness among Navy Submarine School students.

Research

Negative life events in the recent past were related to reports of illness. Although social support by itself was not related to illness reports, the relationship between negative life events and illness was stronger among subjects with low rather than high levels of social support.

Of interest to researchers of social support.

915. "Stress, social support and depression." *American Family Physician* 27, no. 6 (1983): 102, 105.

A brief overview of the general relationship between stress and illness and the ameliorative action of social support.

Editorial

Refers to the results of the Los Angeles community study of life change and illness experience, which showed that participants with higher degrees of social support had less illness independent of their life change scores. Suggestions are made for physicians to influence and provide more social support for their patients.

Helpful to anyone providing care to people, especially physicians, nurses, and allied health professionals.

916. WEST, Malcolm, W. John Livesley, Linda Reiffer, Adrienne
      Sheldon. "The place of attachment in the life events model of
      stress and illness." *Canadian Journal of Psychiatry*   31
      (1986): 202-207.

Discusses the relevance of attachment theory for understanding susceptibility to stress, and individual differences in the use of social
support during times of stress.

Theoretical and Analytical

Attachment is likely to influence the onset of psychiatric illness in
three ways: 1) by giving rise to a nonspecific vulnerability to
stress, which predisposes to the onset of symptoms; 2) by influencing
the individual's ability to establish and utilize social networks,
thereby affecting the availability of support at times of stress; and
3) by influencing the way in which the individual reacts to life
events, and the way in which he or she appraises them.

Of particular interest to pediatricians, child psychologists, and
psychiatrists and specialists in development.

917. WILLIAMS, Ann W., John E. Ware, Cathy A. Donald. "A model
      of mental health, life events, and social supports applicable to
      general populations." *Journal of Health and Social Behavior*
      22 (December 1981): 324-336.

Addresses measurement issues, derives a model of the effects of life
events on mental health, and tests hypotheses regarding the role of
social supports in modifying these effects over time.

Research

Results support the following conclusions: 1) social supports predict
improvements in mental health over time; 2) life events and physical
limitations predict a deterioration in mental health over time; 3) the
negative effects of life events and physical limitations on mental
health do not vary according to the amount of social support; and
4) differences in measurement strategies for life events and social
supports produce some variance in results, but not in conclusions
about whether effects on mental health are additive or interactive.

Of interest to researchers studying stress.

c. Chapters

918. GENTRY, W. Doyle, and Suzanne C. Ouellette Kobasa. "Social
      and psychological resources in mediating stress-illness rela-
      tionships in humans." *In* W. Doyle Gentry (Ed.). *Handbook
      of Behavioral Medicine*   New York: Guilford Press, 1984.

Identifies some of the major psychosocial factors that operate to
protect individuals and groups from various forms of stress, considers

some of the methodological strengths and weaknesses of research studies, and outlines future research objectives.

Review and Analytical

Most of the mediation of stress-illness relationships occurs at the individual psychological level, that is, it has to do with individual perceptions, attitudes, and coping styles. Social factors operate in the main to promote and facilitate psychological resources; thus, their influence is indirect. Research investigating the mediating effects of social and psychological factors on stress-illness relationships in humans has become conceptually and methodologically sophisticated, to the point where model building and the prediction of individual health risk is now possible.

Of interest to social and behavioral scientists and to health professionals interested in stress and social support.

919. SATARIANO, William A., and S. Leonard Syme. "Life change and disease in elderly populations: Coping with change." *In* James L. McGaugh and Sara B. Kiesler (Eds.). *Aging: Biology and Behavior.* New York: Academic Press, 1981.

Reviews and evaluates available evidence regarding the relation between life change and disease in elderly populations, suggests that the effects of life change on health are mediated by a person's network of social contacts, and proposes a research strategy for investigating disease patterns among the elderly.

Literature Review

The authors conclude that the study of life change, social relationships, and social support may help us to understand the relation between aging and susceptibility to disease. This information will be helpful in the design of more effective preventive health strategies for the elderly. It may be possible to encourage the development of supportive relationships to help elderly people moderate the negative effects of change.

Should interest social workers, mental health professionals, and gerontologists.

920. SOLOMON, Susan D. "Mobilizing social support networks in times of disaster." *In* Charles R. Figley (Ed.). *Trauma and Its Wake. Volume 2. Traumatic Stress Theory, Research and Intervention.* New York: Brunner/Mazel, 1986.

Examines the assumption that the impairment of social support networks affects recovery from disaster and increases victim vulnerability to a variety of physical and mental health problems.

Review and Analysis

Defines the terms social support and social network; summarizes findings from the stress literature on the mental health effects of the presence or loss of social support; considers ways in which mental health professionals can intervene in the personal network to preserve and enhance social support in times of emergency; and discusses issues in need of further research.

Of particular interest to researchers of stress and social support, human service workers, and public policymakers concerned with disaster intervention.

d. Dissertations

921. ANDERSON, Laurel A. "The effects of life stress on immuno-competence: The role of social support, health related practices and depression." Ph.D. dissertation, California School of Professional Psychology, Los Angeles, 1982.

A study of the impact of life stress on vulnerability to illness, taking into account psychological, physiological, social, and behavioral variables in a sample of healthy graduate students.

Research

Several interesting findings were reported. For example, positive long-term stress, more than negative or total stress, was associated with immuno-deficiency. Immuno-deficiency was also positively associated with the amount of social contact.

Of special interest to stress researchers.

922. BROWN, Gordon E., Jr. "Stress, social support, and health: A longitudinal analysis." Ph.D. dissertation, University of South Carolina, 1983.

A longitudinal study of the stress-buffering effects of social support.

Research

The study concludes that when appropriate controls are used, little or no buffering effects of social support are maintained. It was suggested that social support basically has a direct, rather than an interactive, effect on the relationship stress-health outcomes.

Should primarily interest stress researchers, and social and be-havioral scientists in general.

923. CARLETON, Cheryl Jean. "The impact of life events and social support networks on adult health." Ph.D. dissertation. University of Pennsylvania, 1981.

A study of the effects of life events and social support on health and demand for medical care using an economic model of human behavior.

Research

Presence of social support networks was strongly related to subjective measures of health, but not to objective health outcomes. Life events did not show a consistent relationship with health outcomes. Social support was also significantly related to demand for health care. Life events, such as retirement and moving increased demand, while other events, such as divorce or becoming widowed, decreased demand.

Should interest social scientists, particularly those concerned with utilization of health services, and health care policymakers/planners.

924. DICKEY, Elizabeth Dunbar. "Life events, social support, and adjustment in women: A field study." Ed.D. dissertation, University of Massachusetts, 1977.

Provides information on the apparent connections between life events (stress) and both physical and emotional illness.

Research

Results supported the relationships between life events (stresses) and adjustment; the high stress values were associated with poor adjustment. The postulated buffering effects of social support did not develop, though they were supported in the interviews.

Of interest to researchers of stress and social support.

925. FARRAN, Carol J. "A survey of community-based older adults: Stressful life events, mediating variables, hope and health." D.N.Sc. dissertation, Rush University, College of Nursing, 1985.

Examines the effects of stress, social support, personal control, and religiosity on hope and health in a sample of 126 older adults.

Research

Mental and physical health were positively associated with hope and personal control; social support was positively related only to mental health; and hope was positively associated with social support, personal control, and religious beliefs.

Useful for social scientists, gerontologists and pastoral counselors.

926. GARDOL, Louis C. "A canonical analysis of the relationship of psychosocial stress, problem-focused coping, and social support to physical and mental health." Ph.D. dissertation, United States International University, 1983.

An attempt to strengthen the psychosocial stress/health outcome relationship by combining measures of physical and mental health and including measures of coping style and social support.

Research

The prediction of health outcomes by stressful life events was improved when physical and mental symptomatology were combined. However, problem-focused coping style and social support did not add significantly to the prediction.

Of interest to social and behavioral scientists, particularly stress researchers.

927. HELRICH, Karen L. "The use of hardiness and other stress-resistance resources to predict symptoms and performance in police academy trainees." Ph.D. dissertation, California School of Professional Psychology, San Diego, 1985.

Examined how moderator variables such as hardiness, coping, and social support affect the relationship between stress and illness and stress and job performance among police academy trainees.

Research

The presence of daily hassles was found to distinguish those who reported symptoms from those who did not, while coping was also associated with levels of psychological symptoms. For extreme groups, it was found that those who experienced higher levels of stress and had good resistance resources (hardiness, coping, social support) had better grades at the academy than those with equal amounts of stress but fewer resistance resources.

Of interest to social and behavioral scientists, in particular stress researchers.

928. MOURY, Randolph L. "Social support, stressful life events, and psychological impairment: A study of deaf persons." Ph.D. dissertation, The University of Tennessee, 1985.

Examined psychological symptoms in relationship to life events and social support among deaf persons, and compared the results with those of a hearing sample.

Research

There were no significant differences between the two groups in levels of current or past symptoms. Deaf subjects reported more events for three of the nine life event variables, and less support on all three social support variables. No significant evidence was found for the buffering effect of social support in either group.

Should interest social and behavioral scientists.

929.   NEULICHT, Ann T.   "The impact of minor and major life events
       as mediated by social support and individual characteristics:
       A study of retarded adults."   Ph.D. dissertation, University
       of Oregon, 1983.

Explores the impact of stressful events on several health outcomes as
well as the buffering role of social support and individual
characteristics.

Research

Social support did not significantly affect any of the stressor/health
relationships.   Minor life effects were found to have a negative
health effect among older persons.   Several personal characteristics
like income, skills, and leisure activities had a positive influence
on emotional problems for the younger females.

Should be of interest to stress researchers and health professionals
working with mentally retarded adults.

930.   PRESTON, Deborah B.   "The effects of marital status, sex
       roles, stress, coping, and social support on the health of the
       elderly."   Ph.D. dissertation, Pennsylvania State University,
       1984.

A study of how a number of social-psychological factors affect health
in a sample of 900 people aged 65 and over.

Research

In general, it was found that not only individual attributes, but also
sex roles, as shaped in the social environment of marriage, affect the
impact of stress and social support on health among the elderly.

Of interest to social scientists and gerontologists.

931.   TIERNANN, Kathleen A.   "Life events, social support, and
       health: An examination."   Ph.D. dissertation, Western
       Michigan University, 1984.

A study of the relationships between life events, social support, and
health, testing a theoretically derived model.

Research

The results focus on the overlap that exists between undesirable
health-related life events and health outcomes.   This suggests a
severe measurement problem in this area of research.

Of interest to stress researchers and social scientists in general.

932. TOWERS, Jane F. "A meta-analysis of the relationships among stress, social supports, and illness and their implications for health professions education." Ph.D. dissertation, University of Pennsylvania, 1984.

A meta-analysis of the stress-social support-illness relationships on 45 samples.

Research

Results indicate a very strong relationship between psychosocial stress and onset of illness, and an almost significant intervening effect of social support in this relationship.

Useful for social scientists, health professionals, and health professions educators.

B. THE MODIFICATION OF STRESS

a. Articles

933. ADAMAKOS, Harry, Kathleen Ryan, Douglas G. Ullman, John Pascoe, Raul Diaz, John Chessare. "Maternal social support as a predictor of mother-child stress and stimulation." *Child Abuse and Neglect* 10 (1986): 463-470.

This study assessed the relationship between maternal social support and two areas: stress in the mother-child relationship, and level of stimulation provided in the home.

Research

Data regarding social support was obtained from 38 urban low SES mothers prenatally and followed up two years later, at which time variables were compiled on stimulation in the home of their two-year-old children. Maternal social support correlated positively with level of stimulation and negatively with level of mother-child stress, and was the best predictor of both, relative to any SES mother or child variables. High stress, low support mothers provided significantly less stimulation to their children. The theoretical implications for social support as a mediator variable, as well as its implications for early identification and prevention of abuse and neglect, are discussed.

Of interest to child welfare workers, social workers, mental health professionals, and researchers of social support.

934. ANASHENSEL, Carol S., and Jeffrey D. Stone. "Stress and depression: A test of the stress buffering model of social support." *Archives of General Psychiatry* 39 (1982): 1392-1396.

In 1979, a large community sample of Los Angeles County adults were interviewed to determine whether effective social support networks lessen the adverse psychological consequences of stress.

Research

Life-event losses and perceived strain were positively related to depressive symptomatology, while close relationships and perceived support were negatively related. In all models tested, these effects were found to be direct, not interaction effects as predicted by the buffering model. Stress had similar effects on depressive symptomatology among those who had both low and high levels of social support. Findings suggest that social support may be important in ameliorating depressive symptoms and that lack of support may contribute to the creation of depressive symptoms.

Should interest social scientists.

935. BILLINGS, Andrew G., and Rudolf H. Moos. "The role of coping responses and social resources in attenuating the stress of life events. *Journal of Behavioral Medicine* 4 (1981): 139-157.

Examines the influence of individual coping responses and of quantitative and qualitative measures of social resources on the negative effects of stressful life events.

Research

Undesirable life events were found to be associated with impairment in personal functioning, particularly among women. However, these negative effects were attenuated by certain coping strategies and qualitative measures of social support. More reliance on active strategies to cope with life events lead to less stress.

A paper for social scientists interested in stress-related phenomena.

936. BLUMBERG, Phyllis, Joseph A. Flaherty, Ann E. Morrison. "Social support networks and psychological adaptation of female and male medical students." *Journal of the American Medical Women's Association* 39, No. 5 (1984): 165-167.

A study of the psychological adaptation of female and male medical students, with special emphasis on social support.

Research

Female medical students encounter more difficulties than male students in regard to number of life changes and general mental health status. However, they are more likely to look for supportive social contacts, which may buffer the potentially negative effects of their greater psychological problems.

Of particular interest to medical educators.

937. CLARKE, Adrienne, and J.M. Innes. "Sensation-seeking motivation and social support moderators of the life stress/illness
relationship: Some contradictory and confirmatory evidence."
Personality and Individual Differences 4 (1983): 547-550.

Describes the relationship between life change and reported physical
and psychological symptoms, the degree of sensation-seeking, and
social support.

Research

Sensation-seeking behavior among firefighters was linked to high life
change and increased illness.   Social support did not reduce the
relationship between life change and illness.

Psychologists and other behaviorally oriented researchers will find
this article of interest.

938. COBB, Sidney. "Social support as a moderator of life stress."
Psychosomatic Medicine 38 (1976): 300-314.

The evidence that supportive interactions among people are protective
against the health consequences of life stress is reviewed.

Review and Analysis

It appears that social support can protect people in crisis from a
wide variety of pathological states.   Furthermore, social support may
reduce the amount of medication required, accelerate recovery, and
facilitate compliance with prescribed medical regimens.

Useful to teachers, researchers, and health practitioners concerned
with stress and its buffers.

939. COHEN, Sheldon, and Harry M. Hoberman. "Positive events
and social supports as buffers of life change stress."
Journal of Applied Social Psychology 13 (1983): 99-125.

Examines both social support and positive events as possible moderators of the relationship between undesirable life events and physical
and depressive symptomatology.

Research

Perceived availability of social support and a number of positive
events moderated the relationship between negative life stress and
depressive and physical symptomatology.

Of interest to mental health professionals and researchers of stress
and social support.

940. COHEN, Sheldon, Drury R. Sherrod, Margaret S. Clark. "Social skills and the stress-protective role of social support." *Journal of Personality and Social Psychology* 50 (1986): 963-973.

Evidence suggests that social skills are related to the development of social support and friendship and provide a stress buffering effect.

Research

A cross-sectional study of a large incoming college freshmen class examined the relationship of social competence, social anxiety, and self-disclosure, as these are related to stress protection and social support development. A prospective study of a sample followed at 11 and 22 weeks served as the study group.

Psychologists, counselors, and other mental health professionals will find this study useful.

941. COHEN, Sheldon, and Thomas Ashby Wills. "Stress, social support, and the buffering hypothesis." *Psychological Bulletin* 98 (1985): 310-357.

Investigates whether the positive association between social support and well-being is attributable more to the overall beneficial effect of support (main or direct-effect model) or to a process of support protecting persons from potentially adverse effects of stressful events (buffering model).

Literature Review and Analysis

Evidence for a buffering model is found when the social support measure assesses the perceived availability of interpersonal resources that are responsive to the needs elicited by stressful events. Evidence for a main effect model is found when the support measure assesses a person's degree of integration in a large social network.

Of interest to researchers of stress and social support.

942. DEAN, Alfred, and Nan Lin. "The stress-buffering role of social support." *Journal of Nervous and Mental Diseases* 165 (1977): 403-417.

Identifies some key empirical, theoretical, and methodological problems in studying social support and suggests some approaches to their resolution.

Theoretical and Review

The authors stress the use of a longitudinal design in future studies so that the cause-effect relationship between variables can be documented.

Of use to social and behavioral scientists and researchers of stress.

943. DIMSDALE, Joel E. "The coping behavior of Nazi concentration
      camp survivors." *American Journal of Psychiatry* 131
      (1974): 792-797.

This study of coping strategies reports on interviews with 19 survivors of Nazi Concentration Camps.

Research

Group affiliation was important in providing information, advice, and
protection. It was also important in reinforcing the person's sense
of individuality and worth. The size of the group was not of key
importance. The two person friendship group was extremely effective
in mediating between the person and stress.

Of interest to mental health professionals and social and behavioral
scientists.

944. EPLEY, Stephen W. "Reduction of the behavioral effects of
      aversive stimuli by the presence of companions." *Psychol-
      ogical Bulletin* 81 (1974): 271-283.

Examines the assumption that the presence of a companion diminishes
behavioral reactions to stressful or aversive stimuli.

Literature Review

No studies, to date, provide unequivocal support for the assumption
that the simple physical presence of a companion is sufficient to
diminish reactions to aversive stimuli.

Of interest to social and behavioral scientists, especially social
psychologists.

945. FINNEY, John W., Roger E. Mitchell, Ruth C. Cronkite,
      Rudolph H. Moos. "Methodological issues in estimating main
      and interactive effects: Examples from coping/social support
      and stress field." *Journal of Health and Social Behavior*
      25 (March 1984): 85-98.

Attempts to clarify points of confusion regarding the issue of
estimating main effects and the relationship between product-term
regression and other forms of analyses in stress research.

Analytical

A paradigm to study the mediating and moderating effects of stress
within a single framework is proposed.

Of use to researchers of stress.

946. FONTAINE, Gary. "Roles of social support systems in overseas
      relocation: Implications   for   intercultural   training."
      International Journal of Intercultural Relations   10 (1986):
      361-377.

Reviews the research literature on social support systems, the roles
such systems can play in overseas relocation, and the implications for
intercultural training.

Literature Review

A primary source of stress in overseas relocation is the disruption of
a person's social support system. A primary strategy for coping with
the stress of overseas assignment is the use of available support
systems, but social support systems are frequently hindered in providing adequate support overseas because they, too, are often under
stress. Three potential roles of social support systems in intercultural training are suggested; a social skills training approach is
presented as a way of usefully providing training in the development
and use of social support systems overseas; and a specific training
model is described.

Particularly useful to administrators and counselors in diplomatic,
military, religious, and professional agencies, organizations, and
businesses which employ overseas personnel.

947. FUNCH, Donna P., and James R. Marshall. "Self-reliance as a
      modifier of the effects of life stress and social support."
      Journal of Psychosomatic Research 28 (1984): 9-15.

Considers the relationships between stress, support systems, and
psychological adjustment to breast surgery due to cancer.

Research

The relationship between social support, stress and outcome is modified by a self-reliance factor. Self-reliance may play a mediating
role in the relationship between stress, support, and adjustment.

Of interest to researchers of stress and social support.

948. GANELLEN, Ronald J., and Paul H. Blaney. "Hardiness and
      social support as moderators of the effects of life stress."
      Journal of Personality and Social Psychology 47 (1984):
      156-163.

This study examined the relation and relative importance of social
support and the hardy personality in reducing the effects of life
stress.

Research

The commitment and challenge dimensions of hardiness were found to be
significantly correlated with social support, whereas the control

dimension was not.   When the interactions among life stress, social support, and hardiness were considered, only the alienation from self scale was found to moderate the effects of life stress.

Of interest to social and behavioral scientists.

949.   HABIF, Valerie L., and Benjamin B. Lahey.   "Assessment of the life stress-depression relationship: The use of social support as a moderator variable."   *Journal of Behavioral Assessment* 2, no. 3 (1980): 167-173.

Investigates whether social support modifies the effects of life stress on psychological distress.

Research

The hypothesis that social support may act as a buffer between life changes and experienced distress was generally confirmed.   The correlations between negative life changes and total life changes were found to be much higher for subjects with low social support than for those with more social support.   It was concluded that the presence of social support may alter vulnerability to stress.

Useful for social scientists interested in stress research.

950.   HUSAINI, Baqar A., James Alan Neff, J.R. Newbrough, Michael C. Moore.   "The stress-buffering role of social support and personal competence among the rural married."   *Journal of Community Psychology* 10 (1982): 409-426.

Examines the effect of the stress-buffering properties of personal competence and social support on depressive symptoms.

Research

Results demonstrate that individuals with high levels of stress and low personal competence have high levels of depressive symptoms, independent of social support.

Researchers and family therapists will find this article useful.

951.   KIECOLT-GLASER, Janice K., and Brian Greenberg.   "Social support as a moderator of the aftereffects of stress in female psychiatric inpatients."   *Journal of Abnormal Psychology* 93 (1984): 192-199.

This study assesses the impact of social support on post stressor cognitive impairment.

Research

Support was found for the stress buffering hypothesis of social support.   Social support was not related to stress reduction in a lab group receiving low stress, but was very important in a similar group receiving high stress.

Experimental psychologists and other empirically oriented personality researchers will find this an interesting study.

952. KISSEL, Stanley.   "Stress-reducing properties of social
      stimuli."   *Journal of Personality and Social Psychology*   2
      (1965): 378-384.

Examines the effect the presence of other people has on stress.

Research

Stress responses were lowered more in the presence of friends than in the presence of a stranger. Affiliation motivation was not found to be related significantly to social stimuli as stress reducers.

Of interest to social and behavioral scientists, especially those studying stress.

953. KRAUSE, Neal.   "Social support, stress, and well-being among
      older adults."   *Journal of Gerontology*   41 (1986): 512-519.

Investigates whether social support buffers the deleterious effects of stressful life events on depressive symptoms in older adults.

Research

Findings reveal that, although social support fails to modify the effects of a global stressful life events indicator, specific types of social support buffer the impact of specific types of stressors (bereavement, crime, and social network crises).

Of interest to gerontologists and social and behavioral scientists.

954. LEFCOURT, Herbert M., Rod A. Martin, Wendy E. Saleh.
      "Locus of control and social support--interactive moderators
      of stress."   *Journal of Personality and Social Psychology*
      47 (1984): 378-389.

A replication and expansion of the work of Sandler and LaKey. Hypothesis was that persons who are internal for affiliation and achievement, low in the need for affiliation, and high in the need for autonomy, will more commonly exhibit moderator effects from social support than will their opposites.

Research

Results corroborated previous findings that persons with an internal locus of control derive greater benefits from social support than do those who have a more external orientation. Furthermore, the moderating effect of social supports largely occurs among those who are less generally affiliative and are more highly autonomous.

Of interest to social and behavioral scientists.

955. LIN, Nan, Mary W. Woelfel, Stephen C. Light. "The buffering effect of social support subsequent to an important life event." *Journal of Health and Social Behavior* 26 (1985): 247-263.

Examines the buffering effect of social support, identifying the most important life event experienced by an individual and tracing the characteristics of the person who helped during and/or after the event.

Research

It was found that individuals showed an increased level of depressive symptoms if they experienced a most important and undesirable event, but the effect was reduced when help came from strong (rather than weak) ties.

Of importance to researchers studying social support and stress.

956. MILLER, Rickey S., and Herbert M. Lefcourt. "The stress buffering function of social intimacy." *American Journal of Community Psychology* 11 (1983): 127-139.

Explores the role of social intimacy in predicting individual response to stress.

Research

Although the accountability between intimacy and individual life stress remains unclear, it is likely that current intimacy enhances self-esteem. The relationship provides an opportunity to share life events and helps the individual resist the effects of stressors.

Of interest to social and behavioral scientists and mental health professionals.

957. NEZU, Arthur M., Christine M. Nezu, Marta A. Peterson. "Negative life stress, social support and depressive symptoms: Sex roles as a moderator variable." *Journal of Social Behavior and Personality* 1 (1986): 599-616.

This study evaluated the moderating function of sex roles on stress-related depressive symptomatology and assessed the relationship of social support to sex-role differences.

Research

Multiple regression analysis, using data from 168 undergraduate students, indicated that the masculinity dimension served as a moderator of both negative life stress and family social support. Subjects high on the masculine dimension scale, even those with low levels of family support, reported lower depression scores under high levels of stress than people who scored low in masculinity. The femininity dimension was found to contribute little to the prediction of depressive symptoms. No differences as a function of sex were found. Implications for stress research and the sex-role literature are discussed.

Of interest to researchers of stress and social support.

958. NORRIS, Fran H., and Stanley A. Murrell. "Protective function of resources related to life events, global stress, and depression in older adults." *Journal of Health and Social Behavior* 25 (1984): 424-437.

Explores the potential protective functions of resources (those relatively stable conditions and supplies that are appraised by the person as available for use in meeting life changes, including, but not limited to, environmental events).

Research

One thousand, four hundred and two older adults were interviewed twice with a six month interval. The direct, indirect, and interactive relationships of resources, life events, global stress, and depression were examined, using multiple regression procedures to isolate the unique contributions of six hypothesized functions of resources. It was found that stronger resources did not reduce undesirable events, but did reduce the degree to which one experienced global stress, and reduced depressive symptoms. Strong resource persons had less global stress than weak resource persons at low levels of events, but (contrary to the prediction) this advantage disappeared as levels of events increased. The buffer hypothesis was not supported--the advantage of strong over weak resource persons held at all levels of events. Strong resource persons, only, had less change in depression than weak resource persons at the higher levels of global stress.

Should be of particular interest to researchers of life events and stress.

959. PARRY, Glenys, and David A. Shapiro. "Social support and life events in working class women: Stress buffering or independent effects?" *Archives of General Psychiatry* 43 (1986): 315-323.

A community survey of 193 working class mothers in which social support, threatening life events, psychiatric symptomatology, and psychological well-being were measured using a standardized interview and case-identification procedure with self-report questionnaires yielding continuous measures of distress and well-being.

Research

The effects of life events and social support were found to be largely independent of one another.

Of interest to mental health professionals.

960. POPIEL, Debra A., and Edwin C. Susskind. "The impact of rape: Social support as a moderator of stress." *American Journal of Community Psychology* 13 (1985): 645-676.

This study investigated 25 victims' reactions to sexual assault and the role of social support in their subsequent adjustment.

Research

The highly elevated scores on both adjustment measures clearly indicated that the assault is far from resolved at 3 months following the trauma. The aftermath of the assault may be particularly problematic in the case of women experiencing attempted rapes. The data indicated that these women received significantly less support than did victims of completed assaults.

Of interest to mental health professionals, judges, and law enforcement officals, and to social and behavioral scientists.

961. SANDLER, Irwin N. "Social support resources, stress and the maladjustment of poor children." *American Journal of Community Psychology* 8 (1980): 41-52.

The effects of the presence of social support resources as moderators of the relationship between stress and maladjustment were investigated.

Research

Results indicate that older siblings and two parents in the family both reduce the negative effects of stress on children. These results were interpreted to be consistent with social support literature. Implications for preventive interventions are discussed.

Of interest to social and behavioral scientists, early childhood teachers and social workers.

962. ———, and Brian Lakey. "Locus of control as a stress moderator: The role of control perceptions and social support." *American Journal of Community Psychology* 10 (1982): 65-80.

Investigates the effects of locus of control beliefs as an individual difference variable on the relationship between negative life events and psychological disorder, perceptions of control over negative life events, and the receipt and impact of social support.

Research

Results replicated the findings of Johnson and Sarason (1978) that the individual difference variable of locus of control beliefs moderates the effects of stress, but failed to provide evidence that locus of control beliefs was related to either perceptions of control over negative events or the effects of such control perceptions on the stressful impact of negative events. There were differences in the receipt and impact of social support for internals and externals.

Of interest to social and behavioral scientists, especially researchers of stress and social support.

963. SOLOMON, Zahava, and Bruce Oppenheimer. "Social network variables and stress reaction--lessons from the 1973 Yom-Kippur war." *Military Medicine* 151 (1986): 12-15.

Evidence suggests that a high level of community integration reduces the risk of combat stress reaction.

Research

Two sets of variables were examined in this study: 1) personal characteristics such as communal settlement background, birth order, and occupation solely as a soldier; and 2) family variables, including immigrant status and membership in a vulnerable family (one with problems). Those soldiers who experienced less combat stress came from vulnerable families in which they held central places; those who were born in Israel, lived in communal settings, and kept in close touch with their families also experienced less combat stress.

Of interest to researchers.

964. THOITS, Peggy A. "Conceptual, methodological, and theoretical problems in studying social support as a buffer against life stress." *Journal of Health and Social Behavior* 23 (1982): 145-159.

Reviews empirical work on the buffering hypothesis, outlines alternate conceptions of support, presents a refined hypothesis and model for analysis, and suggests three theoretical approaches that may be used to explain the interrelationships between support, events, and disturbance.

Literature Review

The relationships between events, support, and psychological disturbance have not been clarified theoretically; thus, the possibility that support itself is an etiological factor has been overlooked. The direct effect of events upon support and the interactive (buffering) effect of events with support have been confounded in many studies, so that results may have been biased in favor of the hypothesis.

Of interest to researchers concerned with stress and social support.

965. ———. "Explaining distributions of psychological vulner-
ability--lack of social support in the face of life stress."
Social Forces 63 (1984): 453-481.

Describes a study of the psychological vulnerability of disadvantaged
persons and their exposure to undesirable life events and low social
support.

Research

A panel study of 1,106 subjects found that vulnerability was not
accounted for by exposure to undesirable life events and that social
support counterbalances, rather than buffers, the impact of life
stress.

Of value to social science researchers.

966. THOMSON, Brian, and Alan Vaux. "The importation, transmission, and moderation of stress in the family system."
American Journal of Community Psychology 14 (1986): 39-57.

To test the importation and transmission of stress in families, a
cross-sectional study involving a survey of family triads was
conducted.

Research

Two measures of distress were related significantly to both macro- and
microstressors, and perceived social support did not buffer this
relationship.

Of interest to psychologists, sociologists, and social workers.

967. WETHINGTON, Elaine, and Ronald C. Kessler. "Perceived
support, received support, and adjustment to stressful life
events." *Journal of Health and Social Behavior* 26 (1986):
78-89.

This study, concerned with the perception of support availability,
indirectly indicates that actual network responses to stressful events
directly promote health adjustment, and that the perception of support
availability directly influences adjustment by modifying appraisals of
the situation.

Research

Analysis showed that perceived support is, in general, more important
than received support in predicting adjustment to stressful life
events. Evidence is also presented that the influence of received
support may be mediated by perceived support.

Of interest to researchers of stress and social support.

968. WILCOX, Brian L. "Social support, life stress, and psychol-
      ogical adjustment: A test of the buffering hypothesis."
      American Journal of Community Psychology 9 (1981): 371-386.

Assesses the influence of social support on the relationship between
stressful life events and psychological judgment.

Research

The hypothesis that social support mediates or serves as a buffer
between life events and psychological distress was tested for each of
two support measures in combination with the life events measure in
predicting psychological distress variables. All hypotheses were
supported.

Of interest to researchers of stress and mental health professionals.

b. Chapters

969. COHEN, Sheldon, and Garth McKay. "Social support, stress,
      and the buffering hypothesis: A theoretical analysis." *In*
      Andrew Baum, Shelley E. Taylor, Jerome E. Singer (Eds.).
      Handbook of Psychology and Health, Volume 4. Hillsdale, NJ:
      Lawrence Erlbaum, 1984.

Discusses the buffering hypothesis and alternative buffering
mechanisms.

Theoretical

A model is proposed that argues the importance of evaluating the
relationship between the coping requirements elicited by the event and
the experience of stress and the coping resources provided by one's
support systems.

Of interest to social and behavioral scientists studying stress and
social support.

970. FLEMING, Raymond, Andrew Baum, Martha M. Gisriel, Robert
      J. Gatchel. "Mediating influences of social support on stress
      at Three Mile Island." *In* Alan Monat, and Richard S.
      Lazarus (Eds.). *Stress and Coping. An Anthology.* Second
      Edition. New York: Columbia University Press, 1985.

Examines one explanation for differential stress at Three Mile
Island--the mediating effects of social support.

Research

The data suggest that social support affects those processes involved
in psychological and behavioral aspects of stress, but does not
appreciably reduce arousal associated with stress. Social support may
bolster Three Mile Island residents' ability to cope and to minimize

the aversiveness of stress, but the nature of the situation does not appear to allow either termination of stress or ready adaptation to it.

Of general interest to health professionals and social and behavioral scientists.

971. GORE, Susan. "Stress-buffering functions of social supports: An appraisal and clarification of research models." *In* B.S. Dohrenwend, and B.P. Dohrenwend (Eds.). *Stressful Life Events and Their Contexts* New Brunswick, NJ: Rutgers University Press, 1981.

A discussion of the functions of social support in stress processes and the interaction between social support and stress.

Theoretical

Several recommendations are offered for future research. The challenge is to redirect attention from evidencing a presumed support effect to documenting the nature of support mechanisms.

Of use to social and behavioral scientists interested in stress and social support.

972. HELLER, Kenneth, and Ralph W. Swindle. "Social networks, perceived social support and coping with stress." *In* Robert D. Felner, Leonard A. Jason, John N. Moritsugu, Stephanie S. Farber (Eds.). *Preventive Psychology: Theory, Research and Practice*. Elmsford, NY: Pergamon, 1983.

Presents a model that links the different aspects of social support to effective coping with stress.

Theoretical and Analytical

Current approaches to the buffering hypothesis that involve cross-sectional correlational studies have taken the literature as far as they can. The resulting ambiguity is both conceptual and methodological. More work needs to be done explicating the different aspects of social support. The structure, function, and quality of relationships with others in one's network; individual competency levels; the nature of environmental demands and whether they can be modified; and how these variables are perceived and appraised all contribute to eventual coping and adjustment and should be studied.

Of interest to teachers and researchers of social support.

973. SARASON, Irwin G., and Barbara R. Sarason. "Life changes, moderators of stress, and health." *In* Andrew Baum, Shelley E. Taylor, Jerome E. Singer (Eds.). *Handbook of Psychology and Health*. Volume 4. Hillsdale, NJ: Erlbaum, 1984.

Describes some of the variables that appear to moderate the stress of life events and shows how they can be taken into account in research on stressful life events. Suggests a theoretical formulation as a basis for conceptualizing the complex interaction of variables observed by researchers in this area.

Theoretical and Analytical

Discusses measures of stressful life events; variables that moderate stress; assessing social support; methodological questions regarding life events, moderators, and health; life changes as part of a theoretical framework; and future directions for research on personality, life experiences, and social support.

Should interest social scientists engaged in research on stress and social support.

974.   THOITS, Peggy A. "Coping, social support, and psychological outcomes: The central role of emotion." *In* Philip Shaver (Ed.). *Review of Personality and Social Psychology 5: Emotions, Relationships, and Health.* Beverly Hills: Sage, 1984.

Offers a theory of stress-buffering processes, with respect to psychological outcomes, that, when tested and refined, may specify the conditions under which, and the mechanism through which coping and supportive responses to stressors are likely to reduce psychological distress and disorder.

Theoretical

Argues that buffering effects are the products of successful emotion-management efforts that are initiated by individuals and sustained by specifiable others in the face of threatening circumstances.

Of particular interest to psychologists and sociologists.

975.   WILLIAMS, David R., and James S. House. "Social support and stress reduction." *In* Cary L. Cooper, and Michael J. Smith (Eds.). *Job Stress and Blue Collar Work.* Chichester: John Wiley & Sons, 1985.

Reviews evidence from a variety of sources on the relationships among social support, work stress, and health, focusing particularly on studies of blue collar populations.

Literature Review

Reviews empirical evidence that focuses on work stress, social support, and health among blue collar populations; discusses the negative aspects of social relationships, and sociocultural variations in the effects of social support; and addresses three issues regarding the enhancement of social support for blue collar workers: creating structural arrangements that facilitate support among workers; using organizational change processes to enhance support, having support enhance the efficacy of these processes; and facilitating supportive supervisory behavior.

Should interest specialists in organizational management and personnel and social and behavioral scientists.

c. Dissertations

976. ATKINSON, Thomas W.   "The effects of life events on social supports: Implications for testing the stress-buffer hypothesis." Ph.D. dissertation, Boston College, 1984.

Investigates the effects of life events on the quality and availability of social support and the implications for the stress-buffering function of social support.

Research

The data indicate that only undesirable stressful events produced negative changes in social support, which effect was basically limited to the support resources in the family. A model was presented, including main and interactive effects of social support, on symptoms and main effects of stressful events on social support.

Interesting for social and behavioral scientists, in particular, stress researchers.

977. BROWNELL, Arlene B.   "Emotional and tangible social support as moderators of the stress-health relationship: A test of the specificity model." Ph.D. dissertation, University of California, Irvine, 1981.

Tests the differential effectiveness of emotional and tangible support, occupational stress, and physical health stress on psychological and physiological symptoms.

Research

The data provided evidence of the moderating influence of social support on the health effects of psychosocial stressors. Results were discussed in terms of the differential main and interaction effects of social support found in the literature.

Of interest to social and behavioral scientists, in particular stress researchers.

978. HANDEN, Benjamin L.   "The effect of social support and stress on the health of community-living elderly." Ph.D. dissertation, University of Massachusetts, 1985.

Examines the stress-buffering effects of social support on health in an active and homebound elderly sample.

Research

Perceived social support had a greater relationship to illness than did actual number of social contacts, and was more predictive of psychological than of physical measures of health.

Useful to gerontologists and social scientists, particularly researchers of stress and illness.

979. IDE, Bette A. "Health change, life change and social network support among low-income elderly." Ph.D. dissertation, University of Arizona, 1973.

A study of the buffering effects of social supports on health among elderly people who are especially vulnerable to stress.

Research

Results indicated that social support factors had a protective effect upon the impact of stressful conditions on subsequent health status in this population. This effect was clearer in objective measures of health change, particularly objective functional health change, than in subjective measures.

Should be useful for gerontologists, but may also interest social and behavioral scientists.

980. KEE, Carolyn C. "Stressful life events, functional health status, and social support in the elderly." Ph.D. dissertation, Georgia State University, 1984.

Investigation of the modifying effect of social support on the relationship between life events and functional health status among the elderly.

Research

Life events were not an important predictor of health status in this sample. Social support had a significant positive effect on health.

Should interest gerontologists and social scientists.

981. MONTGOMERY, Mary Lee. "The impact of psychosocial support on the stress process." Ph.D. dissertation, George Peabody College for Teachers of Vanderbilt University, 1984.

Examines the potentially modifying effects of psychosocial support on the stress process in a six-month follow-up study.

Research

Results indicated that social support may influence the perception of stressful life events and self-reported acute health status.

Psychosocial support did not seem to prevent the occurrence of life events, nor did it ameliorate the chronic effects of stress.

Useful for stress researchers and social and behavioral scientists.

982. WELLS, James A. "Social support as a buffer of stressful job conditions." Ph.D. dissertation, Duke University, Durham, 1980.

Examines whether social support has a buffer effect on health among blue collar workers who experience stressful working conditions.

Research

Support was found for the main hypothesis: high social support, to a certain extent, lead to a reduction in symptoms, buffering the effects of stressful perceptions of objective job conditions. The supervisor at work provided the most important source of support.

Of interest to social scientists, particularly researchers of occupational stress.

C. PREGNANCY, CHILDBIRTH, AND ADJUSTMENT TO PARENTHOOD

a. Articles

983. BOYCE, W. Thomas, Catherine Schaefer, Chris Uitti. "Permanence and change: Psychosocial factors in the outcome of adolescent pregnancy." *Social Science and Medicine* 21 (1985): 1279-1287.

A cross-sectional analysis of perinatal complications and psychological well-being as they relate to a variety of psychosocial variables, including stressful life events, social network support, and a questionnaire measure of the sense of permanence.

Research

Multivariate analysis indicated that while life events and social support had effects in the expected directions, the sense of permanence constituted an important, additional factor in the effects of social experience on pregnancy outcomes.

Of interest to social and behavioral scientists.

984. BROWN, Marie Annette. "Social support, stress, and health: A comparison of expectant mothers and fathers." *Nursing Research* 35, no. 2 (1986): 72-76.

The influence of social support and stress on expectant mothers' and fathers' health was determined by testing and comparing different predictive models.

Research

Results indicated that social support and stress were useful in predicting health. Partner support appeared to be the most important variable in understanding expectant fathers' health, but social support for mothers included a larger domain, and social networks contributed to their health in the same way as partner support. These data suggest that nursing interventions targeted at reducing stress and improving expectant parents' satisfaction with their partner support might enhance their health.

Of interest to obstetricians, nurses, and maternal and child health specialists.

985. CARLSON, Mary L., Katherine Laux Kaiser, Rosalie C. Yeaworth, Robert E. Carlson. "An explanatory study of life-change events, social support and pregnancy decision in adolescents." *Adolescence* 19 (Winter 1984): 765-780.

Focused on the relationship of life-change events and family and social support to decision making in pregnant adolescents.

Research

Suggests that teens electing to continue pregnancies had higher life change scores, lower levels of social support, more disciplinary incidents, and more personal and family problems.

Health professionals working with teens may benefit from this study.

986. COPSTICK, S.M., K.E. Taylor, R. Hayes, N. Morris. "Partner support and the use of coping techniques in labour." *Journal of Psychosomatic Research* 30 (1986): 497-503.

The relationship between partner support, use of pain control techniques, and epidural anesthesia was examined in 80 primiparous women.

Research

The use of psychological 'pain control' techniques did not reduce the intensity of labor pain or enable women to do without an epidural anesthetic. However, the use of these techniques did correlate with reduced frequency of anesthesia when women were consistently supported and encouraged throughout labor, and when labor was relatively short.

Of interest to obstetricians and obstetrical nurses.

987. CRNIC, Keith A., Mark T. Greenberg, Arlene S. Ragozin, Nancy M. Robinson, Robert B. Basham. "Effects of stress and social support on mothers and premature and full-term infants." *Child Development* 54 (1983): 209-217.

Examines the relationships of stress and social support to maternal attitudes and early mother-infant interactive behavior.

Research

Although no group differences were found, when data were pooled, both
stress and support significantly predicted maternal attitudes at one
month and interactive behavior at four months. Mothers with greater
stress were less positive in their attitudes and behavior, while
mothers with greater support were significantly more positive.
Intimate support proved to have the most general positive effects.

Of interest to health professionals in obstetrics/gynecology.

988. CRNIC, Keith A., Mark T. Greenberg, Nancy M. Robinson,
     Arlene S. Ragozin. "Maternal stress and social
     support--effects on the mother-infant relationship from birth
     to 18 months." *American Journal of Orthopsychiatry*
     54 (1984): 224-235.

Investigates the relationship of maternal stress and social support
and their impact on mother-infant bonding and interaction.

Research

Social support and perceived stress were significant predictors of
maternal attitudes and the quality of maternal intervention with
infants. High levels of stress and low social support correlated with
poor behavioral interactions and low infant stimulation.

Child development specialists will find particular value in this work.

989. CRONENWETT, L.R., and W. Kunst-Wilson. "Stress, social
     support, and the transition to fatherhood." *Nursing
     Research* 30 (1981): 196-201.

A paradigm from the field of stress research is adapted to the transition to fatherhood.

Theoretical

The new paradigm organizes and integrates the factors that impact on a
man's experience of becoming a father. Through this process, a better
theoretical understanding of social support, as well as a guide to
future inquiry concerning fatherhood, is acquired.

Of interest to social and behavioral scientists.

990. CUTRONA, Carolyn E. "Social support and stress in the
     transition to parenthood." *Journal of Abnormal Psychology*
     93 (1984): 378-390.

Investigates the components of social support and stress as predictors
of postpartum depression.

Research

Social support was found to predict postpartum depression in the later weeks of the postpartum period. Deficiencies in social integration and reliable alliance were found to be the key components of social support related to depression. These results fail to support the stress-buffering hypothesis of social support.

Mental health researchers will find this an interesting paper.

991. ————, and Beth R. Troutman. "Social support, infant temperament, and parenting self-efficacy: A mediational model of postpartum depression." *Child Development* 57 (1986): 1507-1518.

A model of maternal postpartum depression in which difficult infant temperament was construed as a stressor and supportive interpersonal relationships were construed as a protective resource was tested.

Research

It was hypothesized that both infant temperamental difficulty and level of social support would affect maternal depression. Fifty-five married women were assessed during pregnancy and again three months postpartum. Infant temperament was assessed through observation, maternal crying records, and the Revised Infant Temperament Questionnaire. Path analysis indicated that infant temperamental difficulty was strongly related to the mothers' level of postpartum depression. Social support appeared to exert its protective function against depression. Practical implications for identifying women at risk for postpartum depression and theoretical implications for understanding the mechanisms through which stressful events and social support affect adjustment are discussed.

Of interest to social scientists, obstetricians, and mental health professionals.

992. FARIA, Geraldine, Elwin Barrett, Linnea Meany Goodman. "Women and abortion: Attitudes, social networks, decision-making." *Social Work in Health Care* 11 (1985): 85-99.

Three major research areas are examined: 1) the attitudes and feelings women have about abortion in general; 2) from whom women seek help in deciding to have an abortion; and 3) the specific reasons women give for deciding to have an abortion.

Research

Although women arrive at the decision to have an abortion from divergent pathways, most go through the decision-making process with no apparent difficulty. Women who are non-white, non-Protestant, younger, less educated, of lower economic status, non-contraceptive users, or lack a supportive social network appear to be at risk of encountering severe conflicts in decision-making.

Of interest to nurses, social workers, counselors, physicians, and public health out-reach workers.

993. HOBFOLL, Stevan E., Arie Nadler, Joseph Lieberman. "Satisfaction with social support during crisis: Intimacy and self-esteem as crtical determinants." *Journal of Personality and Social Psychology* 51 (1986): 296-304.

Provides evidence that satisfaction with social support is essential to recovery from normal and medically complicated pregnancy.

Research

A relationship was found between intimacy with spouse and with friends and satisfaction with social support. Self-esteem, social network parameters, and type of pregnancy outcome did not modify the relationship of social support and satisfaction with it.

Those interested in social support, group process, and outcomes of pregnancy as affected by social relations will benefit from this article.

994. LENZ, Elizabeth R., Peggy L. Parks, Louise S. Jenkins, Grace E. Jarrett. "Life change and instrumental support as predictors of illness in mothers of 6-month-olds." *Research in Nursing and Health* 9 (1986): 17-24.

The extent to which life change after birth of a baby and instrumental support of parenting predict the occurrence of illness in mothers of 6-month-olds was studied.

Research

Life change and intensity of support were positively related, and size of the support network was negatively related to illness. There was no evidence of the buffering effect of support. Findings conferred that life change helps predict postpartum illness, and revealed that characteristics of instrumental support differ in their importance as predictors.

Of interest to pediatricians and family physicians.

995. MERCER, Ramona T., Kathryn C. Hackley, Alan Bostrom. "Social support of teenage mothers." *Birth Defects* 20, no. 5 (1984): 245-290.

Reports on the social support perceived to be available by teenage mothers during their first year of motherhood, and on the correlation of perceived social support with maternal role attainment variables.

Research

During early postpartum, the only type of support to correlate with maternal attachment was informational support, and teenagers had received less than older women. There was no significant correlation of any of the support variables with the teenagers' perceptions of their neonate. Teenagers received less emotional support from mates and from parents than older women. Social support variables failed to correlate with maternal role attainment measures of perceptions of the neonate, ways of handling irritating child behaviors, or infants' growth and development. Physical and emotional support correlated positively with feelings of love for the infant. Physical support correlated positively with maternal competency behaviors.

Of particular interest to nurses and social workers.

996. NORBECK, Jane S., and Virginia P. Tilden. "Life stress, social support, and emotional disequilibrium in complications of pregnancy: A prospective, multivariate study." *Journal of Health and Social Behavior* 24 (March 1983): 30-46.

This study used a multivariate approach to determine the effects of selected psychosocial variables on complications of pregnancy in a population of medically-normal women from various racial, marital, and socioeconomic groups.

Research

Life stress and social support (emotional) were significantly related to emotional disequilibrium. A significant interaction of life stress during pregnancy and social support (tangible) was found for all three types of complications, but not for overall complications of pregnancy.

Of interest to social and behavioral scientists, obstetricians, and obstetrical nurses.

997. NUCKOLLS, K.B., John Cassel, B.H. Kaplan. "Psychosocial assets, life crisis and the prognosis of pregnancy." *American Journal of Epidemiology* 95 (1972): 431-441.

A search for a correlation between psychosocial assets and social stresses, as measured by cumulative life change scores, with the prognosis of pregnancy.

Research

Women with high life change scores both before and during pregnancy were less likely to suffer complications if they also possessed high psychosocial assets. Women who were unaffected by life change showed no significant relationship between psychosocial assets and complications.

Of interest to those concerned with maternal health.

998. O'HARA, Michael W. "Social support, life events, and depression during pregnancy and the puerperium." *Archives of General Psychiatry* 43 (1986): 569-573.

A sample of 99 women was studied prospectively from the second trimester of pregnancy until nine weeks postpartum.

Research

Women experiencing postpartum depression reported more stressful life events and less support from their spouses after delivery than did women not experiencing postpartum depression. Women experiencing depression during pregnancy reported somewhat less support from their spouses and more support from their confidants than nondepressed women. The results suggest that different causes may be responsible for prepartum and postpartum depression.

Of interest to obstetricians and mental health professionals.

999. ———, Lynn P. Rehm, Susan B. Campbell. "Postpartum depression. A role for social network and life stress variables." *Journal of Nervous and Mental Diseases* 171 (1983): 336-341.

Investigates the effects of social network variables and experience of life events on postpartum adjustment.

Research

Depressed postpartum women experienced more stressful life events since the onset of pregnancy and since delivery than the depressed control subjects. The depressed mothers also received less social support, particularly that provided by the spouse.

Useful to obstetricians and other health professionals involved in pre- and postnatal care and helpful to social scientists interested in stress-health outcome research.

1000. PANZARINE, Susan. "Stressors, coping, and social supports of adolescent mothers." *Journal of Adolescent Health Care* 7 (1986): 153-161.

Describes the perceived stressors, coping strategies, and social supports of a group of adolescent mothers during their first month at home after delivery.

Research

Findings suggest that puerperium is not a time of major distress for most of these young women. Factors contributing to a relatively smooth transition to motherhood were the adolescents' use of anticipatory coping prior to birth, their extensive reliance on family support once at home, and their past experience with child care.

Of interest to pediatricians, family physicians, and other health care personnel.

1001. PAYKEL, E.S., E.M. Emms, J. Fletcher, E.S. Rassaby. "Life events and social support in puerperal depression." *British Journal of Psychiatry* 136 (1980): 339-346.

Reports on a study of puerperal depression in the milder clinical range. Particular attention was given to assessment of life events and other possible antecedent factors.

Research

A 20 percent prevalence of mild clinical depression was found in 120 women assessed at about six weeks postpartum. The strongest associated factor was the occurrence of recent stressful life events. Social factors were also reflected in the inverse of depression with a poor marital relationship and reduced social support.

Of interest to gynecologists, mental health professionals, and social and behavioral scientists.

1002. PEREZ, Robert. "Effects of stress, social support and coping style on adjustment to pregnancy among Hispanic women." *Hispanic Journal of Behavioral Sciences* 5 (1983): 141-161.

A sample of 107 Hispanic women attending the UCLA Prenatal Clinic were studied to determine the effects of stress, social support, and coping styles on prepartum anxiety and intrapartum processes.

Research

Findings indicated that stress, whether indexed in terms of life changes or anticipation of labor and delivery pain, was significantly related to prepartum anxiety and, especially in interaction with prepartum use of medical personnel for information and reassurance, affected both prepartum anxiety and intrapartum analgesia requirements. The social support and coping style variables failed to consistently predict the intrapartum criterion variables and many stresses by social support or coping style interactions were nonsignificant.

Should be of special interest to social scientists engaged in the study of stress.

1003. PHILIPP, Connie. "The relationship between social support and parental adjustment to low-birthweight infants." *Social Work* 29 (1984): 547-550.

Twenty-four parents of low birthweight infants, were assessed regarding the availability of social support and their capacity to use this support.

Research

Findings show that the availability of social support facilitates the capacity of parents to cope with the hospitalization of their low birthweight infant and is also related to their overall adjustment to the child. The ability to use support following discharge was more highly related to parental adjustment than availability or use of support during hospitalization.

Of interest to physicians and mental health professionsals.

1004. PRIDHAM, Karen F., Kathleen Batato Egan, Audrey S. Chang, Marc F. Hansen. "Life with a new baby: Stressors, supports, and maternal experience." *Public Health Nursing* 3 (1986): 225-239.

This 90 day, longitudinal study explored the nature of the stressors and supports that 62 mothers reported during their infants' first three months, and examined their relationship to maternal experience.

Research

Supports were almost equivalent to stressors throughout the 90 days, and for both stressors and supports, the existential type was more frequent than the social type. Overall, stressors and supports decreased significantly across the six 15-day periods into which the study was organized, but three support classes (activities/plans, behavior of self and others, and conditions) and three stressor classes (tasks/responsibilities, conditions, and events) did not change significantly. The relationship of stressors and supports remained strong and positive throughout the study.

Of interest to researchers of the stresses and supports of new parenthood.

1005. SOSA, Roberto, John Kennel, Marshall Klaus, Steven Robertson, Juan Urrutia. "The effect of a supportive companion on perinatal problems, length of labor, and mother-infant interaction. *New England Journal of Medicine* 303 (1980): 597-600.

The effects of a supportive lay woman ("doula") on the length of labor and on mother-infant interaction after delivery was studied in healthy Guatemalan primigravid women.

Research

Mothers who had a doula present during labor were awake more after delivery and stroked, smiled at, and talked to their babies more than the control mothers.

Of interest to obstetricians, obstetrical nurses, and early child care specialists.

1006. STEMP, Peter S., R. Jay Turner, Samuel Noh. "Psychological distress in the postpartum period: The significance of social support." *Journal of Marriage and the Family* 48 (1986): 271-277.

This panel study examines changes in the psychological distress of 280 new mothers over a one year period.

Research

Regression analyses show that when social support is indexed as the extent of the mother's social network, this variable has no impact on changes in psychological distress. However, the cognitive experience of social support and the degree of marital intimacy make significant independent contributions to changes in psychological distress.

Of interest to obstetricians and pediatricians.

1007. THOMPSON, Maxine Seaborn. "The influence of supportive relations on the psychological well-being of teenage mothers." *Social Forces* 64 (1986): 1006-1024.

Explores the influence of family and peer resources on adaptation to teenage motherhood.

Research

Supports from friends and relatives, particularly female siblings, are associated with higher levels of stress and distress, while support from a male partner is associated with low levels of distress. Results suggest that race and education are also important in explaining variations in the psychological well-being of teenage mothers.

Of interest to counselors, obstetricians, and family planning specialists.

1008. TILDEN, Virginia Peterson. "The relationship of life stress and social support to emotional disequilibrium during pregnancy." *Research in Nursing and Health* 6, no. 4 (1983): 167-174.

One hundred and forty-one normal adult women in their mid-trimester of pregnancy were tested with standardized instruments during a routine prenatal visit. Life stress was measured for the preceding twelve month period, with emotional disequilibrium as the dependent variable.

Research

Emotional disequilibrium in pregnancy decreased as a function of decreasing life stress and increasing social support.

Should interest health care professionals and social and behavioral scientists.

1009. VENTURA, Jacqueline N. "Parent coping, a replication." *Nursing Research* 35 (March/April 1986): 77-80.

Forty seven pairs of parents of two to three month old infants were asked to respond to a questionnaire to determine parent coping in relation to infant temperament and parent psychological responses.

Research

Mothers' and fathers' reports of helpfulness of coping behaviors were similar, but fathers reported more responses of depression and anxiety and focused less on coping by seeking social support and being responsible. Mothers who viewed their infant as of optimal temperament sought social support, maintained family integrity, and reported being religious, thankful, and content.

Of interest to early childhood specialists and pediatricians.

1010. WANDERSMAN, Lois, Abraham Wandersman, Steven Kahn. "Social support in transition to parenthood." *Journal of Community Psychology* 8 (1980): 332-342.

Explores the effects of different types of social support on the adjustment of first time parents in the postpartum period.

Research

Results suggest that the importance of a particular type of support may be different for fathers and for mothers. Implications for the provision of support by the naturally occurring informal networks of family, friends, and of specific group support systems are suggested.

Useful to mental health professionals dealing with adjustment to parenthood.

b. Dissertations

1011. COHEN, David A. "A multivariate regression examination of stressful life events, social support, and the postpartum depression syndrome." Ph.D. dissertation, University of Southern California, 1983.

A study of social stress upon the generation of postpartum depression, and the potentially modifying role of social support.

Research

Only motherhood role stress was a significant predictor of postpartum depression, whereas general stress was not. Support from the husband was very effective in moderating the negative impact of motherhood role stress, but support and help from other family members and friends were of little significance in reducing postpartum depression.

Should interest professionals involved in postnatal care, pediatricians, and health educators, and be informative for young mothers and fathers.

1012. CRAWFORD, Gretchen. "Teen social support patterns and the stress of pregnancy." Ph.D. dissertation, Case Western Reserve University, 1980.

Studies the relationship between patterns of social support and stress in terms of coping responses and pregnancy complications among teenage prenatal patients.

Research

An analysis was performed on sets of structural and social-emotional support factors, but no specific patterns could be determined. Social-emotional support was found to be a stronger predictor of coping responses or pregnancy complications than structural support or control variables.

Helpful for professionals involved in prenatal care.

1013. LAWRENCE, Edith Catlin. "The relationship between husband supportiveness and wife's adjustment to motherhood. Ph.D. dissertation, University of Virginia, 1982.

Examines the relationship between husband support and wife's parenting stress level.

Research

Data analysis revealed a significant inverse relationship between husband support and wife's parenting stress level. The aspects of husband support found to have the greatest relationship with stress were emotional support, acceptance of the father role, and favorable evaluation of wife as mother. The hypothesis that the negative relationship between parenting stress and husband support would be stronger for couples holding an egalitarian sex role ideology was not confirmed.

Of interest to social and behavioral scientists.

1014. NUCKOLLS, Katherine B. "Psychosocial assets, life crisis and the prognosis of pregnancy." Ph.D. dissertation, University of North Carolina, Chapel Hill, 1970.

A major focus of this study is the development and testing of an instrument which will give an index score of the "adaptive potential" for pregnancy, and therefore be predictive of pregnancy complications.

Research

Although the hypothesis that women with higher psychosocial assets will be less likely to have complications of pregnancy is not supported unequivocally, the data indicate that a meaningful association exists if the relationship is considered in the context of life events.

Of use to social and behavioral scientists, health educators, obstetricians, and nurses.

1015. TILDEN, Virginia P. "The relationship of single status during pregnancy to life stress, social support, and emotional disequilibrium." D.N.S. dissertation, University of California, San Francisco, 1981.

Compared the differential effects of life stress and social support on the emotional state during pregnancy in a sample of single and partnered women.

Research

Single and partnered women did not differ significantly in experience of life stress, social support, or depression, although the two groups were different on some of the subfacets of social support. Single women were higher on state-anxiety and lower on self-esteem. Life stress accounted for a major part, and social support for a smaller, but still significant, part of the variance in emotional disequilibrium, beyond the subject's partner status. There was some evidence for the buffering role of social support.

Of interest to social and behavioral scientists, health educators, obstetricians, and nurses.

D. FAMILY RELATED STRESSES

a. Books

1016. McCUBBIN, Hamilton I., Elizabeth Cauble, Joan Patterson (Eds.). *Family Stress, Coping, and Social Support.* Springfield, IL: Charles C. Thomas, 1982.

A basic introduction to historical and contemporary thought on family life in response to stress.

Book of Readings

Divided into one section on family stress and crisis theory, and one on family stressors, coping, and social support. Examines the fundamental nature of life changes, their impact on family life, and how families call upon internal interpersonal relationships as well as the community for support in coping and adaptation.

Should interest students, researchers, and practitioners in the social sciences and mental health professions.

1017. WEISS, Robert S. *Going it Alone.* New York: Basic Books, 1979.

A book based on interviews with over 200 single parents and about 40 children of single parents.

Research

Describes how people became single parents, the household of the single parent, and the way single parents organize their lives. Considers the strengths and vulnerabilities that can be found in parenting alone and the ways in which single parents manage.

Of interest to social and behavioral scientists, social workers, mental health professionals, and single parents.

b. Articles

1018. BELSKY, Jay. "The determinants of parenting: A process model." *Child Development* 55 (1984): 83-96.

Three domains of determinants of parental functioning are identified and discussed--personal psychological resources of parents, characteristics of the child, and contextual sources of stress and support--and a process model of competent parental functioning is offered.

Theoretical, Analytical

Argues that parental functioning is multiply determined; sources of contextual stress and support can directly affect parenting or indirectly affect parenting by influencing psychological well-being; personality influences contextual support/stress, which feeds back to shape parenting; the personal psychological resources of the parent are more effective in buffering the parent-child relation from stress than are contextual sources of support; and contextual sources of support are more effective stress-buffers than are characteristics of the child.

Should interest social and behavioral scientists.

1019. BRANDT, Patricia A. "Social support and negative life events of mothers with developmentally delayed children." *Birth Defects* 20 (1984): 205-244.

This study examined the relationship of social support and its relationship to negative life events experienced by mothers of developmentally delayed children.

Research

A questionnaire-based study of 91 mothers of children, aged six months to three years, with developmental disabilities, showed that mothers with high negative events felt less social support and were less satisfied with the quality of the support they did receive. Both the number and impact of negative life events were correlated with lower support.

Child development and family workers, social workers, and others interested in the single parent will find this a useful article.

1020. ———. "Stress-buffering effects of social support on maternal discipline." *Nursing Research* 33 (1984): 229-234.

The purpose of this study was to investigate whether social support and stress influence maternal discipline of the 6-month to 3-year old child with a developmental delay.

Research

Pearson correlations indicated that social support was inversely related to restrictive discipline for high stress mothers, but not for low stress mothers. The positive influence of social support was also found for mothers of children with three to five delays but not for mothers of children with one to two delays.

Of interest to pediatricians and developmental psychologists.

1021. BURKE, Ronald J., and Tamara Weir. "Maternal employment status, social support and adolescents' well-being." *Psychological Reports* 42 (1978): 1159-1170.

Examines the effects of maternal employment on the well-being of high school adolescents.

Research

Surveys show that maternal employment increased the life stress level of female adolescents. These individuals also showed a decrease in social support from their mothers and a decrease in well-being. Male adolescents showed no significant changes.

Of interest to mental health professionals.

1022. GARRISON, William, and Felton Earls. "Life events and social supports in families with a two-year-old: Methods and preliminary findings." *Comprehensive Psychiatry* 24 (1983): 439-452.

Presents findings on the frequency and types of life events and the characteristics of the social networks of families with two-year-old children who live in a demarcated community.

Research

Although the data illustrate that the amount of stress in families requires much coping and adaptation, they also suggest that the majority of families perceive satisfactory levels of help and support. Perhaps most important, in the context of how events impact on nuclear families, is the degree to which spouses experience a supportive relationship within their marriages.

Of interest to mental health professionals and social and behavioral scientists.

1023. HOWZE, Dorothy C., and Jonathan B. Kotch. "Disentangling life events, stress and social support: Implications for the primary prevention of child abuse and neglect." *Child Abuse and Neglect* 8 (1984): 401-409.

Explores the relationship between stress and child abuse and neglect.

Theoretical and Analytical

The ecological model points the way to redefining interventions for the primary prevention of child abuse and neglect. Existing support systems can be strengthened in order to increase a family's ability to cope with untoward events before these became stressful. In addition, advocacy activities, which support children and families in general, can be major components in the primary prevention of child abuse and neglect.

Of interest to social workers, child development specialists, child psychiatrists, and child advocates.

1024. KAZAK, Anne E., and Robert S. Marvin. "Differences, difficulties and adaptation: Stress and social networks in families with a handicapped child." *Family Relations* 33 (1984): 67-77.

Discusses differences in 100 families with and without a handicapped child with respect to three types of stress and three structural characteristics of their social support networks.

Research

Generally, higher levels of stress and distinct network structures were found for the families with handicapped children. Despite the presence of high levels of stress, the families were found to have successful coping strategies. The results are discussed in terms of recognizing family strengths and incorporating existing adaptational patterns into clinical interventions.

Of interest to social and behavioral scientists.

1025. PETERSEN, Paul. "Effects of moderator variables in reducing stress outcome in mothers of children with handicaps." *Journal of Psychosomatic Research* 28 (1984): 337-344.

A study of factors that help buffer mothers from the stresses of having a handicapped child.

Research

Mothers who experienced a lot of stress as a result of having a handicapped child benefitted significantly from sources of support in their environment. These resources included a variety of emotional and physical supports.

Particularly helpful to stress researchers, but also to health professionals working with handicapped children and their families.

1026. SCHILLING, Robert F., Lewayne D. Gilchrist, Steven Paul Schinke. "Coping and social support in families of developmentally disabled children." *Family Relations* 33 (1984): 47-54.

Personal coping and social supports are presented as resources for parents of handicapped children.

Review

Begins with a description of research on stress in the families of handicapped children, followed by a discussion of coping and social support. Studies on coping and social supports among parents of handicapped children are described. A training model to help parents use personal coping and social supports is presented.

Of interest to psychologists, physicians, and other persons working with handicapped children and their families.

1027. SCHILLING, Robert F., and Steven Paul Schinke. "Personal coping and social support for parents of handicapped children." *Children and Youth Services Review* 6 (1984): 195-206.

This paper discusses stress in families of developmentally disabled children and how parents of special needs children draw on personal and social coping strategies to manage daily challenges.

Literature Review and Analysis

The authors call for prevention strategies to prevent stress-related maltreatment of special needs children.

Of interest to pediatricians and other health professionals working with handicapped children.

1028. SOLOMON, Zahava. "Stress, social support and affective disorders in mothers of pre-school children--a test of the stress-buffering effect of social support." *Social Psychiatry* 20 (1985): 100-105.

This study attempted to assess the stress-buffering role of social support using data from a survey of 436 mothers from two semi-rural regions of Pennsylvania.

Research

Results indicated that women with less adequate social support were at greater risk of psychiatric disorders following the Three Mile Island nuclear accident. However, the role of social support as a stress moderator was not substantiated vis-a-vis affective disorder.

Of interest to mental health and public health professionals, and social and behavioral scientists.

1029. TURNER, R. Jay, and William R. Avison. "Assessing risk factors for problem parenting: The significance of social support." *Journal of Marriage and the Family* 47 (1985): 881-892.

Reports on the extent to which three social psychological variables-- social support, life stress, and personal control--constitute signifi- cant risk factors with respect to maladaptive parenting.

Research

Analyses of case comparisons were used to assess the power of these three variables to distinguish a sample of maladaptors from a sample of comparison mothers. Results indicate that experienced or individu- ally perceived social support effectively distinguishes among women who vary in their adaptation to the parenting role. Life stress and personal control are also significant, but social support may be of dramatic adaptive relevance.

Should interest social scientists engaged in social support research.

1030. WEINRAUB, Marsha, and Barbara M. Wolf. "Effects of stress and social supports on mother-child interactions in single and two-parent families." *Child Development* 54 (1983): 1297-1311.

Social networks, coping abilities, life stresses, and mother-child interaction were studied in 28 mother-child pairs--14 single mothers and their preschool children and 14 matched married women and their children.

Research

Predicting optimal mother-child interaction in single parent families were: fewer stressful life events, reduced social contact, increased parental support, and hours of maternal employment. Predicting optimal interaction in two parent families were: fewer stressful events, satisfaction with emotional support, and the availability of household help.

Of interest to child development specialists and social workers.

c. Chapter

1031. BELLE, Deborah. "The stress of caring: Women as providers of social support." *In* Leo Goldberger and Shlomo Breznitz (Eds.). *Handbook of Stress: Theoretical and Clinical Aspects*. New York: Free Press, 1982.

Directs attention to the health consequences for women of providing social support to others, particularly when it is not reciprocated.

Review

Discusses the traditional role of women as providers of social support and the status-reducing lack of recognition of the support that they provide. Points out the inequities of many support exchanges, particularly those involving young children; the stressfulness of providing support, especially that which is not reciprocated; and the clinical and public policy implications of recognizing the stressfulness of a support gap for many women.

Should interest mental health professionals, public policy providers, and social scientists.

d. Dissertations

1032. D'ERCOLE, Ann. "Stress, strain, coping and social support among single mothers." Ph.D. dissertation, New York University, 1983.

A study of the effect of coping, esteem, and social support on strain experienced by single mothers.

Research

Social support, particularly from friends, was found to have a direct effect on strain and well-being in this population. No buffering effects were noticed. Economic hardship, being the most important predictor of strain, proved to be the major stressor for single mothers.

Of interest to counselors working with single mothers, policymakers, and primary care practitioners.

1033. GREENBERG, Debra Lee. "Support systems and parent stress in families with trainable mentally retarded youngsters." Ph.D. dissertation, University of Pennsylvania, 1983.

Examines, through self-reports, how parents of mentally retarded youngsters perceive various aspects of their support systems and the extent to which this variable relates to levels of parent stress.

Research

Parents rated informal supports as more helpful than formal ones. Spouses and other parents with handicapped children were considered most helpful.   Parents also reported more stress than a normative sample representative of parents with non-handicapped children.

Of interest to social and behavioral scientists.

1034.   HALL, Lynne A.   "Social supports, everyday stressors, and maternal health."   Dr. P.H. dissertation, University of Carolina at Chapel Hill, 1983.

Examines the effect of several types of supports and stresses on mothers of children under six years of age.

Research

Psychological well-being was found to be dependent upon certain life situations, such as income and marital status. Everyday stressors and the quality of the primary intimate relationship were significantly associated with maternal mental health.

Of interest to social scientists, stress researchers and mothers of young children.

1035.   ZIMMERMAN, Jeffrey Leslie.   "The relationship between support systems and stress in families with a handicapped child."   Ph.D. dissertation, University of Virginia, 1980.

Evaluates the relationship between informal social supports and the stress of raising a handicapped child.

Research

Mothers of children with cerebral palsy were, indeed, experiencing significantly more stress than mothers of non-handicapped children. While the overall level of stress on the mothers' personal emotional state was not different between the groups, mothers of handicapped children reported added stresses on their personal health, and seemed to be suffering from the restrictions and social isolation that caring for their handicapped child presented.   They were not, however, more depressed nor did they have more trouble in their marital relationships than mothers of non-handicapped children.

Of interest to social and behavioral scientists.

E. SEPARATION AND DIVORCE

a. Articles

1036.   CALDWELL, Robert A., and Bernard L. Loom. "Social sup-
        port: Its structure and impact on marital disruption."
        American Journal of Community Psychology   10 (1982):
        647-667.

In an effort to learn more about the structure and impact of social
support as it relates to marital disruption, 50 newly separated men
and women were interviewed at two months and at eight months after
their separations.

Research

The structure of social support was found to include: 1) several
important sources of support, including family, friends, and the
larger community; 2) an index of social activity; and 3) a sense of
satisfaction with present marital status. Although the stress associated with separation was positively related to poorer adjustment,
certain aspects of social support were found to moderate this
relationship.

Of interest to family and marital counselors, social workers, and
mental health professionals.

1037.   CHIRIBOGA, David A., Ann Coho, Judith A. Stein, John
        Roberts. "Divorce, stress, and social supports: A study in
        helpseeking behavior." *Journal of Divorce* 3 (1979):
        121-135.

Considers variations in the use of social supports among persons who
are in the process of divorcing.

Research

Three hundred and ten men and women, aged 20 to 79, were interviewed.
Most frequently turned to for help were friends, spouse, and counselors. Men and older respondents were found to seek out supports less
frequently than women and younger respondents. Ethnicity and education influenced the pattern more than the frequency of support utilization. For all respondents, perceptions of the degree of stress
evoked by the divorce appeared to be a major force behind the use of
social supports.

Of interest to sociologists, psychologists, social workers, and family
and marital counselors.

1038.   COLLETTA, Nancy Donohue. "Support systems after divorce:
        Incidence and impact." *Journal of Marriage and the Family*
        41 (1979): 837-846.

Examines the effects of social support on post-divorce family
functioning.

Research

Maternal role performance was found to be related to the amount of available family support. Under extreme adverse conditions, women needed high levels of support in order to maintain adequate maternal functioning. Such conditions occurred particularly among low-income, divorced mothers, who, despite having, on the average, high levels of support, expressed dissatisfaction with the outside help they received.

Especially helpful to family sociologists.

1039. HENDERSON, Monika, and Michael Argyle. "Source and nature of social support given to women at divorce/separation." *British Journal of Social Work* 15 (1985): 57-65.

Thirty divorced or permanently separated women rated 12 different sources of social support according to their importance in providing 17 different types of help or support during the first six months of their separation/divorce.

Research

Friends proved to be the single overall important source of support, but the differential importance of social support as a function of the type of help received points to the multidimensional aspect of social support.

Of interest to family sociologists, marriage counselors, and social and behavioral scientists.

1040. LESLIE, Leigh A., and Katherine Grady. "Changes in mothers' social networks and social support following divorce." *Journal of Marriage and the Family* 47 (1985): 663-673.

Examines whether a mother's network characteristics are associated with the provision of support, and explores how both network characteristics and support may change in the months and years immediately following a divorce.

Research

Thirty-eight mothers were interviewed following their divorces, and again one year later, concerning the structural and interactional characteristics of their social networks and the support available to them. Results indicated that the characteristics associated with the support a mother receives may differ from the characteristics associated with her degree of satisfaction with her network. In the year following divorce, networks become more homogeneous and allow for greater support as they become denser and more kin-filled.

Should interest researchers of social networks and social support.

b. Dissertations

1041. MANELA, Roger W. "With a little help from my friends: Social
       support and health during marital problems, separation, and
       divorce." Ph.D. dissertation, The University of Michigan,
       1981.

Examination of the kind of social contacts people seek during marital
separation and how supportive they are.

Research

The investment in a marriage influenced the effect of separation on
blood pressure and distress levels. Blacks sought more help from
relatives, and whites more from friends. Women were more likely to
discuss marital problems with professionals and relatives than men,
and relatives could only help people who wanted to stay married, but
not those who wanted to get divorced.

Of interest to social scientists and mental health professionals.

1042. PROVENZANO, Frederic P. "Effects of social support in
       mediating adjustment to marital separation." Ph.D. disserta-
       tion, University of Washington, 1983.

Addresses the issues of social support and adjustment after
separation.

Research

Satisfaction with social support had a positive effect on psychological adjustment, more consistently for intangible types of support
than for tangible types. Women, however, also needed adequate
tangible support. In general, there were no significant differences
in levels of distress after separation across the sexes.

Of interest to social scientists, particularly marital counselors.

F. THE STRESS OF ILLNESS

a. Book

1043. GARFIELD, Charles A. (Ed.). *Stress and Survival: The
       Emotional Realities of Life-Threatening Illness.* St. Louis:
       C.V. Mosby, 1979.

Attempts to understand the human capacity for endurance of stressful
situations; to offer insight into the ways that emotional support can
promote the quality of life, longevity, and survival; and to examine
the best methods of providing such support to patients and their
families facing life-threatening illness.

Book of Readings

Divided into sections on the relation of social and psychologic factors to illness, new dimensions in the alleviation of stress, emotional impact on health professional and patient, personal encounters with life-threatening illness, social and psychologic support, the chronically ill child, understanding pain and suffering, and care of the dying patient.

Useful to health care professionals, mental health professionals and any other individuals who may be called on to provide emotional support in time of personal crisis.

1044. STOLL, Basil A. (Ed.).   *Coping with Cancer Stress.*
       Dordrecht: Martinus Nijhoff, 1986.

Reviews the emotional pressures and coping methods of cancer patients and the help currently available to them, the special problems of children and terminal patients with cancer, and the role of the family in coping.

Book of Readings

The three sections of this book are devoted to the impact of cancer on the patient, support of the cancer patient, and personal viewpoints. A critical assessment is made of the defects of health organization, training of personnel, and attitudes to cancer patients in Western society, as well as the growing tendency to self-help, mutual help, and group activities for such patients.

Useful to physicians, nurses, psychologists, sociologists, clergy and interested laypersons.

b. Articles

1045. AHMADI, Kate S. "The experience of being hospitalized--
       stress, social support and satisfaction." *International
       Journal of Nursing Studies* 22, no. 2 (1985): 137-148.

Explores relationships between patient stress, social support, and satisfaction with care in two companion units at a large teaching medical center.

Research

Relationships were found between the potential social support of family, friends, and other patients; family, friends' support, and overall satisfaction level; and other patients' support and stress.

Of interest to nurses and hospital personnel involved in direct patient care.

1046. LINN, J. Gary, and Baqar A. Husaini. "Chronic medical problems, coping resources, and depression: A longitudinal study of rural Tennesseans." *American Journal of Community Psychology* 13 (1985): 733-742.

This analysis examined chronic medical problems as a risk factor for depression using longitudinal survey data from a sample of rural Tennesseans.

Research

Personal resources and social support operated as moderating factors between the stress of medical problems and psychiatric impairment. The buffering effects of both social support and personal resources were explored.

Of interest to mental health professionals.

1047. McCUBBIN, Hamilton I., Marilyn A. McCubbin, Joan M. Patterson, A. Elizabeth Cauble, Lance R. Wilson, Warren Warwick. "CHIP--Coping Health Inventory for Parents: An assessment of parental coping patterns in the care of the critically ill child." *Journal of Marriage and the Family* 45 (1983): 359-378.

Data were collected on 100 families who have a child with cystic fibrosis to determine parental coping patterns when a child has a chronic illness.

Research

Analysis of the Coping Health Inventory for Parents (CHIP) showed three parental coping patterns: a) maintaining family integration; cooperation, and an optimistic definition of the situation; b) maintaining social support, self-esteem, and psychological stability; and c) understanding the medical situation through communication with other parents and consultation with medical staff.

Of interest to health professionals and social and behavioral scientists.

1048. POTASZNIK, Harry, and Geoffrey Nelson. "Stress and social support: The burden experienced by the family of a mentally ill person." *American Journal of Community Psychology* 12 (1984): 589-607.

Examines the burden experienced by the families of mentally ill persons and the relationship between stress and social support.

Research

A study of 56 parents of schizophrenic patients indicated that low levels of burden were associated with small, effective social networks and satisfaction with support, especially that received from self-help groups and when both spouses were involved with the patient.

Will interest social workers, psychologists, and others involved in self-help groups.

c. Dissertation

1049.   McDowell, Jennifer.   "Social support and stress among parents of diabetic children."   Ph.D. dissertation, George Peabody College for Teachers of Vanderbilt University, 1981.

A study of the role of social support in adaptation to stress among parents of diabetic children.

Research

Results showed high intercorrelations among the four social support measures, but no relationships between any of those measures and either perceived physical or mental health or perceived impact on the family.   Possible explanations for the negative results were discussed.

Of interest to social and behavioral scientists, particularly researchers of social support and stress.

G. OCCUPATIONAL STRESS

a. Books

1050.   HOUSE, James S.   *Work Stress and Social Support*.   Reading, MA: Addison-Wesley, 1981.

Focuses on the role of social support in reducing work stress and improving health.

Textbook

The study of work stress, social support, and health is presented as an inherently social psychological problem, involving the interplay between the nature of individuals and the nature of the social environments and social structure in which they are enmeshed.

Useful to teachers, students, and managers desiring an overview of stress and of factors that can buffer it.

1051.   REICHE, H.M.J.K.I.   *Stress aan Het Werk.   Over de Effecten van de Persoonlÿkheid en Sociale Ondersteuning op Strains.*   (Dutch.)   Lisse: Swets & Zeitlinger, 1982.

A study of the effects of personality factors and social support on the stressor-strain relationship among middle managers.

Research

Type A/B personality and rigidity had only indirect effects on strain-outcomes. Support from superiors and colleagues was found to be very effective in the reduction of stressors and the prevention of strains. Other findings related type of organizations to strain-outcomes.

Useful for organizational psychologists and social scientists interested in stress research.

b. Articles

1052. ABBEY, David E., and James P. Esposito. "Social support and principal leadership style--a means to reduce teacher stress." *Education* 105, no. 3 (1985): 327-332.

Demonstrates that the relationship between the leadership style of school principals and occupational stress in teachers is modified by the amount of social support teachers perceive they obtain from co-workers.

Research

Stress levels were lower in teachers who perceived that their major reasons for compliance were referent, expert, and reward supports.

Educators and others interested in occupational stress and social support will find this article useful.

1053. ABDEL-HALIM, Ahmed A. "Social support and managerial affective responses to job stress." *Journal of Occupational Behavior* 3 (1982): 281-295.

Examines the moderating or buffering effects of two social support variables on the relationships of role conflict and ambiguity to intrinsic job satisfaction, job involvement, and job anxiety.

Research

Significant interactions were obtained between the role variables and both social support variables.

Of interest to social and behavioral scientists, especially industrial and occupational psychologists.

1054. ALEXANDER, Dale, John S. Monk, A. Patrick Jones. "Occupational stress, personal strain, and coping among residents and faculty members." *Journal of Medical Education* 60 (1985): 830-839.

Differences in ratings by 155 individuals at four levels of medical experience on measures of occupational stress, personal strain, and availability of coping resources were examined.

Research

No significant differences were detected among the four groups on overall measures of occupational stress and personal strain. There were differences between first-year residents and faculty members on the subscales measuring physical environment stress, physical strain, recreation, and self-care. The findings support the need for residents to employ coping strategies during the residency years, and provide guidance regarding the kind of coping strategies needed.

Of interest to medical faculty, students, and housestaff.

1055. BAMBERG, Eva, Dorothee Rückert, Ivars Udris. "Interactive effects of social support from wife, non-work activities and blue-collar occupational stress." *International Review of Applied Psychology* 35 (1986): 397-413.

Investigates whether family support is an independent moderator variable in the stress process, whether social support is influenced by work, and the extent to which social support is influenced by the work situation.

Research

Although no significant relation was found between job ratings and social support, small, but significant relations were found between job ratings and inadequate wife support and between self-assessment of the work situation and perceived support. It was cautiously concluded that the 'objective' job situation, the perception and appraisal of an individual's job conditions seem to be important for the prediction of different dimensions of spouse support.

Of interest to researchers of social support and occupational stress.

1056. BEEHR, Terry A., and John A. Drexler, Jr. "Social support, autonomy, and hierarchical level as moderators of the role characteristics-outcome relationship." *Journal of Occupational Behavior* 7 (1986): 207-214.

Tests the potential effects of three moderators on the relationships between three role stressors (role conflict, role ambiguity, and role overload) and two types of employee responses (job satisfaction and job search intent).

Research

The moderator effects of social support, autonomy, and hierarchical level on role characteristics and employee outcomes were so weak that they were of no theoretical or practical importance.

Of interest to occupational therapists, corporation managers, and industrial psychologists.

1057. BLAU, Gary. "An empirical investigation of job stress, social support, service length, and job strain." *Organizational Behavior and Human Performance* 27 (1981): 279-302.

Several relationships were evaluated using the job stress model of French, employing bus operators from a midwestern transit authority as the sample.

Research

Results provided only limited support for the model, and length of services was found to be an important variable to consider in future research. In contrast to French's model, no type of social support acted as a buffer between any job stress-job strain relationships.

Of interest to occupational psychologists and managers of organizations.

1058. BRENNER, Sten-Olof, Dag Sörbom, Eva Wallius. "The stress chain--a longitudinal confirmatory study of teacher stress, coping and social support." *Journal of Occupational Psychology* 58 (1985): 1-13.

A conceptual core model of the teacher stress process was tested on longitudinal data.

Research

An attempt was made to incorporate social support from colleagues in the model as an independent variable, but this was rejected as inclusion resulted in significant misfit of the model. Neither did social support substantially interact with the stress process.

Of interest to stress researchers and occupational psychologists.

1059. CHISHOLM, Rupert F., Stanislav V. Kasl, Lloyd Mueller. "The effects of social support on nuclear worker responses to the Three Mile Island accident." *Journal of Occupational Behavior* 7 (1986): 179-193.

Examines what role social support plays in the relationship between a major stressor, job strains and health outcomes.

Research

Social support, especially that of supervisors, seems to have a direct protective effect against stress, even in the presence of a major stressful event. The buffering effects of social support appear to function only under certain conditions.

Very useful to stress researchers, particularly those interested in job-related stress and health.

1060. COOPER, Cary L. "Social support at work and stress management." *Small Group Behavior* 12 (1981): 285-297.

A discussion of the relationship between social support at work, stress management, and coronary heart disease.

Descriptive and Analytical

The individual's work group and social group provide effective social support, which offsets some of the effects of stress and coronary heart disease.

Of interest to social and behavioral scientists.

1061. FIMIAN, Michael J. "Social support and occupational stress in special education." *Exceptional Children* 52 (1986): 436-442.

Presents the results of a study examining the influence of the presence or absence of peer and administrative support on the frequency and strength of stress reported by three state-wide samples of special education teachers.

Research

A majority of the group comparisons indicated stronger and more frequent stress levels for nonrecipients of supervisory support than for recipients. A smaller number of group comparisons also indicated stronger and more frequent stress levels for nonrecipients than for recipients of peer support.

Of interest to special education teachers and supervisors.

1062. FIRTH, Hugh, Jean McIntee, Paul McKeown, Peter Britton. "Interpersonal support amongst nurses at work." *Journal of Advanced Nursing* 11 (1986): 273-282.

Attempts to clarify the nature of effective support from a superior, as perceived by nursing staff working in psychiatric, mental handicap, and medical settings.

Research

'Personal respect,' 'empathic attention,' and 'absence of interpersonal defensiveness' appeared to be important components of support. Staff on the same ward showed a high degree of agreement in judgments of their superior's personal respect and empathic attention, but perceptions of interpersonal defensiveness appeared to be more specific to perceptions or interactions between particular staff. Greater degrees of 'personal respect' experienced by staff were associated with role ambiguity and reduced emotional exhaustion (burn-out).

Of particular interest to nurses and hospital ward personnel.

1063.   GANSTER, Daniel C., Marcelline R. Fusilier, Bronston T.
        Mayes.   "Role of social support in the experience of stress
        at work."   *Journal of Applied Psychology*   71 (1986): 102-
        110.

The present study was designed to examine the role of social support
in the experience of work stress with a sample large enough to provide
statistically powerful tests of models of social support that specify
two-way and three-way interactions.

Research

No support for higher order interaction models was found.   In addition, no evidence emerged demonstrating any buffering effect for
social support.

Of interest to social and behavioral scientists.

1064.   GOPLERUD, Eric N.   "Social support and stress during the
        first year of graduate school."   *Professional Psychology*
        11 (1980): 283-290.

Describes the effects of social interaction on first year graduate
students' reports of stressful events and on their health and
emotional problems during the first six months of school.

Research

The more interactions first year graduate students had with peers and
faculty during the first 10 weeks of graduate study, the fewer
stressful life events, physical, and psychological disturbances they
reported in the first six months of study.   The quality of interactions was also important in the relationship.

Appropriate for a general audience.

1065.   GRAF, Francis A.   "The relationship between social support
        and occupational stress among police officers."   *Journal of
        Police Science and Administration*   14, no. 3 (1986): 178-186.

Investigates the relationship between police officers' perceived
social support, and their perceived job stress.

Research

Findings suggest that police officers who identify greater numbers of
support persons also perceive their occupation as less stressful.   An
examination of the relationship between number of supports at work and
the satisfaction with that support reveals a strong correlation
between the two.

Of interest to stress researchers and police officials.

1066. JAYARATNE, Srinika, and Wayne A. Chess. "The effects of
emotional support on perceived job stress and strain."
Journal of Applied Behavioral Science 20 (1984): 141-153.

Uses a national sample of social workers to examine the relationship
between work stress, strain, and emotional support.

Research

Results indicate negative associations between support and perceived
stress and strain. The authors, however, found no evidence for the
buffering effects of emotional support.

Of interest to social and behavioral sciences.

1067. JAYARATNE, Srinika, Tony Tripodi, Wayne A. Chess. "Perceptions of emotional support, stress, and strain by male
and female social workers." *Social Work Research and
Abstracts* 19, no. 2 (1983): 19-27.

Examines the relationship of emotional support to work-related stress
and strain among male and female social workers. The buffering
hypothesis was tested.

Research

Results indicate negative associations between support and stress and
between support and strain for both male and female workers; however,
no evidence was found to support the buffering hypothesis.

Of special interest to social service workers.

1068. KARASEK, Robert A., Konstantinos P. Triantis, Sohail S.
Chaudhry. "Coworker and supervisor support as moderators
of associations between task characteristics and mental
strain." *Journal of Occupational Behavior* 3 (1982):
181-200.

Several coworker and supervisory support measures are identified and
their buffering effects are tested by using a new model of social
support.

Research

Evidence was found to support the "stress-transfer" aspect of the
authors' social support model. Individuals in low stress personal
job situations report higher psychological strain where social
support is strong. This association supplements its conventionally
described mirror image: "positive buffering" where individuals in
high stressor personal job situations report lower psychological
strain when social support is strong.

Of interest to industrial sociologists and psychologists.

1069. KAUFMANN, Gary M., and Terry A. Beehr. "Interactions between job stressors and social support: Some counterintuitive results." *Journal of Applied Psychology* 71 (1986): 522-526.

Report on a field study of the psychological and physiological strains and organizational consequences of job stressors and social support among 102 hospital nurses.

Research

Contrary to the expected moderation of the relationship between stressors and strains in the presence of strong social support, social support strengthened the positive relationship between stressors and strains in the sample population, contradicting most theories and models of job stress and social support.

Of interest to social and behavioral scientists, and particularly researchers of job stress and social support.

1070. La ROCCO, James M., James S. House, John R.P. French. "Social support, occupational stress, and health." *Journal of Health and Social Behavior* 21 (September 1980): 202-218.

Concerned with the buffering hypothesis that social support ameliorates the impact of occupational stress on job-related strain and health.

Research

Findings support the buffering hypothesis for mental and physical health variables, but fail to support the buffering hypothesis in regard to job-related strains.

Of interest to researchers studying stress and social support.

1071. La ROCCO, James M., and Allan P. Jones. "Coworker and leader support as moderators of stress strain relationships in work situations." *Journal of Applied Psychology* 63 (1978): 629-634.

Evidence supports the notion that stress and support are additive; i.e., high levels of support result in greater self-esteem and job retention, while high stress produces the opposite effect.

Research

A survey of 3,225 Navy enlisted personnel found that coworker and leader support had direct effects on several job satisfaction measures. This correlational study used multivariate methods.

Researchers interested in burn-out/job retention/job satisfaction will find this survey interesting.

1072. MARCELISSEN, Frans H.G., A.N.H. Weel, J.A.M. Winnubst.
       "Organisatiestress en gezondheid. Tussenstand van een
       longitudinaal onderzoeksproject." (Dutch) *Tydschrift voor
       Sociale Gezondheidszorg* 6 (1983): 811-814.

Examines the effect of Type A behavior and social relations on health.

Research

In this longitudinal study, both Type A behavior and social relationships at work were predictive of the occurrence of psychosomatic
complaints. However, the relationship with a boss or manager was a
much more significant predictor of such complaints than were relationships with fellow workers. No significant associations were found
between Type A behavior or social relations at work and blood pressure
or cholesterol.

Of importance to stress researchers, especially those interested in
occupational stress.

1073. MAZIE, Barbara. "Job stress, psychological health, and social
       support of family practice residents." *Journal of Medical
       Education* 60 (December 1985): 935-941.

Seventy-nine family practice residents were studied to test the
hypothesis that the level of job stress and the level, source, and
type of social support affect residents' psychological health.

Research

Analysis of variances showed that high levels of job stress and/or
social support were associated with a high number of reported symptoms
of psychological distress. Low levels of problem-solving and of
emotional support from people at and outside work also were associated
with a high number of reported symptoms.

Of interest to family residents, family practitioners and medical
educators.

1074. NORBECK, Jane S. "Types and sources of social support for
       managing job stress in critical care nursing." *Nursing
       Research* 34 (1985): 225-230.

The theoretical model of occupational stress developed by LaRocco,
House, and French was tested in relation to job stress in critical
care nursing.

Research

Findings supported all the main effects in the model, but none of the
buffering effects. For the married group, a specific type of support
(work support) explained 24% of the variance of perceived job stress,
nearly double that of the overall social support measure for this
group. For the unmarried group, a specific source of support

(relatives) explained 10% of the variance in perceived job stress and 16% of the variance in psychological symptoms.

Of interest to social and behavioral scientists and nurses.

1075. OXLEY, Diana, and Manuel Barrera, Jr. "Undermanning theory and the workplace--implications of setting size for job satisfaction and social support." *Environment and Behavior* 16 (1984): 211-234.

The research described here demonstrates the utility of undermanning theory, particularly its applicability to work settings.

Research

The results provided support for the generalizability of undermanning theory. Relationships among social support, sharing grievances, and other outcome measures in small and large work settings were examined. Findings indicate that social support may be a mediating process in the relationship between setting size and employee attitudes and behavior.

Of interest to organizational and social psychologists.

1076. REVICKI, Dennis A., and Harold J. May. "Occupational stress, social support, and depression." *Health Psychology* 4 (1985): 61-77.

A model of occupational stress, social support, locus of control, and depression among family physicians was developed.

Research

Results indicate that occupational stress exerts a direct effect on depression. This relationship is moderated directly by family, social, and emotional support and indirectly moderated by the influence of locus of control on family social support. Support from peers was not significantly related to depression.

Of interest to health professionals and researchers of social support.

1077. SEERS, Anson, Gail W. McGee, Timothy T. Serey, George B. Graen. "The interaction of job stress and social support--a strong inference investigation." *Academy of Management Journal* 26 (1983): 273-284.

A comparative examination was made of three alternative hypotheses (buffer, coping, no interaction) predicting job outcomes by job stress and social support.

Research

Evidence supporting the coping hypothesis is more consistent than that for the buffer hypothesis, and, in explanation of the stress support interactions, the coping hypothesis is more consistent with the notion that supportive relationships provide a strategy for dealing with job stress. Social support may be of lesser concern to individuals who are not experiencing a significant amount of stress. For such individuals, job satisfaction may simply be a function of other work characteristics.

Of interest to researchers of job stress and social support.

1078. WELLS, James A. "Objective job conditions, social support and perceived stress among blue collar workers." *Journal of Occupational Behavior* 3 (1982): 79-94.

A study of the stress-reducing effects of social support in the work environment.

Research

Social support was found to reduce levels of perceived stress resulting from negative job conditions. The most effective support was provided by supervisors, friends, and relatives.

Helpful to stress researchers, in particular, those interested in job stress.

1079. WESTMAN, Mina, Dov Eden, Arie Shirom. "Job stress, cigarette smoking and cessation: The conditioning effects of peer support." *Social Science and Medicine* 20 (1985): 637-644.

Relationships between questionnaire measures of job stress and smoking intensity and cessation were studied among 560 disease-free smoking males and 310 quitters, all members of 22 Kibbutzim.

Research

The hypothesis that peer support is related to job stress was confirmed. The authors found that peer support was positively correlated with overload and responsiblity and negatively correlated with conflict, ambiguity, low status, lack of participation, lack of influence, and intrinsic impoverishment. Only meager evidence was found of any buffer effect of social support on the relationship between job stress and smoking intensity. The hypothesis that peer support buffers the relationship between job stress and smoking cessation was confirmed.

Of interest to social and behavioral scientists.

1080. WINNUBST, Jacques A.M., Frans H.G. Marcelissen, Rolf J. Kleber. "Effects of social support in the stressor-strain relationship: A Dutch sample." *Social Science and Medicine* 16 (1982): 475-482.

Describes how social support protects the person against the noxious effects of job stress.

Research

Social support buffers the impact of work-related stressors on psychological and behavioral strains, but there is no buffering effect on health strains.

Of interest to social and behavioral scientists.

1081. ————. "Social support as a moderator of stressor-strain relationships in industrial organizations." *Activitas Nervosa Superior* 1982, Supplement 3 (1982): 230-235.

Describes research on the hypothesis that social support protects against the noxious effects of job stress and will keep job strain and negative health effects at a minimum.

Research

This study of 1246 employees of 13 different industrial organizations demonstrates that social support buffers the impact of work related stressors--role strain, role ambiguity, role overload, responsibility, and future uncertainty--on psychological and behavioral strains. No buffering effect on health strains was demonstrated, although threats to job security and personal irritations were connected to mitigating the effects of social support.

Industrial psychologists and other social scientists working in complex organizations may find this work helpful.

c. Chapters

1082. DOEHRMAN, Steven R. "Stress, strain, and social support during a role transition." *In* Vernon L. Allen and Evert van de Vliert (Eds.). *Role Transitions* New York: Plenum, 1983.

A theoretical model was developed to test the effects of a role transition on middle-aged men retiring from the Navy and entering the civilian job market.

Research

Those undergoing a role transition experienced less job stress and less strain as the transition period progressed, and showed no differences from the no transition control group after six months. There was, however, a lingering residue of vulnerability to job stresses among the transition group members. Social support from supervisors, but not from wives, was seen to increase over time. Supportive others were of valuable assistance during the transition.

Should interest social scientists.

1083. HOUSE, James S., and James A. Wells. "Occupational stress,
       social support, and health." *In* Alan McLean, Gilbert Black,
       Michael Colligan (Eds.). *Reducing Occupational Stress:*
       Proceedings of a Conference. DHEW (N1OSH) Publication No.
       78-140, 1978.

A discussion of potential social mechanisms for mitigating the deleterious effects of occupational stress on health.

Research and Analysis

Current evidence suggests that social support can not only contribute
toward reducing occupational stress, it can also help to alleviate the
deleterious health consequences of such stress which we will not or
can not reduce. Amelioration of the effects of occupational stress,
like any disease-inducing or promoting agent, involves some combination of reducing exposure to the agent and increasing resistance to
its efforts. Social support seems uniquely promising in the latter
respect.

Of interest to social and behavioral scientists, health administrators
and individuals interested in occupational health.

1084. PAYNE, Roy. "Organizational stress and social support." *In*
       Cary L. Cooper and Roy Payne. *Current Concerns in*
       Occupational Stress. Chichester, England: John Wiley, 1980.

Reviews what is known about the role of social support in alleviating
life stress.

Review

Explores how different stages of the stress cycle might require
different sorts of interventions and why. Classifies types of supports and discusses strategies by which organizations can create
conditions that facilitate interaction and caring.

Should interest industrial and organizational management personnel as
well as social and behavioral scientists.

d. Dissertations

1085. BARGAGLIOTTI, Lillian A. "The relationship between
       work-related stress, coping, and social support." D.N.S.
       dissertation, University of California, San Francisco, 1984.

Investigates the relationships between environmental demands, personal
resources, and stress outcomes among medical-surgery and critical care
nurses.

Research

Job demands and personal resources, such as coping strategies and social support, accounted for a sizeable, although not major, proportion of the variance in stress outcomes. The highest proportion of the stressors were in the areas of management patient care and communication. Stress experience in this sample was particularly expressed in high levels of anxiety and moderate levels of burnout.

Should interest nurses and stress researchers.

1086. BOYLE, Coleen, A. "Work stress, health practices, and social support as indicators of general health among nuclear power workers." Ph.D. dissertation, University of Pittsburgh, 1981.

Investigates the relationships between stress, health practices, social support, and health.

Research

Perceived work stress was significantly associated with both physical and psychological measures of health. Poor health practices were related to physical health only in men under 35. Poor health practices also seemed to modify the relationship between stress and illness. Absence of a reciprocal confiding relationship with the spouse was found to be associated with presence of an affective disorder.

Very useful for social and behavioral scientists.

1087. DAVENPORT, Michael P. "The health status of psychiatric nurses: Life stress events and social supports as predictor variables." Ph.D. dissertation, University of Arkansas, 1983.

A cognitive-phenomenological study of the relationship between life events and health status with subjective perception of social supports as mediating variable.

Research

Job-related strain was found to be significantly predicted by self-reported burnout and severity of illnesses. Severity of illness was particularly associated with job-related stress, recent life changes, and differentiation of social supports.

Of interest to social scientists and nurses in mental health care.

1088. GAINES, Jean. "Effects of occupational hazards and social support on the emotional and physical health of blue-collar workers." Ph.D. dissertation, University of Florida, 1984.

A study of workplace stressors, different sources of social support, and health outcomes in a sample of 144 blue-collar workers.

Research

In general, it was found that physical danger was an important workplace stressor, that union support was not related to strain, that there was an objective stressor/perceived stressor association in addition to a linkage of perceived stressor and strain feelings, and a direct effect of supervisor and co-worker support on strain.

Should interest stress researchers and occupational health researchers.

1089. PINNEAU, Samuel R. Jr. "Effects of social support on psychological and physiological stress." Ph.D. dissertation, University of Michigan, 1975.

Examines evidence for the role of support from one's work supervisor, from others at work, and from people at home.

Dissertation

Support from supervisor and others at work were the primary sources to influence dissatisfactions with the job. The other psychological strains showed the effect of home support as well as support at work. Depression was the strain most often and most highly related to social support; overall job dissatisfaction and irritation ranked next.

Of interest to researchers of stress and social support.

e. Conference Proceedings

1090. McLEAN, Alan, Gilbert Black, Michael Colligan (Eds.). *Reducing Occupational Stress. Proceedings of a Conference, May 10-12, 1977.* U.S. Department of Health, Education, and Welfare, Public Health Service, Center for Disease Control, National Institute for Occupational Safety and Health, Division of Biomedical and Behavioral Science, DHEW (NIOSH) Publication No. 78-140, April, 1978.

American, British, and Scandinavian methods of dealing with relationships between occupational stress and health are presented in the proceedings of a conference on occupational stress.

Conference proceedings

Analyses of the work environment; social support for workers under stress; effects of computerization on work environment; management, white collar and blue collar stressors; and stress and its relationship to specific health problems such as myocardial infarction, alcohol abuse, and work-related accidents are covered.

Of interest to mental health professionals, occupational health specialists, and behavioral scientists.

1. BURNOUT

a. Articles

1091. CONSTABLE, Joseph F., and Daniel W. Russell. "The effect of social support and the work environment upon burnout among nurses." *Journal of Human Stress* 12 (1986): 20-26.

Presents and discusses research findings on the effects of various aspects of the hospital work environment on burnout among nurses, and evaluates the effects of social support in reducing and/or mitigating the relationship between negative aspects of the work environment and burnout.

Literature Review and Analysis

The major determinants of burnout were found to be low job enhancement, work pressure, and lack of supervisor support, along with the combined effects of job enhancement and supervisor support.

Of interest to nurses and to students of burnout.

1092. CRONIN-STUBBS, Diane, and Carol Ann Rooks. "The stress, social support, and burnout of critical care nurses--the results of research." *Heart and Lung* 14 (1985): 31-39.

Questionnaires were administered to 296 staff nurses working in four specialty areas in three midwestern hospitals in an attempt to identify stressors that are associated with burnout in critical care, psychiatric, operating room, and medical nurses.

Research

Findings indicated that occupational stress was associated with burnout, validating prior research. Intensity or perceived impact, rather than frequency of job stressors, contributed to burnout. Undesirable personal changes were directly related to burnout and, in combination with other variables, were significantly and inversely predictive of burnout. Positive life changes were inversely related to burnout, suggesting that desirable life changes may counteract burnout while undesirable changes may potentiate the effects of work stress. Social support was negatively associated with and predictive of burnout.

Should interest social scientists and nursing administrators.

1093. DAVIS-SACKS, Mary Lou, Srinika Jayaratne, Wayne A. Chess. "A comparison of the effects of social support on the incidence of burnout." *Social Work* 30 (May-June 1985): 240-244.

A survey of female child welfare workers employed in a state department of social services examined the effects of support from fellow workers and spouses.

Research

Social support, particularly from supervisors and spouses, is associated with low levels of burnout and mental health problems resulting from job stress.

Of interest to social workers and mental health professionals.

1094. DIGNAM, John T., Manuel Barrera, Jr., Stephen G. West. "Occupational stress, social support, and burnout among correctional officers." *American Journal of Community Psychology* 14 (1986): 177-193.

Three alternative models of the role of workplace social support in ameliorating the effect of occupational stress on burnout symptoms were tested.

Research

Analyses showed no support for either the direct or buffering models of social support. Rather, the data were consistent with the indirect model of social support in the workplace.

Of interest to social and behavioral scientists.

1095. ETZION, Dalia. "Moderating effect of social support on the stress burnout relationship." *Journal of Applied Psychology* 69 (1984): 615-622.

This study examined the mdoerating effect of social support on the relationship between life and work stresses and burnout.

Research

The relationship between work stress and burnout was moderated by support in life for women and by support in work for men. The relationship of life stress with burnout was not moderated by any source of social support for either men or women. The discussion focuses on the meaning of social support for men and women in the two main spheres of life.

Of interest to social and behavioral researchers of stress and social support.

1096. KAHILL, Sophia. "Relationship of burnout among professional psychologists to professional expectations and social support." *Psychological Reports* 59 (1986): 1043-1051.

Professional burnout was investigated among psychologists of varying experience.

Research

Burnout was not related to experience in the profession or to other demographic variables, but was significantly related to social support from family and friends, to expectations or attitudes about the profession, and, less strongly, to disillusionment. Graduate students reported significantly more disillusionment than practitioners.

Of interest to social scientists.

b. Dissertations

1097. CONSTABLE, Joseph F. "The effects of social support and the work environment upon burnout among nurses." Ph.D. dissertation, University of Iowa, 1983.

A study of the direct and interactional effects of the work environment and social support on burnout among nurses.

Research

Several aspects of the work environment and supervisor support contributed significantly to burnout experiences among nurses. High levels of supervisor support buffered adverse effects of the work environment.

Should interest nurses and social scientists, in particular occupational stress researchers.

1098. CRONIN-STUBBS, Diane. "The relationships among occupational stress, life stress, social support and the burnout experienced by staff nurses working in diverse hospital-based specialty areas." Ph.D. dissertation, Loyola University of Chicago, 1984.

A study of the occupational and personal variables that relate to the burnout of nurses.

Research

A number of occupational setting variables, occupational stress, and emotional support were predictive of burnout experiences. No significant differences in burnout experiences were found for nurses working in four specialty areas.

Useful for nurses, health care professionals in general, and social scientists.

1099. FONG, Carolyn M. "A study of the relationship between role overload, social support, and burnout among nursing educators." Ph.D. dissertation, University of California, Berkeley, 1984.

Examines the effects of role overload and social support on burnout among nursing educators.

Research

The data suggest that job overload is indeed associated with indices of burnout, in particular, emotional exhaustion. Support from a chairperson or from peers was found to prevent burnout experiences, although no buffer effects against overload could be demonstrated.

Should interest nursing educators, health professionals, and stress researchers.

1100. KIMMEL, Mark R. "Coping strategies, social support, and role related problems as predictors of burnout in nurses." Ph.D. dissertation, California School of Professional Psychology, Berkeley, 1981.

A study of the effects of a combination of social and psychological variables on dimensions of burnout among nursing personnel.

Research

Coping was found to be the best predictor of several dimensions of burnout. Other variables predictive of burnout dimensions include status and length of employment. The social support hypothesis was not confirmed by the findings.

May interest nurses and researchers concerned with health status and working conditions of health care providers.

2. UNEMPLOYMENT

a. Articles

1101. ATKINSON, Thomas, Ramsay Liem, Joan H. Liem. "The social costs of unemployment: Implications for social support." *Journal of Health and Social Behavior* 27 (1986): 317-331.

Examines the effect of unemployment on social support, the mediation of this effect, and the stress buffering hypothesis.

Research

Social support was measured in 82 blue- and white-collar men who had recently experienced unemployment. Data was examined on marital and family support, help from outside the family with problems, and number and frequency of contacts with social network members. Following unemployment, a significant decline in marital support was found for all workers. In relation to the number of weeks of unemployment, the quality of the marital relation decreased for white-collar workers, and they experienced an increase in help with problems, while blue-collar workers experienced a decrease in frequency of contact with network members. Analyses indicated that unemployment has a negative effect on marital and family support, in part through its effect on the husband's psychological well-being. The implications of the nonindependence between stressful events and social supports for the stress buffering hypothesis are discussed.

Of interest to researchers of stress and social support.

1102. GORE, Susan. "The effect of social support in moderating the health consequences of unemployment." *Journal of Health and Social Behavior* 19 (1978): 157-165.

It was hypothesized that social supports would modify the relationship between unemployment stress and health responses among men.

Research

The rural unemployed evidenced a significantly higher level of social support than did the urban unemployed, a difference probably due to the strength of ethnic ties in the small community and a more con-cerned social milieu. No differences between the supported and unsupported were found with respect to weeks unemployed or to actual economic deprivation. However, while unemployed, the unsupported evidenced significantly higher elevations and more changes in measures of cholesterol, illness symptoms, and affective response than did the supported.

Of interest to social and behavioral scientists interested in stress and social support.

1103. JACKSON, Paul. "Social support and unemployment: Towards a model and an empirical test." *Bulletin of the British Psychological Society* A106 (1983): 36.

Seeks to determine whether social support acts as a buffer against the impact of unemployment on personal well-being.

Research Abstract

Demonstrates that empirical studies need to distinguish between the size and structure of social networks as well as the quality of the relationships within those networks. The need for longitudinal studies is documented as one way to assess the impact of changes in the perception of social support on an individual's behavior.

Sociologists and others interested in problems of measurement and design in the study of social support may benefit from this work.

1104. ULLAH, Philip, Michael Banks, Peter Warr.   "Social support,
       social pressures and psychological distress during unemploy-
       ment." *Psychological Medicine* 15 (1985): 283-295.

An assessment of the beneficial effects of support for the unemployed
and an attempt to distinguish supportive relationships from other
social relationships.

Research

Two forms of social support--having someone to turn to for help with
money, and having someone to suggest interesting things to do--were
significantly associated with measures of distress, as were perceived
pressure to obtain a job and employment commitment, but not contact
with other unemployed young people. The association between distress
and having someone to turn to for help with money was greater for
those perceiving pressure from others to obtain a job than for those
not perceiving pressure.

Of interest to social and behavioral scientists.

b. Chapter

1105. LIEM, G. Ramsay, and Joan Huser Liem.   "Social support and
       stress: Some general issues and their application to unem-
       ployment." *In* L.A. Ferman, and J.P. Gordus (Eds.).
       Mental Health and the Economy.   Kalamazoo, MI: W.E.
       Upjohn Institute for Employment Research, 1979.

The authors draw on contributions from a larger body of work to raise
several general issues regarding the conceptualization of social
support as a moderator of stress.   Some of the research on social
support is reviewed, in the context of unemployment stress, as a basis
for suggesting conceptual and methodological considerations for
directing future work in this area.

Review

The most straightforward approach when coping with unemployment, might
be to treat social support as a personal resource that is mobilized in
unique ways.   Interpersonal contexts, like the family and neighborhood, may be   affected by economic change independently of the
employment status of a focal individual.   A map of one's network of
ties to others is shaped by macro social structure as well as the
characteristics of more delimited social contexts and one's unique
interpersonal preferences.

Of interest to social and behavioral scientists.

c. Dissertation

1106. GORE, Susan. "The influence of social support and related
variables in ameliorating the consequences of job loss."
Ph.D. dissertation, University of Pennsylvania, 1973.

A longitudinal study of the health and behavioral effects of job loss
among 100 men employed by two companies which were going to close,
leaving all employees without jobs.

Research

Individuals most at risk were those who had experienced considerable
unemployment and were inadequately supported. Rural terminees and
controls evidenced a significantly higher mean level of total social
support than did the urban groups. The importance of social support
lies in its protective nature for populations at risk.

Useful to social and behavioral scientists; professionals in occupational medicine, preventive medicine, and public health; and mental
health practitioners.

CHAPTER 7

SOCIAL SUPPORT STRATEGIES AND APPLICATIONS

1. SOCIAL SUPPORT STRATEGIES

a. Books

1107. GOTTLIEB, Benjamin H. *Social Support Strategies. Guidelines for Mental Health Practice.* Beverly Hills: Sage, 1983.

Translates the empirical research and conceptual formulations on social support into knowledge that can be used by mental health practitioners.

Literature Review and Application

A book full of practical ideas and examples. It ranges broadly over a number of different fields of application, including the role of social support in preventive programs, in medical practice, in the world of work, in delivering care to the elderly, and in addressing the role of human service professionals in mobilizing social support.

Useful to health practitioners, teachers, and administrators.

1108. LITWAK, Eugene. *Helping the Elderly.* NY: Guilford Press, 1985.

Presents an empirical test of the thesis that in a modern society, both large scale formal organizations and small primary groups, such as family, neighbors, and friends, are necessary to provide adequate social support for the aged.

Resource Book

The principle that groups can optimally manage those tasks that match them in structure is applied to nursing homes to show which sorts of services nursing homes can take over from primary groups and which these groups must retain. The book dispels the myth of the collapse of the family, but reaffirms that traditional definitions may vary greatly within/across certain ethnic and cultural groups. Friendships are viewed on a time-based utilitarian model.

Important to social theorists and gerontologists because it deals with the basic social theory that drives social policy.

1109.   MAYERSON, Evelyn Wilde.   *Putting the Ill at Ease.*   New York: Harper & Row, 1976.

Stresses the "two-way street" aspect of physician-patient communication. The dual process of sending and receiving signals of all types is carefully analyzed.

Textbook

In addition to information gathering and giving, the issues of spatial distancing and touching are addressed.

Of interest to all health professionals.

1110.   POWELL, Barbara.   *Alone, Alive, and Well.*   Emmaus, PA: Rodale Press, 1985.

Outlines the danger signs of negative attitudes toward loneliness and provides strategies for accruing them.

Manual

Abounds with numerous tips and techniques for focusing on the advantages of living alone and ways to develop those pluses as a protection against the demoralizing effects of loneliness.

Of interest to laymen and to social and behavioral scientists.

1111.   SARASON, Seymour B.   *Caring and Compassion in Clinical Practice.*   San Francisco: Jossey-Bass, 1985.

States and examines the possibility that caring and compassion are qualities in short supply among clinicians in various professions.

Theoretical and Analytical

The nine chapters cover the training of physicians, teachers, lawyers, and clinical psychologists with respect to caring and compassion.

Intended for physicians in general, psychiatrists, clinical psychologists, teachers, lawyers, and the recipients of clinical services.

b. Articles

1112. BEEMAN, Pamela Butler. "Peers, parents, and partners. Determining the needs of the support person in an abortion clinic." *Journal of Obstetrics, Gynecology, and Neonatal Nursing* 14 (January/February 1985): 54-58.

To ascertain how clinics might better meet the needs of support persons accompanying clients for an abortion, data were gathered through a questionnaire that related 25 statements to Maslow's five categories of need.

Research

Significant differences among categories of support persons were demonstrated on six of the 25 statements, a finding that suggests that abortion clinics should develop and implement counseling programs specific to the needs of each of the different groups.

Of interest to nurses.

1113. CLAYTON, Diane E., Vicki L. Schmall, Clara C. Pratt. "Enhancing linkages between formal services and the informal support systems of the elderly." *Gerontological and Geriatric Education* 5, no. 2 (Winter 1984-1985): 3-11.

Continuing education and consultation for caregivers of the elderly are described.

Review

Closer linkages between the formal and informal caregivers of the elderly are suggested as a means of improving the lives of both caregivers and those they help. A faculty/academic institution approach is offered as a model for emulation.

Academics interested in elders and caregivers will find this an interesting program description.

1114. COLLINS, Alice H. "Natural delivery systems: Accessible sources of power for mental health." *American Journal of Orthopsychiatry* 43 (1973): 46-52.

Describes a method of identifying, recruiting, and maintaining individuals who provide informal services for their neighbors and assisting them to enlarge their sphere of influence without changing their role and status.

Theoretical

Mental health professionals can expand and facilitate the effectiveness of natural helping systems within the community by identifying and collaborating with natural helpers in the population they wish to serve. This approach may have considerable preventive significance and be an effective method of improving community mental health.

Of interest to mental health professionals.

1115. JANIS, Irving L. "The role of social support in adherence to stressful decisions." *American Psychologist* 38 (1983): 143-160.

Describes the conditions under which a supportive other can help a person make and maintain a stressful decision, especially as it relates to health practices.

Research--Review

Creating a supportive relationship between a health counselor and client can provide motivational power to effect changes in health behaviors and practices. Positive feedback and moderate self-disclosure are associated with adherence to the decision to change health practices.

Health professionals involved in health promotion programs will benefit from this article.

1116. NORBECK, Jane S. "The use of social support in clinical practice." *Journal of Psychosocial Nursing and Mental Health Services* 20, no. 12 (1982): 22-29.

Presents key assumptions and research findings that can guide clinicians in thinking realistically about social support, both in assessing their clients and in planning interventions.

Review and Analysis

Although a large body of research has demonstrated a relationship between inadequate social support and various negative outcomes, no single prescription exists to guide clinical practice. Guidance for planning interventions is offered through typology of deficiencies in social support that highlights the deficiencies commonly found in the psychiatric population.

Of interest to health professionals.

1117. ————, and Barbara A. Resnick. "Balancing career and home: How the OIIN can relieve stress to improve employee health." *American Association of Occupational Health Nurses Journal* 34 (1986): 14-25.

A discussion of stress at work and at home and the interrelationship between stress, social support, and health, with suggestions for worksite interventions.

Descriptive

The occupational nurse is in a strong position to develop counseling and referral services to assist women in seeking outside resources, such as support groups, household services, and cooperative child care and transportation arrangement, to enhance their coping with these demands. If possible, worksite support groups can be provided to assist those women workers who carry multiple roles with inadequate support.

Of general interest to laypersons and health professionals.

1118. ROOK, Karen S. "Promoting social bonding: Strategies for helping the lonely and socially isolated." *American Psychologist* 39 (1984): 1389-1407.

Describes various strategies for helping the lonely and socially isolated enhance their social bonds and social support.

Literature Review

A general model for enhancing social bonding by modifying features of the social settings people live in is provided. Focuses on prevention, network building, family support, and educational approaches.

Provides clinicians with an excellent scheme for working with high risk groups and individuals.

1119. SHONKOFF, Jack P. "Social support and vulnerability to stress: A pediatric perspective." *Pediatric Annals* 14 (1985): 550-554.

Discusses social support as a strategy for health maintenance, disease prevention, and the management of chronic impairment in pediatric practice.

Theoretical

A pediatric practice can be a critical source of social support for children and their families. This support can be transmitted by providing information, assisting in the search for needed community services, and extending emotional support.

Of particular interest to pediatricians.

2. SUPPORT GROUPS

a. Books

1120. LIEBERMAN, Morton A., Leonard Borman, and Associates. *Self-Help Groups for Coping with Crisis: Origins, Members, Processes, and Impact.* San Francisco: Jossey Bass, 1979.

Provides a current perspective on self-help or mutual aid groups through the use of empirical research and theory generated from that research.

Book of Readings

Considers the origins, growth, and development of self-help groups; the kinds of needs they serve, for whom, and under what conditions; the factors that make them effective; how effective they are; and the major considerations and methodological problems that must be faced by researchers investigating self-help groups.

Should be of particular interest to mental health professionals and social science researchers.

1121. SILVERMAN, Phyllis R. *Mutual Help Groups: A Guide for Mental Health Workers.* Rockville, MD: National Institute of Mental Health, DHHS Publication No. (ADM) 80-646, Reprinted 1980.

This monograph, part of the Primary Prevention Publication Services, gives emphasis to primary prevention in the field of mental health/ mental illness.

Theoretical and Informational

The following topics are discussed: mutual help, transitions, the characteristics and nature of help, the role of specific mutual help groups, and the role of the mental health worker in mutual help groups. A bibliography provides guidance on further areas of study.

Useful to mental health professionals in all disciplines.

b. Articles

1122. ABLON, Joan. "Al-Anon Family Groups." *American Journal of Psychotherapy* 28 (1974): 30-44.

Describes Al-Anon Family Groups as they function as a fellowship for spouses, relatives, and friends of alcoholics.

Descriptive/Analytical

The Al-Anon groups constitute a remarkable self-help, nonprofessional modality of group therapy and group education for mental health. Sharing experiences with others in similar circumstances provides a basis for comparison of coping strategies and a stimulation of the process of self-examination, leading to new insight in all areas of the participant's life experience.

Of interest to mental health professionals and laypersons.

1123. BACK, Kurt W., and Rebecca C. Taylor. "Self-help groups: Tool or symbol?" *Journal of Applied Behavioral Sciences* 12 (1976): 295-309.

A description of the unique characteristics of self-help groups and their similarity to social movements.

Descriptive

The vague, general sentiment of self-help groups gives them the character of a social movement. What seems to be missing in contemporary society to which these groups respond? With traditional forms of security missing and the goal state relatively undefined, Americans are groping for a replacement and definition of goals and values.

Of interest to social and behavioral scientists.

1124. BARTH, Richard P., and Steven Paul Schinke. "Enhancing the social supports of teenage mothers." *Social Casework* 65 (1984): 523-531.

Describes a group training program that assists adolescent mothers in learning to build, use, and maintain networks of social support.

Descriptive

Measurement prior to and following the program showed that students learned interpersonal and cognitive skills, strengthened their social support networks, and reported satisfaction with the groups.

Of use to social workers and mental health professionals.

1125. BECKER, Grethe. "Social work in a group practice. Group work with the retired elderly in Copenhagen." *Scandinavian Journal of Primary Health Care* 3 (1985): 45-48.

Describes an experiment in social group work in which 13 recently retired men and women between the ages of 60 and 70 were referred by their general practitioners for participation in a mutual support group.

Descriptive and Theoretical

Elderly people, expressing their individual problems to each other in a group, may be stimulated to a better adaptation to their new role as pensioners by compensating for their change in status through engagement in other activities. Guidelines may be developed, as well, for resolving various common problems.

Of interest to social workers and gerontologists.

1126. BERGER, Jeanne Manchester. "Crisis intervention: A drop-in
       support group for cancer patients and their families." *Social
       Work in Health Care* 10 (1984): 81-92.

A drop-in, open-ended, professionally-run support group for cancer
patients and their families is described as a means of crisis intervention for the mobilization and promotion of adaptive processes.

Descriptive

The model is easily generalizable. It offers aid to the cancer family
in crisis, serves as an enhancer of adaptive behavior, and provides
on-going support for individuals in the midst of the crisis of cancer.

Of interest to social workers, oncologists, and other health professionals caring for cancer patients and their families.

1127. BERGMAN, Anne Sturmthal. "Marital stress and medical
       training: An experience with a support group for medical
       house staff wives." *Pediatrics* 65 (1980): 944-947.

Reports on a support group for medical staff wives.

Descriptive

All participants agreed that the group had been a positive experience,
allowing them to express anger in a safe place and not to their
husbands. They also stated that the group validated the fact that
their concerns were, in fact, real and shared by many women. Further
study of the impact of the training experience on both physician and
spouse would be helpful in determining appropriate methods of intervention to reduce feelings of stress and depression for both physician
and spouse during the training period.

Of interest to health professionals, especially physicians who are
married.

1128. BORKMAN, Thomasina. "Experiential knowledge: A new con-
       cept for the analysis of self-help groups." *Social Service
       Review* 50 (1976): 445-455.

Experiential knowledge is introduced as a new analytical concept that
characterizes self-help groups.

Theoretical

The attributes of experimental and professional knowledge are compared. This new concept is useful in considering the theoretical and
practical issues regarding the relationship between self-help groups
and professionals.

Of interest to social workers, psychiatrists, and human service
professionals who work with self-help groups.

1129. BYRNE, Carolyn M., Michelle Stockwell, Susan Gudelis.
"Adolescent support groups in oncology." *Oncology Nursing
Forum* 11, no. 4 (1984): 36-40.

A study of two support groups comprised of adolescent oncology patients identified major themes in the groups.

Descriptive

The themes discussed in both groups demonstrated that these adolescents used the opportunity to discuss and share the experience of
having cancer as it related to their age and development: in physical
appearance, loss of control, over-protection, being different, and
feeling a sense of responsibility to families. The adolescent support
groups were helpful in assisting the group members to identify and
share common concerns about having cancer.

Of interest to pediatric oncologists and nurses.

1130. CAIN, Eileen N., Ernest I. Kohorn, Donald M. Quinlan, Kate
Latimer, Peter E. Schwartz. "Psychosocial benefits of a
cancer support group." *Cancer* 57 (1986): 183-189.

The long-term benefits of a thematic counseling model, used both as a
structure for group support and for counseling patients individually,
are compared.

Descriptive

The women who participated in thematic counseling were significantly
less depressed and less anxious and had more knowledge of their
illness, better relationships with caregivers, fewer sexual difficulties, and more participation in leisure activities. Data confirmed
the model to be equally helpful whether it was used as a structure for
individual counseling or more cost-effective group counseling. This
model is easily adaptable to the needs of persons with other forms of
cancer.

Of interest to oncologists and mental health professionals.

1131. CANTLEY, Caroline, and Gilbert Smith. "Social work and a
relatives' support group in a psychogeriatric day hospital--a
research note." *British Journal of Social Work* 13 (1983):
663-670.

Describes research on the way in which a relatives' group fulfills a
number of very useful functions in terms of providing a service to
relatives.

Research

The main categories of interaction observed and the functions of the
relatives' group are the exchange of information, individual consultation, resource allocation, negotiation, and therapy. The relatives'

group affects relationships between relatives and staff in the hospital and has a significant bearing upon the influence which relatives
are able to exercise over hospital services.

Of interest to social workers and health professionals in hospitals
caring for the elderly.

1132.   CHAMBERLAIN, Jeanette G., and Andrew G. Sparber.   "Can-
        cer: Are support groups meaningful in the workplace?"
        American Association of Occupational Health Nurses Journal
        34 (1986): 10-13.

Describes the establishment of a cancer support group at the National
Cancer Institute.

Descriptive

Three basic assumptions were made by the leaders in forming a cancer
support group: the establishment of a cancer support group in the
worksite would attract affected employees to the group; this constructed group model could be replicated in other worksites; and the
worksite would provide easier access to cancer support groups than the
community.

Of interest to oncologists.

1133.   DeBASIO, Nancy, and Nancy Rodenhausen.   "The group
        experience: Meeting the psychological needs of patients with
        ventricular tachycardia."   *Heart and Lung*   13 (1984): 597-
        602.

Description of the formation of a support group for patients with
ventricular tachycardia.

Descriptive

The group experience provides a forum where clients can share their
problems, fears, concerns, and questions with their peers.   The
presence of knowledgeable staff serves to correct misconceptions, when
appropriate, and to facilitate the group process.   The principles of
group therapy underlie group activities, which have resulted in mutual
client support, camaraderie, and the meeting of social needs.   Mutual
support has been extended to spouses who share similar concerns.

Of interest to nurses and other health professionals caring for
cardiology patients.

1134.   DROGE, David, Paul Arntson, Robert Norton.   "The social
        support function in epilepsy self-help groups."   *Small Group
        Behavior*   17 (1986): 139-163.

Results of a preliminary survey of epilepsy self-help group members
are presented.

Descriptive

Effects relating to stigmatization, reasons for participation, asserted curative factors, and formal versus informal participation in the group process are examined. Societal reaction to people with epilepsy is viewed as a major contributor to problems associated with this disability.

Of interest to social workers, mental health professionals, family physicians, nurses, and social and behavioral scientists.

1135. ELLIS, Peter. "Relative support groups." *Journal of the Royal College of General Practitioners* 36 (1986): 51.

Groups providing support for relatives of the elderly are useful and their formation is to be encouraged.

Commentary

Relative support groups are one example of community health initiatives which include self-help groups, community health groups, or community development health projects. The inclusion of professional workers within relative support groups, which would otherwise be self-help groups, helps break the traditional barrier between the expert professional view and the patient or caring relative.

Of interest to health care professionals.

1136. FLEXNER, Carol, Denise Wray, Thomas Black. "Support groups for moderately hearing-impaired college students: An expanding awareness." *The Volta Review* 88 (1986): 223-229.

Describes the development of the Support-Information Group for Hard-of-Hearing College Students at the University of Akron.

Descriptive

An information-support group was designed by clinical supervisors at the University of Akron to meet the needs of congenitally, moderately hearing-impaired college students, which often go unrecognized and/or unserviced. This article discusses the development of the group, profiles the needs of moderately hearing-impaired students, and discusses group intervention strategies.

Of interest to otolaryngologists, audiologists, speech pathologists, and social and behavioral scientists.

1137. FRIEDLANDER, Stephen R., and C. Edward Watkins, Jr. "Therapeutic aspects of support groups for parents of the mentally retarded." *International Journal of Group Psychotherapy* 35 (1985): 65-78.

Two support groups developed to assist parents in adjusting to their retarded children are described.

Descriptive

Prospective group members were not persons who were seeking psychotherapy; had taken no initiative in searching for formal, professional
help for problems in adaptive living; and had expressed no desire, at
the onset, for engaging in an intense group experience. On the other
hand, they were hurt, confused, and largely isolated from sources of
help. The group experience, designated by the term support group
rather than group therapy, constituted a successful approach for
giving parents the opportunity to meet with others with similar
problems and give mutual support.

Of interest to mental health professionals, social workers, and
professionals working with the mentally retarded.

1138.   FRIEND, Ronald, Yvonne Singletary, Nancy R. Mendell,
        Hazeline Nurse. "Group participation and survival among
        patients with end-stage renal disease." *American Journal of
        Public Health* 76 (1986): 670-672.

All 126 end-stage renal disease patients who entered dialysis between
1971 and 1981 at the Harlem Hospital Center, New York City, were
separated into those who had participated in a patient support group
and those who had not done so.

Research

Patients who engaged in group activities survived considerably longer
than nonparticipants. When 13 psychosocial and physiological
covariates were controlled for, the group participation effect
remained substantial.

Of interest to personnel working with dialysis patients.

1139.   GLOSSER, Guila, and Debra Wexler. "Participants' evaluations
        of educational/support groups for families of patients with
        Alzheimer's disease and other dementias." *Gerontologist* 25
        (1985): 232-236.

Describes an evaluation of educational/support groups for families of
patients with Alzheimer's Disease and other dementias.

Research

Shows educational/support groups generally to be effective in resolving intrafamilial conflicts and providing helpful information on
coping with legal, financial, and social problems of elders suffering
dementia.

Of interest to health professionals who work with the families of
Alzheimer's patients.

1140. GOETZEL, Ronnie Z., Lila G. Croen, Steven Shelov, Jo. I.
Boufford, Gilbert Levin. "Evaluating self-help support
groups for medical students." *Journal of Medical Education*
59 (1984): 331-340.

Support groups were evaluated by 26 medical students who completed a
nine-part questionnaire.

Research

Respondents indicated that they were primarily drawn to support groups
because of a desire for social affiliation and an opportunity to
express their feelings in a "safe" environment. Members shared in the
leadership responsibilities of the group and dealt with external
personal problems of the students rather than with the internal group
dynamics. The gains from participation in these groups included
opportunities for having nonprofessional contact with faculty members,
getting help and support from fellow students, and participating in
stimulating discussions about the medical field.

Of interest to medical students, medical educators, and spouses of
medical students and housestaff.

1141. GUSSOW, V., and G.S. Tracy. "The role of self-help clubs
in adaptation to chronic illness and disability." *Social
Science and Medicine* 10 (1976): 407-414.

Discusses the establishment, growth, services, and programs of self-
help health groups and their relationship with the medical
institution.

Research

Emphasizes that self-help organizations are not social clubs. Few
structures can rival the self-help concept in providing services for
people with long-term adaptive problems when continuing support is
necessary to prevent backsliding.

Should be of interest to all health professionals.

1142. HEPBURN, Kenneth, and Mona Wasow. "Support groups for
family caregivers of dementia victims: Questions, directions,
and future research." *New Directions for Mental Health
Services* 29 (March 1986): 83-92.

Explores both the positive and negative effects of support groups for
the caregivers of Alzheimer's and other dementia victims.

Literature Review and Analysis

Investigates when groups are helpful, when harmful, and what makes the
difference; what different models of support groups accomplish; what
are their stated goals, and for whom. Examines four basic models
of support groups, and proposes three new models designed to meet

different needs of caregivers. Considers five areas of concern that
seldom appear in the literature: sexuality, preparation for the
caregiver's life after the death of the victim, permission for divorce, encouragement to give up care, and the right to death.

Should interest social scientists and public policymakers.

1143. KANAS, Nick. "Support groups for mental health staff and
       trainees." *International Journal of Group Psychotherapy*
       36 (1986): 279-296.

A review of support groups to help mental health staff and trainees
deal with job-related stress.

Literature Review

Three types of support groups are identified: system-oriented, long-
term member oriented, and short-term member-oriented. They are
descriptively and empirically compared and evaluated, and technical
issues regarding their clarity of goals, leadership, and system and
role orientation are discussed.

Should particularly interest mental health professionals.

1144. KATZ, Alfred H. "Self-help organizations and volunteer
       participation in social welfare." *Social Work* 15 (1970):
       51-60.

A theoretical analysis of the dynamics of self-help groups, with
special reference to the dimensions of volunteer participation.

Theoretical

Discusses self-help groups in health and welfare from the standpoint
of organizational or small-group theory, considers the motivations of
their members and their relationships with professionals and professional agencies from a social science viewpoint, and considers them as
a focus of and an opportunity for volunteer participation. An attempt
is made to relate self-help groups to some theoretical formulations in
social science and to place them within the structure of community
organization thinking in social welfare.

Should interest social workers, mental health professionals, and
social scientists.

1145. LEON, Ana M., Rosaleen Mazur, Elba Montalvo, Miriam
       Rodrieguez. "Self-help support groups for Hispanic
       mothers." *Child Welfare* 63 (1984): 261-268.

Hispanic families often confront problems raised by the conflicts
between Hispanic and Anglo cultural systems and values. One successful model for assisting Hispanic parents is a self-help group.

Descriptive

The self-help group serves to include the Hispanic mother as a meaningful participant in human services systems rather than a passive recipient of services.

Of interest to social workers and mental health professionals.

1146. LEVIN, Elaine L. "A support group for midlife students reentering college." *Journal of College Student Personnel* 27 (1986): 371-732.

Describes a group support program at Georgia State University designed to explore the interaction between academic stresses and adult developmental issues.

Descriptive

Adult students returning to college at midlife have concerns about adjustment to academic life, problems relating to younger faculty members and students, and feelings of isolation, all of which are compounded by issues of midlife transition. Participation in a support group helps individuals realistically explore resources and learn stress management techniques and other coping strategies. The group also serves as a forum for midlife issues.

Of interest to college educators, administrators, and counselors as well as adult students.

1147. LIPSON, Juliene G. "Cesarean support groups: Mutual help and education." *Women and Health* 6 (Fall/Winter 1981): 27-39.

This exploratory field study was based on participant observation in regular meetings over a two year period in one Cesarean group and six months in the other.

Research

The group constituted a support system that moderated the effect of a stressful event by encouraging participants to express their feelings and work through them, then to turn their energies to assuming maximum control over a subsequent birth through careful planning. This support system aids in primary prevention and psychological growth for its members.

Of particular interest to obstetricians, gynecologists, and nurses.

1148. LISOSKIE, Shelly. "Supporting each other." *Journal of the American Medical Women's Association* 40, no. 4 (1985): 107, 126.

A brief description of the problems and stresses facing women in medical school and their need to support each other.

Editorial

A description of the effectiveness of support groups for women in medicine.

Of interest to women in medicine and spouses of physicians.

1149. LOCK, Stephen. "Self-help groups: The fourth estate in medicine?" *British Medical Journal* 293 (1986): 1596-1600.

Discusses the role of self-help groups and their contribution to the "greater medical profession."

Review

A general review of the definition, history, and role of self-help groups is followed by a discussion of their advantages and disadvantages.

Of interest to health professionals.

1150. McGUIRE, John C., and Benjamin H. Gottlieb. "Social support groups among new parents: An experimental study in primary prevention." *Journal of Clinical Child Psychology* 8 (1979): 111-116.

Assesses the health-protective effects and social consequences arising from the creation of social support groups among new parents.

Research

Social intervention prompted couples to increase their use of informal resources in their own social networks, but did not alter levels of stress or well-being. Addresses the implications for future efforts to mobilize informal social support on behalf of persons undergoing potentially stressful life transitions.

Psychologists and health professionals dealing with human life change.

1151. McSKIMMING, Josie, Louise Gleeson, Merrianne Sinclair. "A pilot study of a support group for parents of children with eczema." *Australian Journal of Dermatology* 25 (1984): 8-11.

The parents of children with atopic dermatitis often require considerable encouragement and support to help them cope with this distressing and potentially disabling condition.

Descriptive

A supportive self-help group may have an important preventive function in the treatment of eczema, assisting parents to cope in a long-term and realistic way with the management of their child's condition.

Of interest to dermatologists and mental health professionals.

1152. MAIDA, Carl A.   "Social support and learning in preventive
      health care."   *Social Science and Medicine*   21 (1985):
      335-339.

Analyzes social learning processes in mutual support groups that were
developed to facilitate clients' understanding of cardiovascular
diseases and their responsibilities for health maintenance.

Research

Social support groups that professional and paraprofessional staff
organized in the clinic offered clients a model of coping which was
consonant with modern group theory and current research on stress
management.   The social support groups encouraged participants to
reformulate their personal roles and coping strategies through a model
of mutual aid.

Of interest to health professionals involved in direct patient care
and to health educators and researchers in preventive medicine and
public health.

1153. MEILMAN, Philip W.   "Meeting the mental health needs of
      medical students: The effects of a peer support program."
      Journal of College Student Personnel   27 (1986): 373-374.

The implementation of a formal peer support program at a midwestern
medical school, and the process by which it contributed to the creation of a campus mental health facility, is described.

Descriptive

Wiitten comments received from first year students indicated that the
program had a significant beneficial effect.   Almost one-fourth of the
first-year students signed up to be peer support group leaders the
following year.

Of interest to medical school administrators, especially those involved in student affairs.

1154. NEWMARK, Deborah A.   "Review of a support group for
      patients with AIDS."   *Topics in Clinical Nursing*   6 (July
      1984): 38-44.

A description of group meetings with 11 patients, some of whom had
AIDS.   The group was structured to include both inpatients and outpatients, with the intention of bringing together people with
different manifestations of the syndrome and at various stages of the
illness.

Descripture

Members shared a heightened sense of vulnerability and a focus on life and death issues. Benefits were the shared mutual feelings of being understood and comforted by others and the valuable contribution of helping others.

Of importance to health care professionals working with AIDS patients and their families.

1155. NOVACK, Marion, Georgina Bru, Maxine C. Davidoff. "Development of a support group for volunteers in a pediatric oncology setting." *Journal of the Association of Pediatric Oncology Nurses* 2, no. 3 (Summer 1985): 30-35.

Discusses the specific application of a support group approach, which helps volunteers in a pediatric oncology unit increase their effectiveness.

Descriptive

Describes a group program for volunteers and staff. Volunteers gain a better understanding of what the children are experiencing physically and emotionally, and develop better skills to cope with the problems and to support the children during traumatic times. The group meetings have had a positive effect on volunteers, staff, children, and families.

Of interest to pediatricians, pediatric nurses, and oncologists.

1156. PAYNE, Glenda M., and Barbara Harrison. "Reducing stress in renal patients and their families: A nurse managed patient support group." *Journal of Nephrology Nursing* 1 (1984): 138-140.

A description of a support group for renal patients and their families.

Descriptive

Describes a weekly patient and family group formed by the renal transplant nursing staff, and its effectiveness in reducing stress.

Of particular interest to nurses and other health professionals caring for renal transplant patients.

1157. ROBINSON, David. "Self-help groups." *British Journal of Hospital Medicine* 34 (1985): 109-111.

A discussion of the characteristics of self-help groups and their relevance to health professionals.

Theoretical

Self-help groups have become a familiar and much discussed feature of contemporary life, and health workers in many countries have come to realize the value of people with particular problems coming together to help each other to help themselves. Self-help offers most to people when it manages to combine mutual support for those who share a common problem with activities and projects that encourage personal development and enable people to influence the quality of their everyday lives.

Of interest to all health professionals and laymen.

1158. ROY, Philip F., and Helen Sumpter. "Group support for the recently bereaved." *Health and Social Work* 8 (1983): 230-232.

Describes a bereavement group that was designed to help the recently bereaved cope with their problems.

Descriptive

Four discussion themes are described: the issue of time, the emotional state of members, family problems, and the significance of social roles.

Of interest to hospice workers, social workers, and nurses.

1159. SHAPIRO, Robert M., Susan M. Possidente, Kathleen C. Plum, Anthony F. Lehman. "The evaluation of a support group for families of the chronic mentally ill." *Psychiatric Quarterly* 55 (1983): 236-241.

Describes the organization, format, and evaluation of a support group for families of the chronically mentally ill.

Research

Preliminary findings indicate that families participating in this program had a realistic understanding of mental illness and of their important role in support of the patient. Patients' social support networks increased as a result of the program.

Mental health workers, social workers, psychiatrists, and others intervening to effect improved mental health support groups should read this paper.

1160. SHEARN, Martin A., and Bruce H. Fireman. "Stress management and mutual support groups in rheumatoid arthritis." *American Journal of Medicine* 78 (1985): 771-775.

In an attempt to determine the effect of stress management and social support on mortality and psychologic health in rheumatoid arthritics, 105 patients were evaluated for depression, life satisfaction, functional disability, and indications of disease activity.

Research

Patients were randomly assigned to one of three groups: stress management, mutual support, or no intervention. Patients in the intervention groups showed greater improvement in joint tenderness, but did
not differ significantly from the patients in the control group in any
of the other outcome measures.

Of interest to family physicians, rheumatologists, and rehabilitation
specialists.

1161. SPIEGEL, David, Joan R. Bloom, Irvin Yalom. "Group support
for patients with metastatic cancer: A randomized prospective
outcome study." *Archives of General Psychiatry* 38 (May
1981): 527-533.

The effects of weekly supportive group meetings for women with metastatic carcinoma of the breast were systematically evaluated in a
one-year, randomized, prospective outcome study.

Research

Objective evidence that a supportive group intervention for patients
with metastatic cancer results in psychological benefit is provided,
and mechanisms underlying its effectiveness are explored.

Of interest to oncologists and other health professionals providing
services to cancer patients and their families.

1162. TAYLOR, Shelley E., Roberta L. Falke, Steven J. Shoptaw,
Rosemary R. Lichtman. "Social support, support groups,
and the cancer patient." *Journal of Consulting and Clinical
Psychology* 54 (1986): 608-615.

Surveys the literature on social support and cancer, and reports
results from an empirical investigation of the factors that lead
cancer patients to join social support groups.

Literature Review

Although most cancer patients report high levels of social support
following cancer, some patients experience isolated instances of
rejection or do not receive the type of support they want from family,
friends, and medical caregivers. This appears to be one impetus for
joining cancer support groups. In addition, cancer support group
attenders are more likely to be white, middle-class females, to report
having more problems, and to use social support resources of all kinds
than are nonattenders.

Of interest to oncologists, nurses, social workers, family physicians,
and mental health professionals.

1163. THAYER, Virginia B. "The use of a support group for
       borderline mothers of adolescents." *Social Work with
       Groups* 9, no. 2 (1986): 57-71.

Discusses the development of an open-ended long-term group for border-
line mothers of adolescents, and the merits of this modality.

Descriptive/Analytical

Gives a brief history of the group and presents the general background
and problems of its members. Includes a discussion of the leadership,
requirements, problems, and enabling strategies. Focuses primarily on
a discussion of how group process helped change the behaviors and
goals of the group's members and enabled them to separate from their
children.

Of particular interest to social workers and mental health
professionals.

1164. VATTANO, Anthony J. "Power to the people: Self-help
       groups." *Social Work* 17, no. 4 (1972): 7-16.

A discussion of the nature of the challenge presented to professional
practitioners by the increasing emergence of self-help groups and its
implications for professional practice.

Essay

Professional practice and education must adapt to change. A new
partnership with clients may give professionals the understanding they
need to design conceptual models of helping that go beyond the dimensions of problems and methodology.

Of particular interest to social workers and mental health
professionals.

1165. WASOW, Mona. "Support groups for family caregivers of
       patients with Alzheimer's disease." *Social Work* 31 (1986):
       93-97.

Discusses some assumptions, dilemmas, and questions that have arisen
in the literature and in personal experience in the area of Alzheimer's Disease.

Theoretical and Analytical

Suggestions are made for a variety of support group models, as caregivers have different needs and different ways of coping. The author
argues for flexible support for support groups and a variety of
models, giving caregivers a choice.

Of interest to social and behavioral scientists and providers of
patient care.

c. Chapter

1166. COBB, Sidney, and Jessie M. Jones. "Social support, support
       groups and marital relationships." *In* Steve Duck (Ed.).
       Personal Relationships 5: Repairing Personal Relationships.
       London: Academic Press, 1984.

Explores and clarifies a more formal scheme for the definition and
measurement of social support. The scheme is applied to the literature on marriage and related heterosexual relationships.

Theoretical

Social support groups ought not to be seen merely as preventive or
therapeutic. The most important function of a marital growth group is
to support and enhance the relationship, to foster fulfillment--
happiness--which is a great deal more than the absence of pain or
sorrow, just as health is more than the absence of disease. Some of
what we expect of social support rests on empirical evidence; some may
be only a project, an article of faith. It is the authors' belief
that if enough esteem and security support are available, and if
appraisal support can be provided pressure-free, many relationships
can be nurtured.

Of interest to teachers and researchers interested in social support.

3. TREATMENT AND THERAPY

a. Books

1167. BURNS, David D. *Intimate Connections.* New York: William
       Morrow, 1985.

Explains how to overcome loneliness by changing the patterns of
perception that create and perpetuate it.

Manual

The 14 chapters illustrate the application of cognitive behavior
therapy to loneliness, shyness, and sexual insecurity.

Of interest to laymen and to social and behavioral scientists.

1168. WERMAN, David S. *The Practice of Supportive Psycho-
       therapy.* New York: Raven Press, 1984.

A warm, nondoctrinaire treatment of the area of supportive
psychotherapy.

Book

Distinguishes the various schools of thought on psychotherapy and covers the stages of transition through the therapeutic encounter. Transference and counter transference are covered extensively from a social support framework.

Provides mental health clinicians with an excellent perspective on interviewing to provide enhanced social networks and resources for support.

b. Articles

1169. ADSETT, C. Alex, and John G. Bruhn. "Short-term group psychotherapy for post-myocardial infarction patients and their wives." *The Canadian Medical Association Journal* 99 (September 23, 1968): 577-584.

Description of a group therapy program for 10 male patients who were having difficulties in adjusting to a myocardial infarction.

Research

Patients and their wives appeared to achieve an improved psychosocial adaptation. The clinical follow-up was too brief to evaluate the long-term effect of group therapy.

Of interest to mental health professionals and physicians caring for coronary patients.

1170. DYCK, Ronald J., Anthony S. Joyce, Hassan F.A. Azim. "Treatment noncompliance as a function of therapist attributes and social support." *Canadian Journal of Psychiatry* 29 (1984): 212-216.

Premature termination of short-term psychotherapy was examined as a function of therapist and social support variables.

Research

Although few of the social support variables were related to the mode of treatment termination, continuers were found to be more likely than terminators to have discussed attendance at the clinic with others, especially family members.

Of particular interest to mental health professionals, especially psychiatrists, psychologists, and social workers.

1171. GOLDBERG, Richard J., and Margaret S. Wool. "Psychotherapy for the spouses of lung cancer patients: Assessment of an intervention." *Psychotherapy and Psychosomatics* 43 (1985): 141-150.

A randomized prospective clinical trial tested the effect of a professionally provided program of social support counselling on newly diagnosed lung cancer patients and their families.

Research

Over the six months of the intervention, there was no differential change by experimental status for either the patients or their principal support persons in outcome measures of emotional, social, or physical function.

Of interest to oncologists, social workers, and mental health professionals.

1172. HEAP, Kari Killen. "Families with abused children: A follow-up study of post-crisis support." *Child Abuse and Neglect* 8 (1984): 467-472.

Treatment provisions that had been planned and executed were studied in a follow-up of 14 abused or neglected children three years after discharge from the hospital.

Research

There is a need for combination of use of well qualified and experienced workers with extensive and creative use of voluntary and other network resources. This is important in order to break the isolation of these families and to prevent their having solely professional people for identification objects.

Of interest to social workers and mental health professionals.

1173. HILTZ, S. Roxanne. "Helping widows: Group discussions as a therapeutic technique." *Family Coordinator* 24 (1975): 331-336.

Examines the nature and difficulties involved in the group discussion technique as applied to widows.

Research

The group discussion can be an effective modality of treatment if the woman is able to relate to the other members and to the leader. A well trained discussion leader, who is able to deal effectively with the emotional problems of widowhood, is essential.

Of interest to mental health professionals and sociologists.

1174. LEVINSON, Boris M. "Nursing home pets. A psychological adventure for patients." (Part 1). *National Humane Review* 58, no. 4 (1970): 14-16.

A discussion of how nursing homes can provide for the need for companionship of older people.

Descriptive

The introduction of pets into nursing homes is part of a carefully planned and structured method of therapy for the aged. Pet programs for the total community are a subject of growing interest for humane agencies.

Of interest to gerontologists and nursing home administrators.

1175. MALOTT, James M., Russel E. Glasgow, H. Katherine O'Niell, Robert C. Klesges. "Co-worker social support in a worksite smoking control program." *Journal of Applied Behavioral Analysis* 17 (1984): 485-495.

Evaluates the addition of social support to a smoking control treatment program.

Research

One of two treatment groups received partner support in the program, which did not result in significant changes in smoking reduction or cessation rates.

Of interest to health behavior researchers and occupational health professionals.

1176. PATTISON, E. Mansell, Donald DeFrancisco, Paul Wood, Harold Frazier, John Crowder. "A psychosocial kinship model for family therapy." *American Journal of Psychiatry* 132 (1975): 1246-1251.

Presentation of a model of family therapy, based on family sociology that includes the total primary psychosocial system.

Theoretical

Argues for the extension of family therapy, which was originally limited to members of the nuclear family, to include individuals who play a significant role in the psychosocial environment of the patient. The concept of psychosocial kinship is introduced, and an inventory is described which measures this concept.

Useful for psychiatrists, especially those interested in family therapy.

1177. RIESMAN, Frank. "The 'helper' therapy principle." *Social Work* 10 (1965): 27-32.

Calls attention to the aid that helpers receive from being in the helper role.

Theoretical

In a wide variety of self-help "therapies," it appears that the people giving help are more certain to benefit from their role than are those receiving help. Conscious planning directed toward structuring self-help groups for the widest possible distribution of the helper role may be a decisive therapeutic intervention, a significant leadership training principle, and an important teaching device.

Of interest to social workers and mental health professionals.

1178. TATTERSALL, Robert B., David K. McCulloch, Mark Aveline. "Group therapy in the treatment of diabetes." *Diabetes Care* 8 (1985): 180–188.

Reviews the need for psychosocial support in the treatment of diabetes.

Literature Review

Group psychotherapy has been used in adjunctive treatment of numerous medical conditions. This review suggests its value in the care of patients with diabetes, although issues are not resolved regarding which patients benefit most, who should serve as group leader, and how to assess the efficacy of this approach.

Health professionals who care for diabetic patients will find this an interesting article.

1179. TELCH, Christy F., and Michael J. Telch. "Group coping skills instruction and supportive group therapy for cancer patients: A comparison of strategies." *Journal of Consulting and Clinical Psychology* 54 (1986): 802–808.

Compares the relative efficacy of comprehensive group coping skills training and supportive group therapy for enhancing cancer patients' adjustment to their disease.

Research

Forty-one cancer patients exhibiting a marked degree of psychosocial distress were randomly assigned to a group receiving group coping skills instruction, a group receiving supportive group therapy, or a no-treatment control group. Support group sessions were nondirective and emphasized mutual sharing of feelings and concerns. Coping skills training included instruction in relaxation and stress management, assertive communication, cognitive restructuring and problem solving, feelings management, and pleasant activity planning. Patients exposed to coping skills training achieved positive treatment gains in a number of different measures, whereas those receiving supportive group therapy showed little improvement in psychological distress and those in the no-treatment control group evidenced significant deterioration in psychological adjustment.

Of interest to social scientists and mental health professionals.

d. Dissertations

1180. EAGLESTON, Jean R. "Measuring and altering social support
       in chronically stressed women."   Ph.D. dissertation,
       Stanford University, 1982.

A methodological study of the construct of social support, conceptualized within a framework of cognitive social learning theory,
and an intervention study to alter social support in a sample of 15
chronically stressed women with sleeping problems and low social
support.

Research

Using a multitrait-multimethod matrix, confirmatory evidence was
provided for the construct validation. The group receiving treatment
to increase their social support showed changes in the desired direction in most of the social variables of interest, and did better than
two control groups.

Of particular interest to scientists concerned with measurement
problems regarding constructs used in social stress research.

1181. ROBERTS, Nancy Ellen. "The effects of a control and social
       support intervention on nursing home residents." Ph.D.
       dissertation, Rutgers University, The State University of
       New Jersey, 1983.

An intervention study providing nursing home residents with more
information and social support and improving their mental and physical
health.

Research

The results indicated that treated residents improved their self-
reported mental and physical health, had greater levels of positive
effect, and shorter lengths of stay than nontreated subjects. Some
differences were found in the quality of social supports utilized by
the two groups.

Should particularly interest mental health care professionals and
gerontologists.

A. SOCIAL NETWORK THERAPY

a. Books

1182. BIEGEL, Donald E., Barbara K. Shore, Elizabeth Gordon.
       *Building Support Networks for the Elderly: Theory and
       Applications*. Beverly Hills: Sage, 1984.

Attempts to stimulate an appreciation for the need to develop and strengthen informal supports for the elderly and to develop innovative informal support strategies.

Resource Book

Gives background information about social networks; definitions, roles, and functions of support systems; and existing knowledge about social support and the elderly. Provides materials and tools for assessing strengths and weaknesses of networks of individuals and communities, and discusses strategies for evaluating intervention programs. Presents a typology of social network interventions with the elderly, and thoroughly discusses each of the specific modalities in the typology, citing examples of projects utilizing each interventive modality and discussing professional roles and implementation issues.

Intended for practitioners in the human services.

1183.   CAPLAN, Gerald, and Marie Killilea (Eds.).   *Support Systems and Mutual Help*. New York: Grune & Stratton, 1976.

An exploration of the mutual-help aspect of support systems.

Book of Readings

Deals with the concepts of support systems and mutual help; empirical studies of the operation of natural societal or organizational support systems that involve mutual help; and recent attempts to make use of support system concepts in organizing helpful intervention programs.

Of particular interest to community mental health workers as well as social scientists.

1184.   GARBARINO, James, S. Holly Stocking, and Associates.   *Protecting Children from Abuse and Neglect: Developing and Maintaining Effective Support Systems for Families*.   San Francisco: Jossey-Bass, 1980.

Based on the view that child abuse and neglect are problems not only of individuals, but also of environments.

Book of Readings

The contributors to this volume come from a variety of perspectives, and differ in the vocabularies they use to describe personal social networks. They sometimes suggest different strategies for creating and supporting social networks, but, together, they provide the rationale for a social network approach to combating child maltreatment and highlight many of the issues that practitioners and policymakers must face in adopting this approach.

Of interest to social and behavioral scientists and health professionals, especially practitioners.

1185. PANCOAST, Diane L., Paul Parker, Charles Froland (Eds.).
        Rediscovering Self-Help: Its Role in Social Care.   Beverly
        Hills: Sage, 1983.

Attempts to explore the area of overlap between informal, private
caring relationships arising out of family, community, and other
social ties and professional, governmentally financed services.

Book of Readings

Illustrates ways in which professional caregivers can exploit natural
support networks. Divided into three sections: initiatives in informal care, professional relationships with self-help groups, and
prospects for policy.

Of interest to social workers, mental health professionals, and social
and behavioral scientists.

1186. RUEVINI, Uri.   *Networking Families in Crisis.*   New York:
        Human Services Press, 1979.

The processes and techniques of helping families in crisis to assemble
and mobilize the extended social network. The material is based on
personal clinical experiences in efforts to help families in emotional
crises reconnect with their family, friends, and others in the social
support system.

Research

The nine chapters in this book include: the network intervention
process, network intervention with difficult family crises, issues in
family networks, training the network interventionist, family networking intervention techniques, adaptation and application of the
networking process.

Of interest to individuals in the field of crisis intervention.

b. Articles

1187. ALCALAY, Rina.   "Health and social support networks--a case
        for improving interpersonal communication." *Social Networks*
        5 (1983): 71-88.

An analysis of research findings documenting the hypothesis that
people need one another and that interruption or modification of
social ties often affects health and well-being.

Research and Analysis

Discusses ways in which social support networks contribute to health,
and societal characteristics that inhibit the development of such
networks.   Suggests approaches that emphasize the importance of
networks.

Should interest social scientists.

1188.   CHRISTEN, Arden G.   "Developing a social support network
        system to enhance mental and physical health."   *Dental
        Clinics of North America*   30, no. 4 Supplement (October
        1986): S79-S92.

Explores the dynamics of a social support system, stressing that the
giving and receiving of social support are skills that can be learned.

Review

Provides an in-depth review of social support, explains the dynamics
and importance of a viable social network system, and discusses its
limitations. Special consideration is given to the social isolation
of dentists, social support provided by one's spouse, some social
aspects of women dentists, the individual's need for privacy, and
personal space and loneliness.

Of particular interest to dentists.

1189.   GOTTLIEB, Benjamin H.   "The contribution of natural support
        systems to primary prevention among four social subgroups
        of adolescent males."   *Adolescence*   10 (1975): 207-220.

Natural support systems in the community, which aid the coping efforts
of adolescents, are examined.

Research

Mental health professionals must re-examine their assumption that
community gatekeepers are in need of further education through consultation in mental health helping skills. A closer collaboration
between professional and lay helper would benefit the professional.

Of interest to mental health professionals.

1190.   JASON, Leonard A., Max Abbott, James Dalton et al.   "Facili-
        tating social support among community psychologists."
        Journal of Community Psychology   13 (1985): 83-89.

Describes key organizing principles for creating viable social support
networks, using one created by a group of community psychologists as a
model.

Review

The principles leading to this professional support network include
active involvement with members, definition of success, resource
exchange, political sensitivity, and fostering the emergence of
alternative support systems. Benefits to the community psychologists
were better social support, more educational opportunities, and
resource exchange.

Community psychologists and others interested in developing professional social support resources will benefit from this paper.

1191. SPECK, Ross V. "Psychotherapy of the social network of a schizophrenic family." *Family Process* 6 (1967): 208-214.

An initial report on the validity of psychotherapy of the extended social network of a schizophrenic person and his family.

Theoretical

The purpose of therapy for members of the social network of the schizophrenic family is discussed. Therapy sessions are attended by the nuclear family of a schizophrenic person, as well as by relatives and friends. The therapy attempts to modify the human environment of the schizophrenic person by changing the relationships between individuals in his immediate social network.

Particularly useful for psychiatrists.

1192. ————, and Uri Rueveni. "Network therapy--a developing concept." *Family Process* 8 (1969): 182-190.

Discusses the rationale and the procedure of network therapy of the social network of the schizophrenic person and his family, kin, neighbors, and friends.

Theoretical

An outline of a network therapy is given, which included a variety of sensitivity training techniques. The therapy is supposed to be successful in modifying the relationships in the schizophrenic's family, in improving their social network, and in providing a viable social structure for continuing positive effects like employment and avoidance of hospitalizations.

Primarily helpful for psychiatrists treating schizophrenics and their social environment.

1193. TRIMBLE, David W., and Jodie Kliman. "Community network therapy: Strengthening the networks of chronic patients." *International Journal of Family Psychiatry* 2 (1981): 269-289.

A description of the authors' use of community network therapy in a chronic psychiatric patient population.

Description

Social network therapy techniques were adapted to the needs and circumstances of chronic patients in a community over a three year period. This experience demonstrated that the network therapy approach was compatible with the networking approach of the case

manager of the NIMH community support program.   Integration of these
two practical applications of the concept of social networks provides
a wide range of strategies for addressing the multiple and complex
problems of deinstitutionalization.

Of special interest to mental health professionals.

1194. WELLS, Lilian M., and Carolyn Singer.   "A model for linking
        networks in social work practice with the institutionalized
        elderly."   *Social Work*   30 (July/August 1985): 318-322.

Describes a demonstration project established by social work students
and faculty in long-term care facilities in Toronto.

Research

Results emphasize the importance of developing and maintaining social
supports and the reciprocal benefits in linking kinship, friendship,
formal caregiving, and mutual-aid networks.   Six key processes used in
the project are provided, illustrating the efficacy of the network
approach.

Of interest to social workers and mental health professionals.

c. Chapters

1195.   BRAMMER, Lawrence M.   "Nonformal support in cross-cultural
        counseling and therapy."   *In* Paul Pederson (Ed.).   *Hand-
        book of Cross-Cultural Counseling and Therapy.*   Westport,
        CT: Greenwood Press, 1985.

Reviews nonformal support from a cross-cultural perspective, and
discusses its role in counseling and therapy.

Review

Reviews three basic forms of nonformal support--family and friends,
community self-help programs, and occupational networks--giving
examples to show how each functions in the context of nonformal
counseling in different cultural settings.   Reviews traditional
assumptions about the universal benefits of social support and discusses some evidence to the contrary.   Presents methods for teaching
nonformal support networking skills, and discusses future directions
for cross-cultural support research.

Should interest social scientists and mental health professionals.

1196. EGAR, Ruth, Wendy Sarkissian, Dorothy Brady, Leslie Hartmann. "Reviewing the Australian suburban dream: A unique approach to neighborhood change with the family support scheme." *In* Marilyn Safir, Martha T. Mednick, Dafne Israeli, Jessie Bernard (Eds.). *Women's Worlds*. New York: Praeger, 1985.

Examines the Family Support Scheme, an innovative, federally funded neighborhood development program in an isolated suburb of Adelaide, Australia.

Descriptive

The scheme described in this chapter provides the link between suburban women—who are often isolated—and the wider community. It encourages more extensive use of services and facilities and promotes self-help initiatives whereby social development can begin.

Of interest to community planners and social and behavioral scientists.

1197. PEARSON, Richard E. "The recognition and use of natural support systems in cross-cultural counseling." *In* Paul Pederson (Ed.). *Handbook of Cross-Cultural Counseling and Therapy*. Westport, CT: Greenwood Press, 1985.

Concerned with the necessity for counselors, working with clients from cultural groups that differ from their own, to recognize and appreciate the contributions and styles of operation of their clients' natural support systems and take advantage of the possibilities for furthering their clients' growth by reinforcing, strengthening, or collaborating with those systems.

Theoretical

Considers the types of social support that are appropriate for particular life issues, the varying actions through which social support is delivered, the sources from which particular individuals normally receive support for specific concerns, and how counselors can strengthen and cooperate with the natural support systems of clients.

Useful to counselors and other mental health professionals.

4. HEALTH EDUCATION AND BEHAVIOR MODIFICATION

a. Articles

1198. BARANOWSKI, Thomas, Philip R. Nader, Kay Dunn, Nathalie A. Vanderpool. "Family self-help: Promoting changes in health behavior." *Journal of Communication* (Summer 1982): 161-172.

Reviews research on the relationship between health and family communication and support systems, and reports on a pilot project that attempted to influence this relationship.

Research

Documents the very low frequency of naturally occurring social support behaviors. A family-based intervention can influence patterns of social support for dietary and exercise change, promote more emotional than informational or material support, and seems to be more effective in influencing dietary than exercise support.

Useful to social and behavioral scientists, pediatricians, and family physicians.

1199. INTAGLIATA, James, and Nancy Doyle. "Enhancing social support for parents of developmentally disabled children: Training in interpersonal problem solving skills." *Mental Retardation* 22 (February 1984): 4-11.

A description of the rationale for and implementation of Interpersonal Problem-Solving Skills Training with parents of developmentally disturbed children.

Description

A training program for enhancing parents' support networks by improving their interpersonal problem-solving skills is described. The program seemed to be effective and provided a needed supplement to the package of helpful services available to parents of the developmentally disabled.

Of interest to child care workers and others working with developmentally disabled children.

1200. KING, Abby C., and Lee W. Frederickson. "Low-cost strategies for increasing exercise behavior--relapse preparation training and social support." *Behavior Modification* 8 (1984): 3-21.

An investigation of the frequency of participant-controlled exercise episodes that occurred outside the context of any formal, ongoing program. Two procedures were studied--social support and relapse preparation.

Research

Results showed that relapse preparation training, alone, and social support, alone, resulted in the initiation of nearly twice as many jogging episodes as were initiated in the controlled condition.

Of interest to rehabilitation, physical fitness, and sports medicine specialists.

1201. MINKLER, Meredith. "Applications of social support theory to health education: Implications for work with the elderly." *Health Education Quarterly* 8 (1981): 147-165.

Three major hypotheses are presented concerning the precise mechanism of action through which social support may work to maintain health and decrease susceptibility to illness.

Descriptive

The particular relevance of social support theory for work with the elderly is discussed. The concept of social marginality, and such network properties as strength of ties, reciprocity, and network size are examined in light of their implications for the design of programs aimed, in part, at fostering social support among the elderly. Several examples of innovative health education programs are used to illustrate the relevance of different theoretical principles in practice settings.

Of interest to social and behavioral scientists and health educators.

1202. MORISKY, Donald E., Nancy M. DeMuth, Marion Field-Fass, Lawrence W. Green, David M. Levine. "Evaluation of family health education to build social support for long-term control of high blood pressure." *Health Education Quarterly* 12 (Spring 1985): 35-50.

An educational program was designed to improve family support for compliance to medical regimens by hypertensive patients.

Research

Reoults showed a strong statistically significant difference between the experimental and control groups, with the experimental group demonstrating higher levels of appointment-keeping behavior, weight control, and controlled blood pressure. Analysis of the main effects of the educational program demonstrated that family support intervention accounted for the greatest decrease in the variability of diastolic blood pressure.

Of interest to internists, other health professionals caring for hypertensive patients, and health educators.

b. Chapter

1203. SIMPSON, Miles E. "Societal support and education." *In* I.L. Kutash, L.B. Schlesinger, and Associates (Eds.). *Handbook on Stress and Anxiety.* San Francisco: Jossey-Bass, 1980.

Outlines societal sources of stress and anxiety so that interventions can be more successful.

Review

More effective prevention efforts are emphasized through educational activities aimed at improving coping skills.

Of interest to social and behavioral scientists, educators, and community interventionists.

c. Dissertations

1204. KENNETH, Hester Young. "The benefits, costs, and sources of social support associated with establishing and maintaining physical activity among employed adults." D.N.S. dissertation, University of California, San Francisco, 1984.

Explores the process by which employed adults establish and maintain leisure time physical activity.

Research

The results indicate that peer social support, in particular, is important for adherence to a physical activity program, whereas total costs have a significant negative influence on adherence. The study concludes that specific social support functions and sources may be important for adherence to programs.

Of particular interest to health educators.

1205. RODGERS, Mary P. "The effect of social support on the modification of smoking behavior." Ph.D. dissertation, University of Michigan, 1977.

Explored the effects of varying degrees of social support on the termination of smoking behavior.

Research

The group support condition demonstrated significantly higher percent reduction over the total support group at certain time periods, but did not significantly differ on final rates. Group support had an immediate impact on quit rates with a significantly larger number of subjects quitting after treatment and maintaining abstinence as long as support continued. Upon termination of support, this group returned to approximately the same quit rates as participants in the other two groups.

Of interest to health educators, health professionals, and program interventionists.

5. SOCIAL SUPPORT SERVICES, PROGRAMS, AND PROJECTS

a. Articles

1206. ABRAHAMS, Ruby Banks. "Mutual help for the widowed." *Social Work* 17, no. 5 (September 1972): 54-61.

Describes a telephone mutual help program in Boston.

Case Report

Describes the characteristics of the users of this telephone reassurance service, identifies the problems they report at different stages of widowhood, and documents the value of the service in helping address loneliness and isolation.

Social workers and others interested in self-help, and facilitators of mutual help programs will benefit from this paper.

1207. BARNARD, Kathryn E., Charlene Snyder, Anita Spietz. "Supportive measures for high-risk infants and families." *Birth Defects* 20, no. 5 (1984): 205-244.

The experience of providing a three-month nursing program of care to infants and their families with physical, health, and social-environmental risks is presented.

Research

Differences emerged in the mothers' involvement in the exploration phase, which involves goal setting. Families with incomplete progression through the helping process not only participated in less mutual decision-making, but were also less open to the initial assessment phase and had higher social risk. The nurses had less total contact with the uninvolved families.

Of particular interest to nurses.

1208. BARSH, Elizabeth T., Judith A. Moore, Leo A. Hemerlynck. "The foster extended family: A support network for handicapped foster children." *Child Welfare* 62 (1983): 349-359.

A program is designed to support the placement of handicapped children using a service model that eases family isolation.

Description

Foster families benefited from increased home programming and increased attention from additional adults. Extended family members experienced a new, worthwhile, and effective role. In fact, the bonds created among them were maintained, even as the program ended. More important, foster families have experienced the rewards of a family network and are better equipped to handle future problems and needs through developing and utilizing their own extended families.

Of interest to social workers and child welfare workers.

1209. BENNETT, Ruth.   "Social isolation and isolation-reducing programs." *Bulletin of the New York Academy of Medicine* 49 (1973): 1143-1163.

Explores the factors associated with social isolation among the elderly, and describes several model programs which are effective in reducing loneliness.

Literature Review

Evidence is provided linking role loss, social isolation, and social-ization within nursing home and long-term care facilities, as well as independent live alone situations. Mental and physical health status are shown to be affected by support programs aimed at reducing isolation. Case histories and vignettes are used effectually to illustrate approaches.

Those working with similar programs, especially for the elderly, should benefit from this article.

1210. BERNARD, Miriam.   "Voluntary care for the elderly mentally infirm and their relatives: A British example." *Gerontologist* 24 (1984): 116-119.

Describes the Potteries Elderly Support Group, an organization in Stoke-on-Trent, which aims to provide support to families caring for an elderly, mentally infirm relative.

Descriptive

The Potteries Elderly Support Group is staffed and supervised by a qualified psychiatric social worker and uses trained volunteers to offer day care, sit with relatives at home, provide support, and offer some relief to relatives before the stress of caring becomes impossible to bear. The organization's rationale, financing, staffing, and activities are discussed in detail.

Should interest health care planners and providers, as well as lay persons concerned with care of the elderly.

1211. BUCKLEY, Susan.   "Parent aides provide support to high risk families." *Children Today* 14, no. 5 (1985): 16-19.

Describes the Parent Aid Support Service (PASS), a project of the Nebraska Department of Social Services in Lincoln.

Descriptive

PASS volunteers offer nurturance, acceptance, and support to families under stress that are at high risk of child abuse or neglect. The project aims at reducing families' social isolation, improving parenting and interpersonal skills, enhancing parents' self-esteem, increasing their ability to solve day-to-day crises, and otherwise lessening the problems associated with child abuse and neglect. Aides are carefully matched with families, supervisors are always available to provide assistance and encouragement, and support groups for aides meet regularly.

Should interest social workers, social service administrators and planners, and lay persons interested in volunteer services.

1212. CARR, Donna, and Samuel F. Knupp. "Grief and perinatal loss. A community hospital approach to support." *Journal of Obstetrics, Gynecology, and Neonatal Nursing* 14 (1985): 130-139.

A hospital team developed a written protocol with support measures to use when a stillbirth occurs.

Descriptive

The protocol has been used for three years and the staff has seen dual benefits. Staff members find constructive ways of offering support, and parents derive a sense of comfort and direction from the approach.

Of interest to obstetrical nurses.

1213. CASTELLANI, Paul J., Nancy A. Downey, Mark B. Tausig, William A. Bird. "Availability and accessibility of family support services." *Mental Retardation* 24, no. 2 (1986): 71-79.

Results of a study of nine family support services delivered by a sample of 133 public and private agencies in New York State are reported.

Research

Problems of service identification and definition and variations in the location, type, auspice, size, and structure of service agencies are shown to affect the availability and accessibility of family support services state-wide. The provision of family support services as groups of services is shown, and the impact of a lack of separate budgeting and existing eligibility criteria for these services, described. Implications for design and implementation of family support service programs is discussed.

Of interest to social workers, public health professionals, and family physicians.

1214. CHANEY, Richard W., Ronald N. Bennett, R. James Kellogg, Rue Morrison, John Ognibene, V.J. Shorty. "AIDS: Community concerns, support services and resources." *Journal of the Louisiana State Medical Society* 137, no. 9 (1985): 62-63.

A description of what volunteer and community organizations in New Orleans and in Louisiana are doing to assist in the AIDS crisis.

Descriptive

Volunteers from the New Orleans AIDS Task Force offer emotional, human, and financial support to persons with AIDS. Along with clerical groups, social service groups provide counseling and care. Legal assistance is available through the Legal Defense Fund. The Louisiana Medical program assists with medical expenses.

Of interest to AIDS workers, health professionals, and the lay public.

1215. CUTLER, David L., Joseph D. Bloom, James H. Shore. "Training psychiatrists to work with community support systems for chronically mentally ill persons." *American Journal of Psychiatry* 138 (January 1981): 98-101.

Presents a training design that integrates the principles and skills associated with this model into a four year residency training program.

Descriptive

While many trainees may not be involved, throughout their career, with the everyday aspects of working in the natural environment of chronically ill patients, it is important for them to be exposed to community support system training.

Of interest to psychiatrists, especially those on medical school faculties.

1216. DOUGLAS, Jeanne A., and Leonard A. Jason. "Building social support systems through a babysitting exchange program." *American Journal of Orthopsychiatry* 56 (1986): 103-108.

The process of developing a babysitting exchange program is described.

Descriptive

There was a steady increase in use of the exchange as women formed small groups and compatible pairs. About half the participants indicated that they found the exchange useful and would continue to use it. Participation was not found to have a differential impact on high-stressed and low-stressed mothers. Implications for the development and evaluation of social support networks are discussed.

Of interest to mental health professionals and laypersons.

1217. ELLIS, June B. "Love to Share: A community project tailored
       by oldsters for "latch-key" children." *American Journal of
       Orthopsychiatry* 42 (1972): 249-250.

Describes the Love to Share Project, a program in which elderly
persons (aged 55 to 82) care for elementary school children with
working parents between the time school lets out and their parents
come home.

Descriptive

"Love to Share" Centers, situated in areas with a high incidence of
working mothers, are staffed by 44 oldsters who feed and care for 100
latch-key children until their parents return home from work. The
project is suitable for large scale application to counteract despon-
dency and feelings of uselessness in old people and withdrawing
behavior in children and to foster healthy emotional behavior.

Should interest social workers and mental health professionals.

1218. FELNER, Robert D., Melanie Ginter, Judith Primavera. "Pri-
       mary prevention during school transitions: Social support
       and environmental structure." *American Journal of Com-
       munity Psychology* 10 (1982): 277-290.

A primary prevention project to facilitate students' coping during the
transition to high school. The project sought to increase the level
of available social support as well as to reduce the degree of flux
and complexity in the school setting.

Research

Participants showed significantly better attendance records and grade
point averages, as well as more stable self-concepts, than controls.
By the final evaluation point, project students also reported perceiving the school environment as having greater clarity of expectations
and organizational structure and higher levels of teacher support and
involvement than did the nonproject controls.

Of interest to school teachers, administrators, and counselors.

1219. GRAHAM, R. Scott. "Employee support systems in a
       psychosocial rehabilitation setting." *Psychosocial Rehabilita-
       tion Journal* 6 (1982): 12-19.

Explains how employee support systems were developed in a psychosocial
rehabilitation setting to maintain positive employee attitudes and a
high level of quality in the provision of services to the chronically
mentally ill.

Descriptive

Two objective measures--a satisfaction survey of staff members and low
employee turnover--indicate the success of employee support systems.

Of interest to management and personnel officers in rehabilitation institutions and to social and behavioral scientists.

1220. GUERNEY, Louise, and Leila Moore. "Phonefriend: A prevention-oriented service for latchkey children." *Children Today* 12, no. 4 (1983): 5-10.

A description of a prevention-oriented community service for latch-key children.

Descriptive

An evaluation of the service found that it was used by both parents and children and that it was an effective way of providing emotional and instrumental support to children alone after school.

Of general interest to lay public and social service professionals.

1221. HERSEY, James C., Leonard S. Klibanoff, David J. Lam, Robert L. Taylor. "Promoting social support: The impact of California's 'Friends Can be Good Medicine' campaign." *Health Education Quarterly* 11 (1984): 293-311.

Reports on the effectiveness of a community intervention aimed at promoting social support.

Research

When comparisons were made of exposed unexposed residents of the Fresno metromedia market area, the campaign appeared to have had an impact on knowledge, attitudes, intentions, and support enhancing behavior. The campaign was most effective when it utilized multiple channels of communications and with residents who had experienced the death of someone close to them during the past year, especially those with below average social support.

This is an important work and should be read by social support researchers.

1222. HUTCHISON, William J., Priscilla Searight, John J. Stretch. "Multidimensional networking: A response to the needs of homeless families." *Social Work* 31 (1986): 427-430.

A six-year study of homeless families who received treatment at the Salvation Army Emergency Lodge in St. Louis, Missouri was carried out to determine how human service agencies can respond to the problem of homelessness.

Research

Professionals assisted families or individuals by facilitating linkages to their natural support systems and to other professional services or agencies in the community. Findings of the study clearly show that partnerships among agencies are required to meet the multiple needs of the homeless. Government, corporate, and voluntary sectors must work together to share this responsibility. A four-stage model of treatment is presented and discussed.

Of interest to social workers, other social services professionals, and social policy planners.

1223.   JENSON, Jeffrey M., J. David Hawkins, Richard F. Catalano. "Social support in aftercare services for troubled youth." *Children and Youth Services Review*   8 (1986): 323-347.

Evaluates programs in which social support strategies are used to facilitate the community adaptation of troubled adolescents.

Review

The development of supportive relationships and prosocial networks in a youth's community, school, and workplace and among parents and family members is important to success in community reentry for the institutionalized adolescent. Research is outlined to advance the development and application of aftercare interventions for youths returning to the community from residential or institutional treatment facilities.

Particularly useful to mental health researchers interested in disturbed adolescents.

1224.   KENKEL, Mary Beth. "Stress-coping-support in rural communities: A model for primary prevention." *American Journal of Community Psychology*   14 (1986): 457-478.

Discusses rural stressors, coping strategies, and support systems, and describes prevention programs directed toward each of these areas.

Theoretical

A stress-coping-support framework, which delineates the aspects of community life that must be assessed and outlines several different intervention goals, is proposed as a guide for developing community programs. The model generally proposes that prevention activities should reduce stress, increase coping, and build support. While it can be applied to any target group, in this article the framework is elaborated to address the unique physical, occupational, and societal characteristics of rural communities.

Of interest to planners and providers of mental health services, particularly in rural communities.

1225. KIRKHAM, Maura A., Robert F. Schilling, II, Kristine
Norelius, Steven Paul Schinke. "Developing coping styles
and social support networks: An intervention outcome study
with mothers of handicapped children." *Child Care, Health
and Development* 12 (1986): 313-324.

Describes an intervention program, evaluation procedures, and results
from a study of skills training for reducing stress with parents of
handicapped children.

Descriptive/Research

Four mothers of developmentally disabled children participated in an
eight-week pilot training program designed to teach parents ways to
enhance their coping skills, increase their social support networks,
and collectively make changes in their environment. Post-test data
indicate that the program shows promise for teaching coping and social
support enhancement skills to parents. Studies of larger samples and
more sophisticated designs are needed to further test preventive
interventions for families of developmentally disabled children.

Of interest to social workers and mental health professionals.

1226. LEVINE, Irene Shifren, Anne D. Lezak, Howard H. Goldman.
"Community support systems for the homeless mentally ill."
New Directions in Mental Health Services 30 (June 1986):
27-42.

Suggests how the framework of the federal Community Support Program
for the chronically mentally ill can be adapted to assure comprehensive care for the homeless among them.

Analytical

The homeless and seriously mentally ill are among the most vulnerable
and disenfranchised clients of the health care system. The approach
of the Community Support Program, which provides grants to state
mental health agencies for the development of community support
systems, assumes that the needs of this population extend beyond
mental health treatment to include a broad number and range of social
supports. With some modification, community support systems can
provide a useful planning tool for creating necessary services and
opportunities for homeless mentally ill persons, but before they can
be implemented nationwide, major structural barriers must be overcome.

Should interest mental health planners, providers, and policymakers.

1227. McCOURT, William F., Ruth D. Barnett, Jean Brennen, Alvin
Becker. "We help each other: Primary prevention for the
widowed." *American Journal of Psychiatry* 133 (1976): 98-
100.

Highlights the need for services at different stages of bereavement.

Review

Describes the inception and evaluation of a program of primary prevention for widows.   The program focuses on the telephone line of the
widowed, home visits, social gatherings, and community seminars.   A
follow-up survey shows a benefit to participants.

Of interest to mental health professionals.

1228. MINKLER, Meredith.   "Building supportive ties and sense of
      community among the inner-city elder: The Tenderloin Senior
      Outreach Project."   *Health Education Quarterly*   12 (Winter
      1985): 303-314.

A case study of an attempt to address the problems of poor health,
social isolation, and powerlessness by social support and social
action organizing among elderly residents of San Francisco's Tender-
loin hotels.

Case Study

The project's theoretical base and the genesis and growth of the
project into a privately incorporated community-based organization is
described.   Examples of individual and community improvement are
presented, and problems in the areas of indigenous leadership development and community versus funding agency agendas are examined.   The
project demonstrates the potential role of enhanced social support in
increasing the sense of control and self-reliance among low income
elders.

Of interest to community organizers, public health professionals,
social workers, and social and behavioral scientists.

1229. MITCHELL, S.F., and J.L.T. Birley.   "The use of ward
      support by psychiatric patients in the community."   *British
      Journal of Psychiatry*   142 (1983): 9-15.

Describes a program which makes ward facilities and staff available on
demand to psychiatric patients living in the community.

Descriptive

Evidence suggests that this type of crisis oriented, patient referred
use of psychiatric services is related to the amount of social interaction with the staff that takes place prior to discharge to the
community.   Those using the program most were schizophrenics with
early onset of disease and poor or scant social networks.

This study may interest professionals planning support programs in
mental health.

1230. PATTERSON, Shirley L., and Esther E. Twente.   "Older
       natural helpers: Their characteristics and patterns of
       helping." *Public Welfare* 29 (Fall 1971): 400-403.

Examines the helping activities of a group of 15 persons, 60 years of
age and older, in a rural Kansas county. It is based on the first
year of a three year research and demonstration project.

Descriptive

Clarification of helper classifications, characteristics, and patterns
will enable helpers to delineate and define the kind of help and the
ways of helping that are most effective. Understanding and application of this knowledge in education and practice will mutually enrich
collaborative and cooperative mental health efforts between local
helpers and social workers.

Of interest to gerontologists, social workers, and the aged and aging.

1231. PENNY, Jean T. "Spotlight on support for impaired nurses."
       American Journal of Nursing 86 (June 1986): 688-691.

A description of the Florida Impaired Nurse Program for nurses with
addiction problems.

Descriptive

The program has been shown to be cost-effective. A state-wide cadre
of qualified volunteers to serve as support persons helped to relieve
the strain on aftercare services. Placing nurses in the same agency
that regulates nurses' licenses has enhanced compliance.

Of particular interest to nurses and day rehabilitation counselors.

1232. PILISUK, Marc, Susan Chandler, Carole D'Onofrio. "Reweav-
       ing the social fabric: Antecedents of social support facili-
       tation." *International Quarterly of Community Health
       Education* 3 (1982-1983): 45-66.

Seven different models of intervention, which address the problem of
augmenting supportive relationships, are examined.

Theoretical

Noticeable similarities among the seven models are: the importance of
listening; the avoidance of a pathology model and its replacement by a
systems model or growth model; prior preparation in interpersonal
relationship skills; and a definition of the task by the client
groupings.

Of interest to social and behavioral scientists.

1233. PINKSTON, Elsie M., and Nathan L. Linsk. "Behavioral family intervention with the impaired elderly." *Gerontologist* 24 (1984): 576-583.

Describes the Elderly Support Project, a study designed to evaluate intervention procedures derived from behavioral parent training research and adapted to teach families better home care of the impaired elderly.

Research

Twenty-one elderly persons and their caregivers took part in this study in which behavioral family training procedures were applied with families and other caregivers of elderly persons. Findings supported the procedures, which offered the caregivers alternative positive responses for use with their older relatives, as valuable for promoting continuing home care, better mental status, and improved behavior of elderly clients.

Should interest social workers, mental health professionals, and gerontologists.

1234. PYNOOS, Jon, Barbara Hade-Kaplan, Dorothy Fleisher. "Intergenerational neighborhood networks: A basis for aiding the frail elderly." *Gerontologist* 24 (1984): 233-237.

Describes Project LINC (Living Independently Through Neighborhood Cooperation) a three-year research and demonstration project designed to organize residents of all ages into neighborhood-based helping networks for frail, elderly community residents and to link those networks to community agencies for access to additional resources when needed.

Descriptive

Intergenerational networks were formed in which the elderly served as donors as well as recipients. Evaluation of the project indicated that frail older persons were provided with needed services, acted as volunteers, developed new friendships, participated in more social activities, and increased their life satisfaction.

Of interest to social workers, health planners and policymakers, health care professionals, and social scientists.

1235. QUAM, Jean K. "Natural helpers: Tools for working with the chronically mentally ill elderly." *Gerontologist* 24 (1984): 564-567.

Describes a program, designed for a board and lodging home, that maximizes the use of natural helpers and takes into consideration the unique needs of the chronically mentally ill.

Descriptive

Residents of Sentinal House, a community based residential care facility, were encouraged to make use of existing informal activities and supports within and outside the facility; natural leaders were given formalized roles and responsibilities in order to support their value to the program; necessary daily activities, such as cooking and cleaning, were gradually turned over to the residents; and program activities were designed to meet their specific developmental needs. These programmatic ways of strengthening and supporting natural helping systems have led to sustained involvement of the residents in the facility and created an atmosphere of trust, relatedness, and consistency.

Should interest mental health care planners and administrators and gerontologists.

1236. RAINEY, Lawrence C. "Cancer counseling by telephone help-line: The U.C.L.A. Psychosocial Cancer Counseling Line." *Public Health Reports* 100 (1985): 308-315.

Describes a communications project that explored the feasibility of providing psychological support to cancer patients and their significant others by telephone.

Descriptive

Callers frequently requested referrals to support groups or discussed anxiety with the disease or its treatment, family problems associated with illness, and difficulties in doctor-patient relations. A telephone counseling service can provide important psychosocial services, including provision of information, needs assessment, linkage to health professionals, psychological interventions during intervals between personal contacts, continuing emotional support, and outreach to psychologically underserved populations.

Of special interest to health professionals.

1237. REUBEN, David B., Dennis H. Novack, Tom J. Wachtel, Steven A. Wartman. "A comprehensive support system for reducing house staff distress." *Psychosomatics* 25 (1984): 815-820.

Describes a program aimed at reducing stress among medical residents by providing a forum for their views and individual counseling.

Case Report

Offers guidelines for implementing support programs to reduce stress in medical residents. The program is suggested to reduce depression, impaired patient care, and poor professional attitudes.

Of interest to health professions students, and medical educators.

1238. RHOADES, Cindy M., Philip L. Browning, Elizabeth J. Thorin. "Self-help advocacy movement: A promising peer-support system for people with mental disabilities." *Rehabilitation Literature* 47 (1986): 2-7.

A description of an international voluntary organization which is a self-help advocacy group run by and for persons with mental retardation.

Descriptive

It is suggested that participation in a self-help advocacy group may improve the self-identity of persons with mental retardation, as well as provide them with an opportunity for developing meaningful friendships with their peers.

Of interest to rehabilitation counselors, especially those working with the mentally retarded.

1239. ROY, Carol A., and Esther Atcherson. "Peer support for renal patients: The Patient Visitor Program." *Health and Social Work* 8 (1983): 52-56.

The authors describe a peer support program for renal patients.

Descriptive

The Patient Visitor Program enables newly diagnosed renal patients facing dialysis or transplantation to meet with someone who has experienced that stress and dealt with it constructively.

Of interest to renal specialists, nurses, social workers, and mental health professionals.

1240. SEITZ, Victoria, Laurie K. Rosenbaum, Nancy H. Apfel. "Effects of family support intervention: A ten year follow-up." *Child Development* 56 (1985): 376-391.

The delivery to impoverished mothers of a coordinated set of medical and social services, including day-care for their children, had effects that were evident a decade after the intervention ended.

Research

The results suggest that family support procedures, including quality day-care, have considerable promise as a general model for intervention programs. Intervention children had better school attendance, and boys were less likely to require costly special school services than were corresponding control children.

Of interest to child development specialists, family sociologists, and social workers.

1241.   SILVERMAN, Phyllis Rolfe.   "The widow as a caregiver in a
        program of preventive intervention with other widows.
        Mental Hygiene 54 (1970): 540-547.

Discusses the Widow to Widow Program, a caregiving group in preventive
intervention.

Descriptive

A group of widows who had recovered from their bereavement were
recruited to reach out to recently widowed women and offer support in
helping them adjust to their new life.   They were very helpful to the
widows they reached, in large part because they shared the same
disability.

Of interest to social workers and mental health professionals.

1242.   TAYLOR, Robert L., David J. Lam, Charles E. Roppell, James
        T. Barter.   "Friends Can Be Good Medicine: An excursion
        into mental health promotion."   *Community Mental Health
        Journal* 20 (1984): 294-303.

Describes *Friends Can Be Good Medicine*, a multi-media, mental health
promotion campaign conducted in 1982 throughout California.

Descriptive

Evaluation findings revealed that *Friends* was most effective when
campaign elements reinforced one another.   Resulting changes in
knowledge, attitudes, and intentions among those reached by *Friends*
were maintained after one year.   It is contended that mass media is
part of the health care system.

Of interest to health educators and mental health professionals.

1243.   THIEL, R., J. Knispel, Hedwig Wallis.   "Entwicklung,
        strukfur und erste auswertung umfassender psychosozialer
        betreuung krebskranker kinder und ihrer familien."
        (German) *Monatsschrift Kinderheilkunde* 133 (1985): 22-27.

Development of a comprehensive care program for children with cancer
and their families.

Research

A procedure was developed and tested to provide comprehensive, preventive psychosocial care for children with cancer and their families.
The procedure is based on the identification of problems in the family
and involves the introduction of psychosocial support schemes.

Of special interest to pediatric oncologists and psychologists and
rehabilitation professionals working with children with cancer.

1244. VERSLUYS, Hilda P. "Thuishulpcentrale: A Dutch model for practical family assistance." *Rehabilitation Literature* 47, no. 3-4 (1986): 50-59.

Describes the interweave of organizations that provide support for families with disabled children.

Descriptive

A review of the rehabilitation, education, and development needs of children with disabilities is presented, comparing supportive programs in The Netherlands and the U.S. Family and social support, independent living, and integration into the community are key concepts underlying Dutch social agencies serving families with disabled children.

Of interest to cross cultural and family researchers interested in childhood disabilities and programs aimed at assisting them.

b. Dissertations

1245. MALONE, Judy A. "An alternative community care program for the chronic mentally ill: An in vivo approach to social skills training and social support utilizing nonprofessional staff." Ph.D. dissertation, University of Texas at Austin, 1984.

A community study of the effects of staff-client interactions on adaptation of mentally ill to independent community living.

Research

Social skills training and social support, both usually provided by traditional psychiatric programs, were shown to be important factors for the rehabilitation of the chronic mentally ill.

Should interest rehabilitation professionals, mental health professionals, and social workers.

1246. REGAN, Joseph M. "Services to the families of alcoholics: An assessment of a social support system." Ph.D. dissertation, Brandeis University, 1978.

Attempts to determine the degree to which family-oriented alcohol abuse services have been translated into the actual practice of service delivery and to identify the key factors that promote or hinder their implementation.

Research

Family-oriented alcohol abuse services are underrepresented and poorly developed in the overall system of service delivery in spite of the increased awareness of the needs of families and the policy declarations that such services must constitute an essential element in service delivery. The reasons for this appear to lie in the lack of a clear sense of professional responsibility for the needs of the family, the way alcohol abuse is interpreted by service providers, and the training and staffing patterns of service programs.

Of special interest to health professionals providing direct services to alcoholics and their families.

c. Conference Proceedings

1247. U.S. Department of Health and Human Services, Public Health Service, Alcohol, Drug Abuse and Mental Health Administration. *A Network for Caring. The Community Support Program of the National Institute of Mental Health.* Summary Proceedings of Four Learning Community Conferences and One Conference on Manpower and Development Training, January 1978-November 1979, DHHS Publication No. (ADM) 81-1063, 1982.

Summarizes and distills the proceedings of four learning conferences designed to improve the quality of life for adults with severe and chronic mental or emotional disorders.

Conference Proceedings

The eight sections include discussions of the federal role in developing community support systems, approaches to local development of community support systems, organizational models for community support services, involving consumers in community social support development, and manpower development and program evaluation issues and approaches.

Of special interest to mental health professionals, social and behavioral scientists, public health nurses, and social workers.

AUTHOR INDEX

SUBJECT INDEX